Unwinding Bone

Unwinding Bone

A Complete Guide to Biodynamic Skeletal Therapy
for Myofascial and Manual Therapists

Scott Sternthal, D.O.

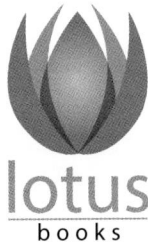

lotus
books

Library of Congress Cataloging-in-Publication Data

Names: Sternthal, Scott, 1974- author
Title: Unwinding bone : a complete guide to biodynamic skeletal therapy for
  myofascial and manual therapists / Scott Sternthal.
Description: Champaign, IL : Lotus Books, [2026] | Includes bibliographical
  references and index.
Identifiers: LCCN 2025026602 (print) | LCCN 2025026603 (ebook) | ISBN
  9781718245020 paperback | ISBN 9781718245037 epub | ISBN 9781718245044
  pdf
Subjects: LCSH: Craniosacral therapy | Myofascial pain syndromes--Treatment
  | Osteopathic medicine
Classification: LCC RZ399.C73 S74 2026 (print) | LCC RZ399.C73 (ebook)
LC record available at https://lccn.loc.gov/2025026602
LC ebook record available at https://lccn.loc.gov/2025026603

ISBN: 978-1-7182-4502-0 (print)

Anatomical Illustrations Amanda Williams
Photographer Emily Gan
Text Design Medlar Publishing Solutions Pvt Ltd., India
Cover Design Keri Evans
Printer Versa Press

Books from Lotus Books are available at special discounts for bulk purchase. Special editions or book excerpts can also be created to specification. For details, contact the Special Sales Manager at Human Kinetics.

Printed in the United States of America   10   9   8   7   6   5   4   3   2   1

The paper in this book is certified under a sustainable forestry program.

Lotus Books
An Imprint of Human Kinetics
1607 N. Market Street
Champaign, IL 61820
USA

United States and International
Website: **US.HumanKinetics.com/pages/lotus-books**
Email: info@hkusa.com
Phone: 1-800-747-4457

Human Kinetics' authorized representative for product safety in the EU is Mare Nostrum Group B.V., Mauritskade 21D, 1091 GC Amsterdam, The Netherlands.

Email: gpsr@mare-nostrum.co.uk

For
Tasha, Frida, and Sarah

Show me slowly what I only know the limits of.

—Leonard Cohen, "Dance Me to the End of Love"

Contents

Preface

When I began my osteopathy practice in 2012, I possessed hundreds of shiny new techniques in my therapist's toolbox, freshly gleaned from school. My tools were sharp and ready for action. They included osteoarticular thrusts and myofascial mobilizations, functional maneuvers like muscle energy and Hoovers, counterstrain holds and cranial V-spreads. I could treat eyeballs and deltoids, thyroid glands and pericardial ligaments. Every tiny bone in each finger and in each foot, each tooth and sinus, every nerve and nodule long and round had its very own technique. But then something surprising occurred:

My toolbox suddenly seemed too big for the job.

After simplifying my practice, I soon realized that I didn't need all of these tools. All that was required was a principle to guide me, and once the principle had been established, the right techniques naturally flowed from it. In a way, this principle became the fulcrum from which the techniques emerged and upon which they then balanced. For me, this principle was (and is) to find and treat intraosseous dysfunction—zones within bone tissue with diminished elasticity and vitality—before doing anything else.

In 2023, I self-published a book called *Melting Bone, Healing Tide*, which discussed this. The ideas in the book were not new, per se. Manual therapists had been treating intraosseous dysfunction for a long time, but instructional information on the subject still remained scarce. Since intraosseous work had become so foundational in my practice, I thought that my perspective could be of some value. While I had first learned about intraosseous dysfunction from my teachers at the Collège d'Etudes Ostéopathiques (CEO) in Montreal, I tweaked the approach and called my variation *biodynamic skeletal therapy* (BST), since it keys off the biodynamic rhythms within skeletal (bone) tissue.

Surprisingly, immediately after publishing *Melting Bone, Healing Tide*, encouraging feedback from readers around the world began to roll in. From this correspondence, I learned that the same principle—finding and treating intraosseous dysfunction *first*—was important for others, too. Furthermore, we were observing similar phenomena unfold.

In February 2024, ConTact CARE practitioners Greg Jamiesson and Rubina Schäfer reached out from Germany and New Zealand, respectively, to say how much BST resonated with their own approach to treating intraosseous dysfunction. ConTact CARE was conceived in New Zealand in 2004 after founder Dale Speedy developed the approach while treating his horse. The protocol uses a "flinchlock release" method to release trapped pressure from bone in both animals and humans. Greg and Ruby believe that the compacted parts of bone that I described in my book were what they refer to as "flinchlocks." According to them, by holding and releasing flinchlocks in a specific way, the pressure from the bone dissipates, and the skeleton returns to a more balanced state, allowing the surrounding soft tissue to unwind on its own. Curiously, similar phenomena occur during BST.

Another reader contacted me to ask if I had heard of Sharon Wheeler. I had not, so I looked her up. I learned that in 1970, at 23 years of age, Sharon began her training with Dr. Ida Rolf, the founder of Structural Integration. Sharon was one of Rolf's youngest students and enjoyed a unique connection with her teacher. Rolf believed that Wheeler could "see bodies in the same way as her." From Sharon's studies, two methodologies eventually emerged: ScarWork and BoneWork. According to Sharon, BoneWork "molds the shape and contour of damaged bones" and restores the way in which bone serves as an anchor within the osseofascial continuum. Curious to know more about Sharon and BoneWork, I made myself a note to reach out to her—but then she beat me to it!

In June 2024, Sharon sent me a meticulously crafted message introducing herself and her approach. She said that she had read my book and was elated that someone else was working with bones in similar ways. In her email, Sharon explained that by using both hands, she transmits an equal amount of compression into the area, what she calls a "field of pressure." Next, she dialogues with the bone until it begins to "dissolve and move—like dancing." She then "follows" the movements, until the bone "feels right." Remarkably, these stages of BoneWork correspond almost perfectly to the cocooning, compression, dialogue, and augmentation stages of BST. I was excited and honored that Sharon—a pioneer in intraosseous manipulation who had developed her approach before I was born— not only appreciated but confirmed the validity of my work nearly 50 years later.

It's worth repeating that I only learned of ConTact CARE and BoneWork *after* I developed BST. It's compelling how these approaches—and others, I'm sure— developed *independently* of each other and then converged. This convergence is significant, since it substantiates our respective findings about the behavior of bone, a tissue many consider too rigid to treat this way.

In July 2023, I received an email from Jon Hutchings of Lotus Publishing (now called Lotus Books) in the United Kingdom. Jon had not only read my book but saw in it the potential for something bigger. Together, we decided that I should write a more in-depth version of *Melting Bone, Healing Tide*—a complete guide to BST—to be published and distributed by Lotus Books' new parent company, Human Kinetics. Roughly two years later, *Unwinding Bone* was born.

This book is everything *Melting Bone, Healing Tide* is and more. My aim here was to compile a text that was scientifically based yet inspirational and fun. A text both grounded and surprising, and informative enough for practitioners like us without being too dense. *Unwinding Bone* is a step-by-step, hands-on study guide generously sprinkled with (what

I hope are) thought-provoking questions and stories. Apart from a few refinements, the nuts and bolts of BST have remained unchanged, and the basic principles of the BST evaluation and treatment protocols still apply. Going above and beyond my first book, *Unwinding Bone* includes precise descriptions of how to find and treat *each* bone, not just a few. Also, besides the local applications of BST, this book introduces and explains the entire series of regional BST techniques. The text also includes hundreds of beautiful photographs and images, which should help you learn the approach more easily.

I like short chapters—they make me feel like I'm getting somewhere in life. But (sigh) longer chapters are useful, too. For this reason, *Unwinding Bone* includes both. This fluctuation is intentional: it reflects the unpredictable nature of manual therapy. As you probably have experienced in your own treatment room, just when we have it all figured out, things change, expanding before us into wide-open vistas, contracting back again into shadow, then reappearing brightly once more. Cycles of certainty, doubt, acceptance, and learning continuously bubbling up and over one another, revealing the ephemeral nature of therapeutic dialogue. While this unpredictable evanescence can be dizzying, I think it also sparkles our work, keeping it fizzy and fresh.

Despite the contributions from people like Greg, Ruby, Sharon, myself, all of those who you'll meet in the pages that follow (and all of those who I may have accidentally left out!), we still know very little about how living bone behaves and how to treat it.[1] For this reason, even this expanded book is but a starting point.

May *Unwinding Bone* light our way forward as we learn more.

---

[1]According to Sara Imari Walker, professor in the School of Earth and Space Exploration at Arizona State University, as of 2023 there is still debate within the scientific community on what it means for human tissue and other objects to be "living" at all.

Introduction

Unwinding Bone is a complete guide to biodynamic skeletal therapy (BST), a comprehensive resource to help you develop your practice.

For some of you more familiar with craniosacral therapy or treating intraosseous dysfunction, the book may serve more as a review, or maybe a synthesis of information you've received in parts. For others from different bodywork backgrounds that have traditionally involved only myofascial work, this book will hopefully provide some accessible and exciting new insights into treating bone tissue.

Simply put, BST helps us find and treat bones that have lost their natural elasticity and vitality. The approach focuses less on the movement *of* bones, and more on the movement *within* them, and is as simple as it is powerful. Similar to how a primer coat of paint prepares an artist's canvas for color, BST "primes" the skeleton for further manual treatment. It opens a window of opportunity through which we can elicit profound change with our hands.

Biodynamic skeletal therapy can be learned and practiced by anyone who uses their hands to help people: massage therapists, craniosacral therapists, physiotherapists, chiropractors, and osteopaths.

The first half of the book discusses the theory behind the approach. We'll review bone anatomy and composition, including bone development, remodeling, and mechanical behavior. Then, we'll see how bone and fascia blend together, forming an "osseofascial continuum." The concepts of biotensegrity and potency will be explored, as will fulcrum-lever systems and the rhythms and textures of primary respiration. Finally, before diving into actual practice, we'll learn about the history and foundations of BST, and outline the generalities of BST treatment and evaluation. As you go through this first section, you may notice a few open-ended questions here and there. As I alluded to in the preface, this is because we have not (yet) been able to explain everything that we feel with our hands. In my opinion, this only makes our brave endeavor more fascinating.

The second half of *Unwinding Bone* serves as the practical guide. Here, we'll walk through a step-by-step procedure for finding and treating osseofascial compactions in nearly every bone in the body, and then discover how to integrate our local work back into the human system.

ENJOY!

Silence

A silence opens.

What does it open?

Stillness

Silence is the garden, stillness is the rain.

—James Jealous

Sensing

At an osteopathy conference in the 1970s, Rollin Becker replaced a speaker who had announced his absence at the last minute. As the assistant assigned to the talk, Becker had to quickly decide what to teach. He asked the group of 50 or so osteopathic physicians to form into pairs, and then take turns assessing their partners. Instead of testing for motion, which would have been their normal routine, they were instructed to *sense* for motion. Becker watched the doctors work in a new kind of silence. At the end of class, two things occurred, both of which Becker found surprising. First, half the class approached him to say that they had experienced the finest treatment of their lives, despite the fact that no treatment had ever been given. Second, not a single one of those who had approached him had any interest in learning why.

How could this be?

CHAPTER 4

Osseofascia

The term *osseofascia* refers to the uninterrupted continuum of bone and fascia otherwise known as the skeleton. A quick note: in the following pages, I will sometimes refer to bone as "bone" and other times as "osseofascia." This is usually just to avoid jargon fatigue, but for all intents and purposes, the terms are interchangeable here. I will revisit this interplay again later when we discuss the osseofascial continuum.

To begin our journey into BST, we'll get to know the osseofascial continuum by reviewing osseofascial anatomy, physiology, and behavior. We'll also learn about what happens when osseofascial tissue becomes dysfunctional, and about how interstitial fluid may be involved in both the formation and resolution of the dysfunction.

BONE ANATOMY

Bone is fascinating! Bone structure and function have been under investigation for hundreds of years and still captivate our imagination. Bone tissue is unique: rigid and elastic and able to support and sustain us. Bones are intertwined with flexible connective tissue passing from their surface to their inner compartments and back to the surface again, connecting all parts. A dynamic, living tissue, bone is capable

of continuous transformation and renewal. It provides shape and structure, permits movement, helps with breathing, transmits sound (through the auditory canal), produces blood cells, and more. Bone not only protects organs, it *is* an organ, with an array of crucial endocrine functions. Furthermore, bone is in direct communication with the central nervous and digestive systems, transmitting and receiving vital information via the gut-brain-bone axis. If the gut is our second brain, bone could very well be our third. Bone keeps busy, playing a starring role in our drive toward homeostasis, health, and evolution.

There are approximately 270 bones in infants, but with the fusing of some as the skeleton develops, adults are left with just over 200. Different authors report different counts, but according to Gray, adults have 204 bones: 26 in the vertebral column, including the sacrum and coccyx; 8 composing the cranium; 6 bones in the auditory canal; 14 bones in the face; and 26 bones in the rib cage, including the ribs, sternum, and hyoid. There are also 64 bones in the upper extremities and 60 in the lower extremities. I think that adds up to 204.

A cross-section of bone reveals an inner surface of trabecular, or spongy, bone and an outer layer of cortical bone (figure 4.1). The cortical bone is made up of cylindrical

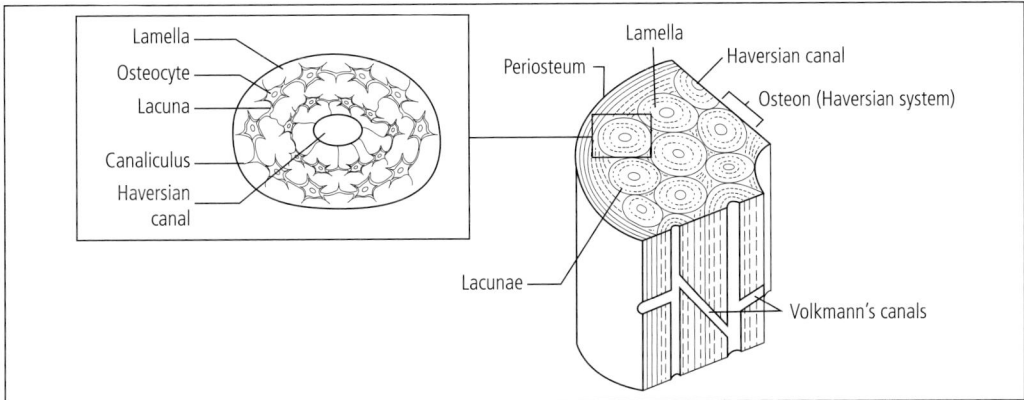

Figure 4.1. Cross-section of bone.

lamellae, arranged in bundles called osteons. During bone development, bone-building cells called osteoblasts deposit new bone around blood vessels, forming Haversian canals. Other passageways, known as Volkmann's canals, run perpendicularly to the Haversian canals, connecting the latter to the blood supply coming through the periosteum. The periosteum is a fascial sheath attached to the surface of bone by tiny collagenous expansions, called Sharpey's fibers, which penetrate the underlying bone tissue (see page 41). Via Sharpey's fibers, the periosteum is linked directly to the bony matrix and even to the endosteum, a second, inner fascial membrane. Together, the periosteum, Sharpey's fibers, and endosteum sustain a cohesive dynamic between the inside and outside of bone, known as the periosteum—Sharpey's fibers—endosteum (PSE) continuum.[2]

Our 200-or-so-piece bone collection consists of bones of all shapes and sizes: long, short, flat, irregular, and sesamoid bones. The long

bones are the clavicle, humerus, radius, ulna, femur, tibia, fibula, metacarpals, metatarsals, and phalanges.

Long bones are tubular and longer than they are wide, and have three distinct zones: the epiphysis, metaphysis, and diaphysis. The epiphyses are the terminal ends, which join with other bones. The metaphyses contain the epiphyseal plates (or growth plates) in children, which remain cartilaginous until after puberty. The diaphysis, or shaft, houses the medullary canal, and in it, the bone marrow. The ends of long bones are covered with slippery hyaline cartilage to ensure smooth articulation with other bones. The short bones are those of the feet (calcaneus, talus, cuboid, navicular, and three cuneiforms) and hands (scaphoid, lunate, cuneiform, pisiform, trapezium, trapezoid, hamate, and triquetral).

Short bones are nuggets of trabecular bone covered by a thin crust of cortical bone. They have no diaphysis and are designed for strength and support. They also have names that are hard to remember (for me, at least).

Irregular-shaped bones include the sacrum, coccyx, temporal, sphenoid, ethmoid, superior maxillary, mandible, palate, inferior turbinates, hyoid, and vertebrae.

---

[2]We can't discuss bone anatomy without giving due mention to bone's fatty "guts." Bone marrow is a red or yellow gelatinous goop responsible for making new red blood cells. Until the age of seven or so, all bone marrow is red. Then, fatty tissue replaces (most of) the red marrow, turning it yellow.

Flat bones are located in the cranium and elsewhere, and are the occipital, parietals, frontal, nasal, lacrimal, vomer, sternum, scapulae, ribs, and both ilia. As the name implies, these bones are flat or sheetlike to provide protection for important stuff inside of them (like the brain) and a large surface area for muscular attachments.

The sesamoid bones are a special group. The word "sesamoid" comes from the Greek word *sēsamoeidēs*, translating to "sesame," since many sesamoid bones resemble small seeds. Sesamoid bones are small bones commonly found within muscles or tendons near joint surfaces. They generally function as pulleys to alleviate mechanical stress. Unlike standard bones, which are connected to others by ligaments, sesamoid bones connect to muscles via tendons. In the hands, two sesamoids are located in the distal portions of the first metacarpal bones within the tendons of the flexor pollicis brevis and adductor pollicis muscles, one sesamoid appears within the interphalangeal joint, and two more are present in the distal portion of the second metacarpal bone and the distal portion of the fifth metacarpal joint. In the wrist, the pisiform bone is a sesamoid located within the tendon of the flexor carpi ulnaris.[3] In the lower extremities, the largest and most famous of all sesamoids is the patella. Other lower-extremity sesamoids include the fabella (often found near the lateral head of the gastrocnemius), cyamella (snuggled within the popliteus tendon), os peroneum (located within the peroneus longus tendon), and the hallux sesamoid pair, one on each side of the plantar surface of the first metatarsal bone. Another sesamoid bone exists within the ear, called the lenticular process of the incus, often known as the fourth ossicle of the middle ear.

The idea that sesamoids often "float" within a muscle or tendon has implications about how other bones behave. In the 1970s, Stephen Levin made a neat observation while performing knee surgery. He noticed that the femur and tibia had a natural space between them, and by tightening up the cruciate ligaments of the knee, the bones moved *further apart*, not closer together. He called this phenomenon the "floating bone principle," which suggests that other bones, too, may act like floating sesamoids.

BONE COMPOSITION AND BEHAVIOR

Even in 2024 as I write this, and despite the phenomenal gains we've made in biomedical research, we still know surprisingly little about how living bone tissue actually behaves inside of us. This makes sense since it's difficult to experiment on bone tissue while it's being used! Let's piece together what we *do* know so we can better understand how bone composition and behavior relate to manual therapy and BST.

The extracellular matrix of bone tissue, also known as the bone matrix, surrounds and supports the bone cells, nerves, and blood vessels nestled within it. The remarkable composition of the bone matrix gives bone tissue many of its unique characteristics. It's made up of 40 to 60 percent hydroxyapatite crystals (the very rigid stuff), 30 to 40 percent collagen and other non-collagenous proteins (the gooier viscoelastic material), and about 20 percent bone water. Each of these components deserves further examination.

Collagen

Collagen is the most widespread structural protein in the human body. There are (at least) 28 types of collagen, but types I through IV

---

[3]There is ongoing debate about whether or not the pisiform is a true sesamoid.

are the most common. Type I is the most abundant, and is found in skin, tendons, ligaments, teeth, and bones, while type II is only found in cartilage. Type III is often present alongside type I, as well as within the walls of the hollow internal organs and blood vessels. Type IV collagen is predominantly found in the extracellular basement membranes of the skin. All of these types of collagen play a vital role in maintaining the strength and flexibility of connective tissues.

Collagen is a viscoelastic material. Viscoelasticity is a property of materials that possess both viscosity *and* elasticity. Such materials are able to stretch and bounce back like an elastic band, while also having some resistance to deformation like a piece of taffy. In fact, collagen is kind of like the taffy in our bones. If your femur were plunged into a tub of acid (please don't), the hydroxyapatite crystals would dissolve, and the remaining collagen "taffy" would retain the shape of the bone and could be cut with a knife, even tied into knots.

Research by orthopedic surgeon Jean-Claude Guimberteau shines a light on the role of collagen in bone and throughout the body. Through his work, Guimberteau revealed an organized network of collagen fibers that permeates all structures. The network extends from the surface of the skin to the nucleus of each cell. This viscoelastic web is self-adjusting and all-pervasive: it links all structures and all systems—including bones—to one another.[4] We will revisit Guimberteau's work soon.

Collagen has a unique hierarchical structure. At the lowest level, collagen consists of three

---

[4]Guimberteau's collagen network is permanently hydrated, and hydration plays a major role in the structure and behavior of collagen. In fact, it has been shown that the dehydration of collagen fibrils leads to fibril shrinkage, negatively impacting collagen function.

left-handed polypeptide chains, which coil up to form the collagen molecule, known as tropocollagen. The twisty triple-helix formation allows the tropocollagen molecules to bend and stretch under strain. Forming the next, larger hierarchical level are the collagen fibrils, which consist of bunches of collagen molecules assembled into tiny ropelike structures. The fibrils then combine to form the next-larger hierarchical level, the collagen fibers, which in turn make up whole tissues like tendons, ligaments, blood vessels, and bones (figure 4.2).

Hydroxyapatite

Hydroxyapatite is a naturally occurring mineral composed mainly of phosphorus and calcium. In bone, hydroxyapatite crystals reinforce the softer collagen matrix. The crystals do this by populating gaps within the collagen fibrils, overlapping into staggered arrangements (figure 4.3). Hydroxyapatite and collagen have a synergistic relationship. Collagen gives bone its tensile strength— it enables a finger to be pulled without snapping. Hydroxyapatite gives bone its compressive strength—it allows you to jump up and down without your leg bones buckling when you land. Logically, the more crystals bound to the collagen, the more rigid the structure. Bone and teeth, for example, have a higher hydroxyapatite-to-collagen ratio than softer connective tissues such as tendons and ligaments.

In reference to collagen in bone, Stock describes collagen as "bending" around the hydroxyapatite crystals, with the embedded crystals preventing excessive distortion of collagen under load. Stock also suggests that some collagen distortion in bone is not only present but necessary for optimal load transfer to occur. This is important. We'll see how the ability of collagen in bone to distort

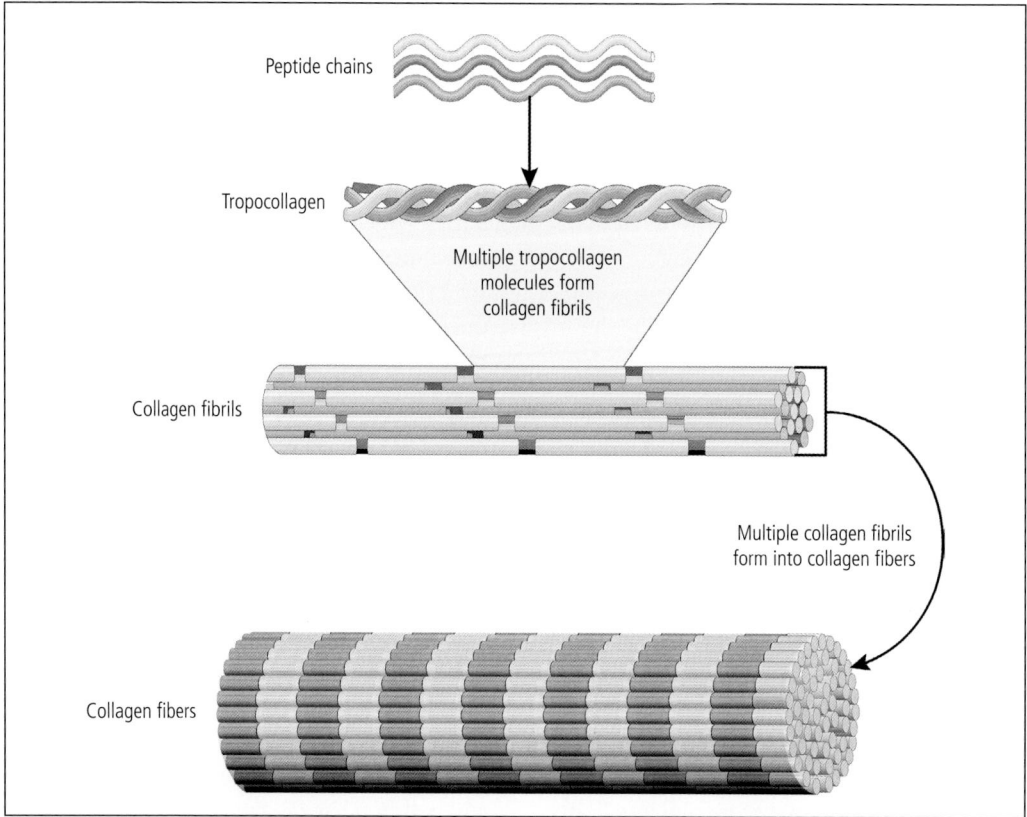

Figure 4.2. The hierarchical structure of collagen.

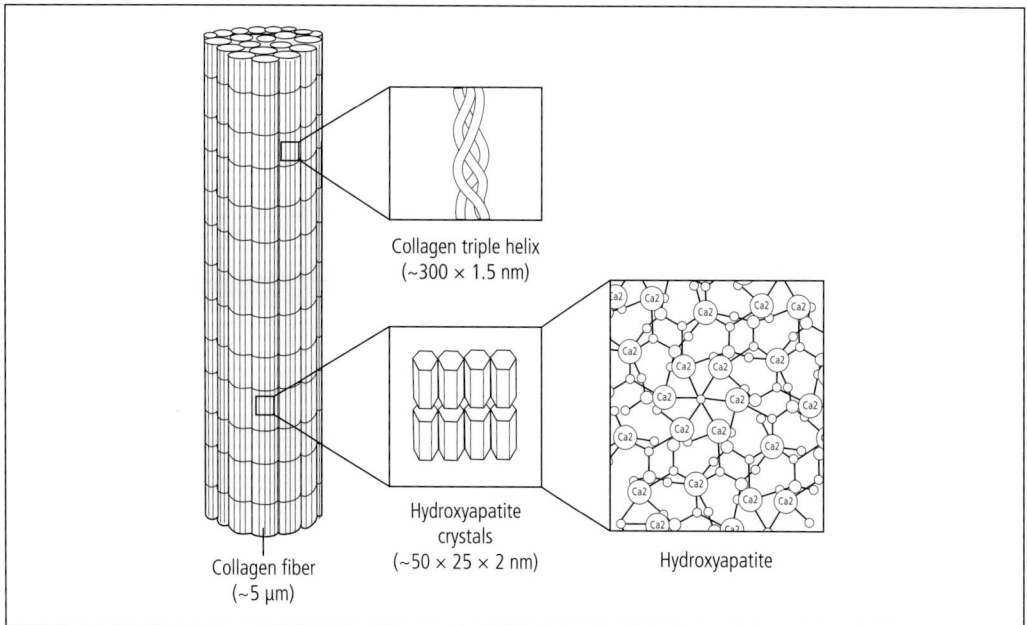

Figure 4.3. Hydroxyapatite crystals populating gaps within the collagen fibrils.

under pressure—even just a little bit—will help us with our work.

Even with the rigid hydroxyapatite reinforcements, bones are anything but lifeless pegs. Some even consider bones to be more like soft-matter gels that can shape-shift between rigid and compliant phases. According to Stephen Levin, a pioneer in biotensegrity science, the apparent solidness of all our tissues—including bone—may be just an illusion.

Bone Water

Bone water is a fundamental component of bone structure and function. Bone contains three types of fluid—blood, interstitial fluid, and lymphatic fluid—and water is found in all three. These three fluids work together to keep bone healthy.

Like all tissues, bone needs a robust blood supply to survive. Blood enters bone tissue through nutrient arteries, which branch into smaller vessels. Together, these blood vessels supply the cortical and trabecular bone, as well as the bone marrow. Blood exits bone through veins that accompany the nutrient arteries. Veins collect deoxygenated blood and metabolic waste from bone tissue and bone marrow, draining into larger veins that return blood to the heart.[5] As you know,

blood is composed mostly of blood plasma (which itself is made mostly of water) and red and white blood cells, along with blood platelets and a selection of electrolytes, proteins, hormones, and waste products.

Separate from (but closely related to) the bloodstream, interstitial fluid is found within the extracellular fluid and surrounds cells. In addition to electrolytes, proteins, and waste products, interstitial fluid is also made mostly of water. In bone, interstitial fluid facilitates the exchange of substances between osteocytes and the bloodstream. It also contributes to the overall hydration of bone, and it's well-known that fluctuations in bone hydration impact the mechanical properties of bone tissue (Bicalho 2020; Granke, Does, and Nyman 2015; Pearson and Lieberman 2004; Surowiec, Allen, and Wallace 2021; Verzella et al. 2020). Without fluid, bone just wouldn't be bone. Bone water is always found in interstitial fluid, but interstitial fluid doesn't contain all the water found in bone. Bone water is also found *outside* of the interstitial fluid, within the tiniest porosities of the bone matrix. As is beautifully depicted in figure 4.4, as adapted from Granke, Does, and Nyman, bone water exists at four hierarchical levels: as pore water within the canals and pores of the vascular-lacunar-canalicular network (within the interstitial fluid), as loosely bound water at the surface of the collagen fibrils and between the collagen and the crystals, as tightly bound water wrapped inside the collagen triple-helix molecule, and as structural water embedded within the hydroxyapatite crystals. Interstitial fluid only flows so far—it exists in the larger spaces of the vascular-lacunar-canalicular network, but doesn't seem to penetrate the smallest spaces between and within the collagen and hydroxyapatite. Bone water, on the other hand, is located throughout: in the larger pores of the lacunae and canaliculi, between

---

[5]Bone also contains nerves, of course. Sensory and autonomic nerves snuggle up alongside blood vessels. Regions of bone subjected to the most mechanical load are also the most vascularized, and not surprisingly, also have the highest density of innervation. Sensory nerves in bone are involved in bone development and remodeling as well as in transmitting information about painful and nonpainful stimuli, body movement, and position. Autonomic nerves are also responsible for bone remodeling, with sympathetic nerve fibers promoting removal of old or damaged bone and parasympathetic fibers favoring new bone formation.

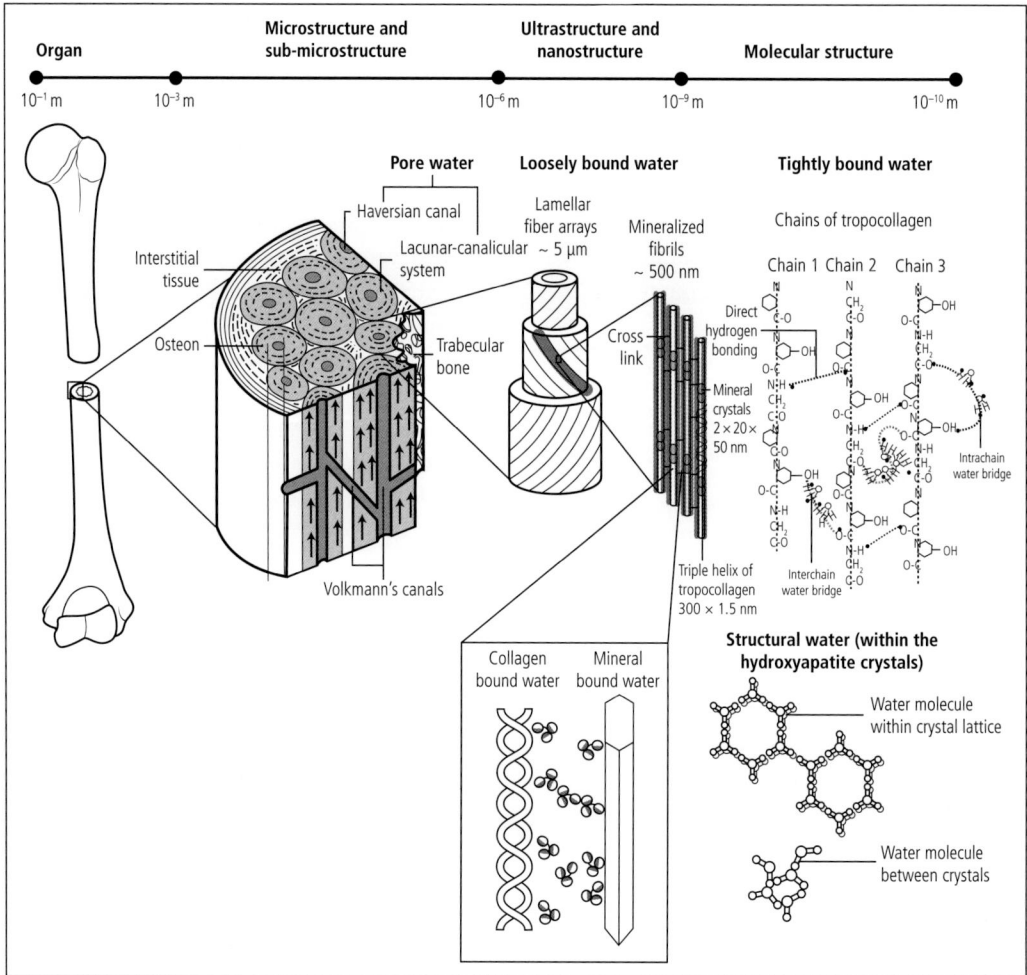

Figure 4.4. The four levels of bone water. Adapted from Granke, Does, and Nyman 2015.

the collagen fibrils and hydroxyapatite crystals, and within the collagen molecules and hydroxyapatite crystals.

Pore water has various functions. When mechanical loads are applied to bone, pore water helps absorb and transmit these forces, helping bone manage stress and strain. Pore water also facilitates the transport of nutrients and metabolic waste products between bone cells and the bloodstream. This is essential for maintaining the health and function of osteocytes, osteoblasts, and other bone cells. Pore water can also influence mechanotransduction and bone remodeling

(both to be discussed soon) via its movement around osteocytes. By detecting the movements of pore water, osteocytes influence the activity of osteoblasts and osteoclasts involved in bone formation or resorption, respectively.

Along with pore water, bound water plays an important role. Loosely and tightly bound water influences the load transfer between collagen and hydroxyapatite by allowing sliding at their interfaces, lowering the stress between them when bone is subject to load or trauma. Bound water also increases bone toughness, or the amount of energy bone can withstand before fracture.[6] Bound water also gives collagen viscosity, allowing us to enter into a special therapeutic relationship with osseofascial tissue. More on viscosity soon.

Lymphatic fluid completes the bone fluid trifecta. Lymphatic fluid circulates through the lymphatic system and drains excess interstitial fluid from bone, transporting it through lymphatic vessels, eventually returning it to the bloodstream. Lymphatic fluid is not contained within interstitial fluid, but interstitial fluid is contained in lymphatic fluid (along with other stuff, like pathogens, lymphocytes, proteins, and lipids).

As we can see, blood, interstitial fluid, and lymph live and flow within and throughout every nook and cranny of every bone. Biodynamic skeletal therapy allows us to dialogue with these fluids, helping us rebalance and reanimate the osseofascial continuum from within.

BONE DEVELOPMENT AND REMODELING

How and when do bones actually become bones? And once bones develop, how do they remain healthy throughout our lives? Both good questions. And while the answers here do not directly pertain to the practical applications of BST per se, this quick review may be of some interest for the extra-curious reader.

Bone formation begins around the sixth or seventh week of embryological development and continues until about 25 years of age. Bones arise from different embryonic lineages; namely, from cranial neural crest cells, prechordal mesodermal cells, paraxial

mesoderm cells (otherwise known as somites), and lateral plate mesodermal cells. Cranial neural crest cells give rise to the dentin of teeth and to the bones and cartilages of the anterior part of the skull. Prechordal mesodermal cells produce the cartilages and bones of the posterior skull. Somites generate the vertebrae, sacrum, and coccyx, the rest of the skull, and the ribs and sternum. Lateral plate mesodermal cells form the limbs and the shoulder and pelvic girdles. Bone development begins when mesenchymal cells migrate from these lineages to future bone sites. Then, after condensing to outline the shapes of bones, they differentiate into either chondrocytes, which form the cartilage of endochondral bones, later converted into bone (endochondral ossification), or osteoblasts, which form bone directly (intramembranous ossification). Endochondral ossification occurs in the base and the posterior part of the skull and the axial and appendicular skeleton, while intramembranous ossification is responsible for the formation of the flat bones of the cranium and parts of the clavicle.[7]

Bone formation happens as part of human differentiation, the process of cells developing

_____

[6]Historically, age-related increased fracture risk was thought to result from lower bone mass and density, but recent research shows that bound water also plays a crucial role.

_____

[7]The period of ossification varies for different bones, and the general timeline for ossification, according to Gray (2010), is as follows: in the second month of fetal development, the clavicle, lower jaw, vertebrae, humerus, femur, ribs, and cartilaginous part of the occipital bone develop. At the end of the second month and beginning of the third, the frontal bone, scapula, radius, ulna, tibia, fibula, and maxilla appear. During the third month, the rest of the cranial bones (with a few exceptions), metatarsals, metacarpals, and phalanges ossify. Month four brings with it the iliac bones, and the tiny bones of the inner ear, the ossicula auditus, while the fourth through fifth months sees the ossification of ethmoid, sternum, pubic bone, and ischium. The sixth and seventh months deliver the calcaneus and astragalus (or talus) in the feet, and during the eighth month, the development of the hyoid bone occurs.

into specific structures. Differentiation is how a liver becomes a liver and not a thyroid gland, or a bone becomes a bone and not a ligament, for example. According to Erich Blechschmidt, embryologist and founder of the Blechschmidt Collection of embryologic reconstructions at the Anatomical Institute of Göttingen University in Germany, bone formation is not based solely on genetics, but also on the movement of embryonic fluids. Blechschmidt emphasized that genes do not only act but also *react* to external *biodynamic* forces (much more on biodynamics soon). According to Blechschmidt, hereditary factors are important in human differentiation, but "the origin of the species and the origin of the organs" involve different processes (Blechschmidt and Gasser 2012, xviii). In other words, genes do not contain the final blueprint for how a heart valve or fibula will look when fully formed—it's actually the extragenic (outside of genetic control) fluid flow that drives human differentiation.[8]

Consider Blechschmidt's view on the development of an embryological leg. As the limb develops, fluidic pressure gradients cause it to bend. This bending squeezes fluid from the limb bud, creating a hardened condensation of cells, leading to the formation of bone. Here, it's the movement of fluid from within the mesenchymal cells toward the periphery that densifies the connective tissue, differentiating it from softer tissues. These biodynamic movements continue to impact skeletal change via bone remodeling throughout life.

Bone remodeling involves the removal of old or damaged bone by osteoclasts, coordinated with the deposition of new bone by osteoblasts. Similarly to how bones are initially formed, bone remodeling occurs by osteoclasts tunneling into old bone and by osteoblasts depositing new bone within the excavated tunnels. Much of the stimulus that leads to bone remodeling is derived from the mechanical load to which bones are subject. Wolff's law says that a bone will adapt to the loads placed upon it—an increase in load leads to the strengthening of the bone; a decrease in load will cause it to weaken.[9] This explains how the bones of the racquet-holding arm of a professional tennis player will be larger and stronger than those in their non-racquet arm.

The mechanism that converts mechanical load to bone remodeling is called mechanotransduction, a process where cells sense mechanical stimuli and then translate the information into signals, which elicit a response. Mechanotransduction in bone occurs via different mechanisms, including the movement of interstitial fluid as it flows over the osteocytes in their lacunae.[10] When everyday levels of mechanical load are applied to bone—like playing tennis or weight lifting or just walking— forces temporarily deform the matrix of the bones involved in the activity. This deformation compresses and stretches the interstitial spaces and the interstitial fluid within them. The deformation creates pressure gradients within the porosity of the bone matrix, causing interstitial fluid to move through the lacunar-canalicular network. As interstitial fluid flows, it exerts shear stress on osteocytes. Osteocytes detect the changes in shear stress through

---

[9]Micromodeling, a subcategory of bone remodeling, can even determine the orientation and direction of new bone deposition based on the direction of the forces acting upon it.

[10]Bone innervation also plays a part in mechanotransduction, as does piezoelectricity (the inherent ability of materials to generate electric fields in response to external strain) within collagen molecules.

---

[8]Fluid flow isn't the only extragenic influence over growth and development. Bioelectricity may also govern the genome in planaria, deer—and through evolution—humans (S. Walker 2024).

mechanosensitive ion channels and cell-surface receptors. This stimulates the osteocytes to regulate bone remodeling by biochemically signaling osteoblasts to build new bone or osteoclasts to resorb old bone. The important take-away here is that bones—despite being quite rigid—adapt and change.

BONE, STRESS, AND STRAIN

We just saw how Wolff's law describes how bone tissue responds to forces of everyday life. Now, let's look at how bone tissue behaves in response to the (much smaller) forces used during BST. Before we do this, let's review some basic physics.

Viscosity is the thickness of a liquid. Some liquids are thick and gooey like honey, others are thin and runny like water. When we move something through a thicker, gooier liquid, it's more difficult than moving it through a thinner, runnier one. The thick liquid offers more resistance to being deformed, and this resistance represents the viscosity of the liquid. The higher the resistance, the higher the viscosity. Shear thickening (sometimes referred to as dilatancy) is when fluid exhibits a drastic increase in viscosity with a sudden application of force. Materials like a cornstarch and water mixture exhibit shear thickening; they behave like a solid under stress and then return to a liquid state once the stress is removed.

The term *elasticity* describes how materials like springs and rubber bands return undamaged to their original shape after being stretched or compressed. Viscoelastic materials like collagen and bone combine the properties of an elastic material with those of a viscous fluid.[11] Elasticity, however, is

not the same as *plasticity*. Elasticity differs from plasticity in that the latter refers to the *nonreversible* deformation of a material. For instance, if the intensity of the stretch applied to the elastic band or tendon increases beyond the material's elastic capabilities, the deformation becomes plastic. During plastic deformation, a tendon or bone won't go back to its original form even if we stop stretching it. If the stretch continues to increase, the tissue may rupture. In the body, viscoelastic tissues only exhibit plasticity if the force applied to them surpasses their viscoelastic capabilities.

Moving from the intrinsic qualities of materials to the extrinsic forces exerted upon them, *compression* is when forces push an object inward on itself. Applying a compressive force is when we squeeze something. *Tension*, on the other hand, refers to a pulling force transmitted in the opposite direction to the compressive force. Applying a tensile force is when we pull something apart.

When compression or tension act upon a material and lead to deformation, *stress* is the measurement that describes the forces present during the deformation. *Strain* is the term used to describe the *amount* of deformation. (To remember this, I imagine the "train" in "strain" extending along train tracks.) An object being stretched, such as an elastic band or tendon or bone, is subject to tensile stress and undergoes elongation strain. The same object being pushed together or crushed experiences compressive stress and undergoes shortening strain. Soon, we'll see how collagen in bone exhibits tiny amounts of strain under tiny amounts of stress, and this behavior is essential to our work.

Speaking of compression, and according to clinical anatomist Peter Abrahams, when

[11]As Currey says about bone, "Although elastic, [bone] can flow a little bit, but not indefinitely" (Currey 2008, 41).

compressed, joints between bones relax under pressure, permitting more movement. During a recent email exchange with Sharon Wheeler, a student of Ida Rolf and developer of the BoneWork approach in the 1970s, she described a similar experience while working with bone tissue. Wheeler explained that when gently compressing bone, a kind of "dancing" sensation occurs. The "easing" described by Abrahams and the "dancing" described by Wheeler corroborate well with my own clinical experience. It seems that when compressing bone tissue with just the right amount of force and at just the right angle, a slippery, easing/dancing/melting sensation occurs, almost as if two ice cubes are being pressed together, squirming and slipping as they melt. But how? While we must be careful in assuming that pure collagen outside bone acts the same way as collagen does *inside* bone, the stress and strain responses of the pure collagen fibril (outside of bone) may help explain.

The Collagen Fibril as a Twisted Nanoscale Rope

The collagen fibril is built like a twisted nanoscale rope, and like actual rope or string, the fibrils are loaded with tension and prone to buckling when compressed. We've all experienced this, haven't we? Ever tried to lace up a shoe with a frayed shoelace? The reason this is so difficult (and frustrating) is because the substrands at the frayed end of the lace have separated, making the tip too wide to easily thread through the lace hole. Or when we counterwind and compress that thick piece of rope in the backyard and the strands separate in our hands? When we counterwind a piece of rope or shoelace—untwisting and compressing it—the rope gets wider as the strands unwind, creating more space between them. If you look closely at

the tip of that frayed lace that you can't fit back into the lace hole, there is *more* space between the strands. If you try to force the tip into the hole (compressing it even more), it gets wider still.

The same phenomenon seems to occur in collagen. During axial compression (when the ends of the fibril are approximated) pure collagen is weak. It will buckle and curl. The fibril expands, like the shoelace. Bozec and his team demonstrated this when they showed how collagen under compression displays "birdcaging," a phenomenon shared with twisted ropes and cables (and yes, shoelaces), which is the separation of the smaller individual substrands (figure 4.5).

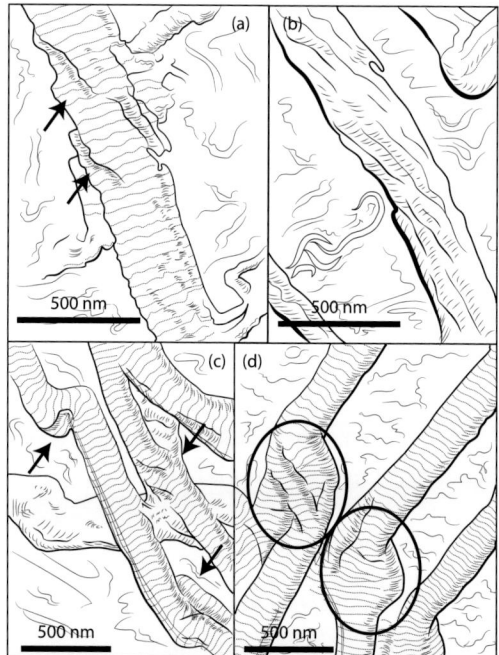

Figure 4.5. Birdcaging of collagen fibrils. (a) A collagen fibril is somewhat unwound. (b) The fibril is more unwound and has the appearance of a twisted rope with linear substructures. (c, d) The arrows indicate the presence of birdcaging along the length of the fibril, a phenomenon seen in ropes or cables that have been counter-wound or placed under compressive force. Adapted from Bozec, Van der Heijden, and Horton 2007.

In collagen, instead of axial compression closing the system it *opens and widens* it, creating pockets of new space. Is the new space created by collagen birdcaging responsible for the dancing sensation that we feel when compressing bone as described above? Perhaps.

Of course, due to the hydroxyapatite crystals within the collagen fibrils in bone, there is much less room for collagen to buckle and squirm than pure collagen would in a lab or even in softer tissues. In bone, the crystals do a great job of resisting compressive load—if they didn't, bone just wouldn't be bone. But as we learned, some collagen distortion in bone is not only present but necessary for optimal load transfer to occur. This tells us that there is still room for collagen in bone to act like pure collagen.

Back to physics (everyone's favorite subject) for a moment. Figure 4.6 depicts a typical stress/strain curve of compressive force applied to bone. We can see that under lower compressive loads, bone exhibits an elastic response: if the load is removed, the bone bounces back to its original shape. As the compressive load increases, the bone

undergoes a plastic deformation where microcracks eventually form. At this point, even if the load is removed, the damage is done (until the bone heals, of course). But what's going on in the stress/strain relationship at the very, very beginning of the curve, under compressive loads more consistent with those applied during BST?

To learn more, let's look at this from the opposite angle, from what happens to pure collagen under tension. It's well known that when a *tensile* force is applied to pure collagen, it undergoes three basic phases of strain: relaxation, elasticity, and plasticity (Bose et al. 2022; Bozec, Van der Heijden, and Horton 2007; Hart et al. 2017; Peacock et al. 2020; Stecco et al. 2020). Stecco explains this multiphasic behavior well. On a typical stress/strain curve, the relaxation phase occurs under very low tensile stress, where an "unkinking" of the collagen molecules takes place (figure 4.7, stage I). If the intensity of the stretch continues to increase, the stress is transferred to the collagen fibrils and then to the fibers themselves, where they undergo elastic strain (figure 4.7, stage II). If the intensity of the stretch is increased even more, the collagen fibers reach a yield point,

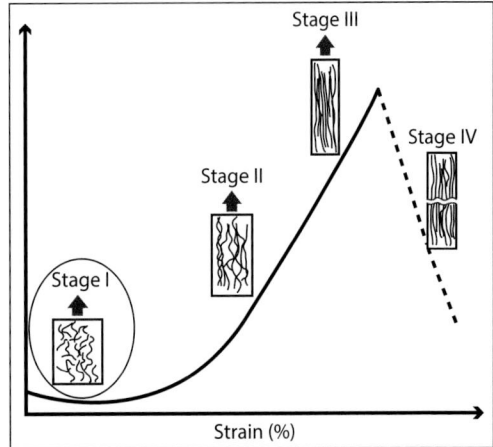

Figure 4.6. Stress/strain curve depicting bone compression. Adapted from Morgan, Unnikrisnan, and Hussein 2018.

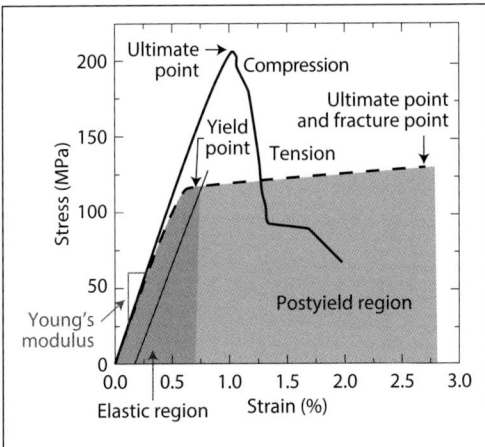

Figure 4.7. Stress/strain curve depicting pure collagen under tension.

after which plastic deformation takes place, leading to irreversible damage (figure 4.7, stage III). Of all three phases, it's the relaxation or toe phase—the very, very beginning of the curve—that interests us most. In this phase, the unkinking of collagen described by Stecco and others involves the collagen molecule's unique relationship with *water*.

According to Shen, the viscoelastic properties of a pure collagen fibril depend on the rearrangement of collagen and water molecules, and this can happen in several ways. First, in the presence of water, collagen molecules themselves could unwind and straighten. Second, facilitated by water molecules, collagen molecules could slide in relation to one another. Third, water molecules could rotate or translate within the fibril, or even be expelled from the fibril completely. Other research by Andriotis confirms that, indeed, the viscoelastic behavior of pure collagen fibrils under tension is due to a kind of "molecular hydroplaning" as water mediates the collagen molecules slipping against each other. This hydroplaning especially happens during the toe or relaxation phase under *very low tensile forces* and results in a sort of rearrangement of the collagen water network. If the tensile force continues to increase, the load is then carried entirely by the solid components of the matrix. In short, it seems that low forces act on fluids; higher forces act on solids. We'll see later why this matters.

When bone (not just pure collagen) is subject to a tensile force (and compared to pure collagen) less strain occurs for a given amount of stress. It deforms less under the same amount of force than a tendon would. This makes sense, of course, since bone is much more rigid. But when bone is subject to very low tensile forces, *we still feel change*. Why is that? Well, remember that some collagen distortion in bone is not only present but necessary for

optimal load transfer to occur. This teeny tiny bit of bone distortion seems to open that small window of opportunity for our therapeutic dialogue and (perhaps) allowing for that micro-birdcaging of collagen discussed earlier.

If bone strain at very low *tensile* stress happens within the viscoelasticity of the collagen, it seems reasonable that the same range of *compressive* bone strain happens within the viscoelasticity of collagen on the way back in. Whether or not this is actually the case remains to be seen (or investigated), but at the very least it's a helpful visualization for us to use. During BST, we move back and forth within this viscoelastic "cushion"—dialoguing with the twisty and fluidic nature of collagen and bone—twisting and squishing out and twisting and squishing back in again. This image reminds me of a musician skillfully playing an accordion, moving the bellows of the instrument back and forth to produce the music.

The Spring-Loaded Accordion: Compression and Tension in Bone

My spring-loaded accordion analogy may help illustrate this. This wonky little accordion has springs housed within a collapsible outer casing. The springs represent the collagen molecules, and the outer casing represents the hydroxyapatite crystal reinforcements. The whole accordion is twisted to replicate a torsional pattern within the bone. Imagine holding the accordion in both hands. As we spread our hands just a bit, challenging the twisty resistance of the torsional pattern, the accordion opens, and the springs begin to straighten. As the accordion opens more, the folds in the hydroxyapatite-reinforced outer casing begin to stiffen and then eventually lock, stopping the accordion from opening anymore. Now, if we bring the accordion back to neutral, going back into the ease of the twist (imagine the counterwinding of the rope here, with the separating substrands of collagen) and allowing the springs to return to resting length, and then continue to move our hands closer together, the folds in the outer casing begin to close. As our hands continue to approximate, the folds in the outer casing eventually shut, stopping the compression altogether.

At first, when the springs begin to straighten—but before the stiffness of the hydroxyapatite casing kicks in—*there is deformation*. Then, when the springs begin to collapse—but before the stiffness of hydroxyapatite casing kicks in—*there is, again, deformation*.

Now, picture moving in and out this springy cushion between the limits of compression and tension, playing the twisted accordion within its range of springiness, challenging and then counterwinding the twists in each direction, staying within the squishiness of the system. This is where the music happens (apologies to the neighbors), and this is a pretty good visualization of how BST might play out in bone.

OSSEOFASCIAL CONTINUUM

Together, the skeleton (bone) and the ligaments (fascia) that hold it together make up the osseofascial continuum, a living ecosystem of collagen-rich connective tissue. We've already discussed bone, but what about fascia?

Medical professionals have been contemplating the definition of fascia for a long time. Apparently, the debate began back in Egypt in 2500 BCE and has been going on until now. Let's pick it up in mid-2014, when the Fascia Research Society, a group of clinicians and researchers, established the

Fascia Nomenclature Committee. In 2019, the committee devised the following two-part definition of fascia:

Anatomical definition:
A fascia is a sheath, a sheet, or any other dissectible aggregations of connective tissue that forms beneath the skin to attach, enclose, and separate muscles and other internal organs. (Schleip et al. 2019)

Functional definition:
The fascial system consists of the three-dimensional continuum of soft, collagen-containing, loose and dense fibrous connective tissues that permeate the body. It incorporates elements such as adipose tissue, adventitiae and neurovascular sheaths, aponeuroses, deep and superficial fascia, epineurium, joint capsules, ligaments, membranes, meninges, myofascial expansions, periostea, retinacula, septa, tendons, visceral fasciae, and all the intramuscular and intermuscular connective tissues including endomysium/perimysium/epimysium. The fascial system surrounds, interweaves between, and interpenetrates all organs, muscles, bones, and nerve fibers, endowing the body with a functional structure, and providing an environment that enables all body systems to operate in an integrated manner. (Schleip et al. 2019)

End of story, right? Wrong! In 2022, another nonprofit organization, the Foundation of Osteopathic Research and Clinical Endorsement, a group of physicians, surgeons, chiropractors, and physiotherapists, redefined fascia as:

... any tissue that contains features capable of responding to mechanical stimuli. The fascial continuum is the result of the evolution of the perfect synergy among different tissues, liquids, and solids, capable of supporting, dividing, penetrating, feeding, and connecting all the districts of the body: epidermis, dermis, fat, blood, lymph, blood and lymphatic vessels, tissue covering the nervous filaments (endoneurium, perineurium, epineurium), voluntary striated muscle fibers and the tissue covering and permeating it (epimysium, perimysium, endomysium), ligaments, tendons, aponeurosis, cartilage, *bones*, meninges, involuntary striated musculature and involuntary smooth muscle (all viscera derived from the mesoderm), visceral ligaments, epiploon (small and large), peritoneum, and tongue. The continuum constantly transmits and receives mechano-metabolic information that can influence the shape and function of the entire body. These afferent/efferent impulses come from the fascia and the tissues that are not considered as part of the fascia in a bi-univocal mode. (Bordoni et al. 2022; emphasis added)

Wait: bone *is* fascia? Maybe! And here's why. First, bone and fascia are linked via their embryological beginnings. From this view, if the human body were a nuclear family, bone and fascia are part of the same offspring. Since bone and fascia have a common origin from cells of the embryonic mesenchyme, they could be considered "mutually dependent specializations of the same tissue" (Armstrong 2021). As we saw earlier, bones arise from the mesoderm, but the mesoderm shares a lineage with the ectoderm, which leads to the development of the skin, neurons, and organs. Some cranial bones arise from the mesoderm, others from the ectoderm, and some from both the mesoderm and ectoderm. And to muddy the waters even more, some bone-forming cells lead to the development of other tissues altogether. Based on this embryological splicing, the delineation between fascia and bone becomes murky at best.

Secondly, clinical anatomist John Sharkey points to the continuity of the bone-fascia relationship and the floating bone principle mentioned earlier and championed by Levin and fellow biotensegrity researcher Graham Scarr. The floating bone principle claims that bone floats within muscles and softer connective tissues, all blended inseparably into one collagen-rich modular flow system. Biotensegrity, an idea we'll explore in more detail soon, refutes the view that the skeleton is just a coatrack of levers and hooks from which softer tissues hang. A more modern view is that our skeleton behaves more like a myofascial ecosystem of stiffer compression struts continuous with a network of softer tension cables, all of which can spontaneously switch between compression and tension roles based on demands and circumstances. For this reason, both Levin and Scarr consider all tissues (including bone) to be more like soft-matter gels. According to Scarr, the question is not *if* bone and fascia are rigid or compliant, but when. The unique ability of bones and fascia to switch roles may be further proof that bone is really just mineralized fascia.

The third argument why bone may be considered to be fascia is that the two share the ability to convert load into action via mechanotransduction. We saw how Wolff's law applies to bone tissue: bones adapt to stresses exerted upon them by remodeling themselves. Fascia also uses mechanotransduction to remodel itself, and Davis's law, developed by orthopedic surgeon Henry Davis, describes a similar phenomenon in softer connective tissues.[12]

---

[12]There are other arguments that make the case for bone to be included within the definition of fascia, including that bone is an organ complete with parenchyma and its own autocrine and paracrine functions, and that fibroblasts, osteoblasts, and chondrocytes all contain similar contractile smooth-muscle-like proteins.

Fourth, and perhaps most relevant to our work, Levin reminds us that the underlying structure of both bone and fascia is the same: a soft collagen network. Sharpey's fibers, tiny expansions of ligaments and tendons (both fascia) that connect bones to other bones and muscles, are not only continuous with the periosteum (also fascia) but also penetrate deep into the bony matrix, blending with it, and essentially becoming the endosteum (also fascia).

For these reasons, bones appear less and less like rigid pegs and knobs tied together with ligaments. Bone and fascia seem to be less like two separate tissues and more like a seamless tapestry of rigid/less-rigid/rigid/less-rigid parts of the same collagen-rich tissue.

OSSEOFASCIAL COMPACTIONS

In 1982, Philippe Druelle founded the Collège d'Etudes Ostéopathique (CEO) in Montreal. Through his teachings, Druelle passed on his treatment philosophy to his students, many of whom became teachers at the college themselves. When I was a student there from 2009 to 2014, Druelle and his colleagues taught us a precise treatment protocol, which ranked osteopathic lesions from most to least disruptive. Regardless of the symptom, we were taught to evaluate the entire body and then treat the highest-priority dysfunctions first.

The approach was logical and effective. In the 1980s and 1990s, young osteopaths graduating from the CEO essentially rewrote the definition of manual therapy in Quebec. Legend has it that in those years, fifth-year students who had opened their calendars in advance of graduation became so overwhelmed with bookings that their practices were full before they had even begun!

As word spread of this new generation of highly sought-after "super physios" (as they were sometimes referred to), aspiring students signed up in droves. The explosive success of traditional osteopathy in Quebec led to the eventual expansion of the CEO across Canada and overseas. Today, the CEO remains the largest private osteopathy college in Canada, with Montreal regarded as an international hub of traditional osteopathy.

What made Druelle's school so successful and his approach so impactful? Many factors, of course. But the curriculum taught there was (and is) unique. First, carrying the torch of traditional osteopathy, Druelle's methodology takes into account the whole person, not just the symptom. Second, his method requires sensing (listening with the hands), an essential first step to evaluation and treatment. Third, at the very top of Druelle's list of most disruptive lesions sits intraosseous dysfunction—and more specifically, intraosseous compaction—which always held extra-special interest to me.

An intraosseous compaction is a kind of bony somatic dysfunction. It refers to a zone within bone that has lost its elasticity and vitality. When palpated, these zones feel more like concrete-hard bone than like wood-hard bone. Intraosseous compactions feel less "alive."

"Traite en decompaction!" Druelle would often say in French, or "treat by decompacting!" We did this through an informal combination of compressive dialogue and direct tension application to the tissue. When the bone tissue softened, the technique was over. I once asked for Druelle's advice on treating the first cervical vertebra of a patient, which was stuck in a translated position. I explained that I had tried everything to no avail. "Traite en decompaction!" he advised me. The next time I saw my patient, I grasped C1 between my thumb and fingers, with my hand cupped underneath the base of the skull and upper neck. Following Druelle's advice, and with pressure into the rigidity of the bone, I felt the bone begin to soften as its elasticity and vitality returned. It was an important moment for me.

Throughout our training, decompacting bone tissue was promoted as a simple yet crucial step. But I thought: if this is so important, why was there not a more detailed evaluation and treatment methodology available? My persistent curiosity in this regard led to the explorations described in these pages.

Druelle and others have described intraosseous compactions as areas within bone with an altered texture. Texture changes in bone can occur following trauma. Acute trauma can cause bone to distort by disrupting the collagen-hydroxyapatite matrix and/or the tiny fluid-filled spaces of the vascular-lacunar-canalicular network contained within it. According to Bicahlo, if there is no fracture following the insult, the bone will recoil but still retain a degree of distortion. That traumatic "imprint" seems to create a palpable change in the texture of the bone. Unless treated, the imprint can remain indefinitely.[13] According to Verzella and Sharma, tissue texture may also be altered *in the absence* of acute trauma, via low-grade inflammation and the concurrent behavior of biological water. In either case, it seems that bone-tissue texture changes involve fluidic phenomena. More on biological water soon.

Before going any further, let's revisit those "bone versus osseofascia" semantics mentioned earlier. Since compactions exist within and between bones, and since bone and fascia can be considered one and the same, we can also refer to intraosseous compactions as *osseofascial* compactions. In my opinion, this term more aptly addresses both types of compactions at once: some osseofascial compactions exist within bone, and some osseofascial compactions live between bones.

Within bone, an osseofascial compaction is a bit like an internal bone scar. On skin, scars contain disorganized patterns of collagen. Bone tissue doesn't always heal from fracture or injury with a permanent or visible scar like skin does, but we can still sometimes feel the traumatic imprint. In nature, wind and water currents are invisible, but we can still feel them. Like these natural currents, the bone "scar" is invisible, but we can often feel its altered texture.

Texture change is a defining characteristic of somatic dysfunction. Dysfunctional fascial tissue feels and behaves differently than normal fascial tissue, and the STAR acronym is an easy way to remember how:

S = sensitivity increased
T = texture changes
A = asymmetry
R = range of motion decreased

There is general consensus that if fascial tissue displays any of these characteristics, the tissue is dysfunctional in some way. But Verzella suggests that the other three STAR signs often depend on tissue texture, so the "T" is an especially reliable indicator of dysfunction. This perspective falls in line nicely with the principles of BST, and champions the benefits of testing and treating texture first.

---

[13]Acute trauma can also lead to inflammatory responses and the subsequent release of collagen-degrading enzymes, disrupting the matrix even further.

Far more research has been done on fascial somatic dysfunction (often referred to as *adhesions* or *fibrosis*) and how to treat it (Armstrong 2021; Chaitow 2014; Cyron and Humphrey 2017; Lesondak 2022; Liem 2016; Tozzi 2015a, b; Verzella et al. 2022) than on bony osseofascial compactions. Due to the behavior of pure collagen in softer collagen-rich connective tissues, however, elements of this research may apply to bone, as well.

Fluid Behavior and Osseofascial Tissue Texture

Some of the earliest testimonies emerging from the manual therapy community claimed that osseofascial tissue texture—the texture of both fascia *and* bone—correlated strongly with the behavior of fluid. In 1899, Andrew Taylor Still, the founder of osteopathy, said that "the soul of man, with all the streams of pure living water, seems to dwell in the fasciae of his body" (Armstrong 2021). William Garner Sutherland, Still's most famous student, carried this idea forward and described how fluid is transported throughout the body via the fascia; how a "tide" that travels throughout the body creates a flow of interstitial fluid that bathes every cell. Still and Sutherland both perceived the fluids as an organizing force through which profound healing occurred. Ann Wales, a former student of Sutherland's, passed on this perspective and spoke of "an intensified interchange between all of the fluids of the body," and said that "it is evident that the reaction is systemic and includes the whole body, even within the bones" (Armstrong 2021). Then, in 2018, new technologies helped Benias and his team confirm these early reports, when they uncovered the existence of a body-wide system called the *interstitium*.

Earlier, we learned of Guimberteau's collagen network. The interstitium is a network of fluid-filled interstitial spaces that runs *within and throughout* Guimberteau's collagen network, bathing and nourishing collagen in both fascia and bone. The interstitium consists of "macroscopically visible ... dynamically compressible and distensible sinuses through which interstitial fluid flows around the body" (Benias et al. 2018). Thanks to these discoveries, we now have evidence of two interconnected, permanently hydrated systems at work, weaving in and around each other throughout our bodies and our bones.[14]

In osseofascial tissue, these fluids seem to impact the behavior of collagen and (perhaps) the texture of bone itself. I mentioned earlier that low-grade inflammation and interstitial fluid behavior have been linked to fascial fibrosis. In contrast to "normal" inflammation, low-grade inflammation can occur in the absence of trauma and without the tell-tale symptoms like heat, pain, redness, and swelling. Low-grade inflammation just sort of lives within us, rising and falling in response to everyday stressors. When there's an increase in stress, low-grade inflammation rises. As it does so, it can impact the nature and behavior of proteins, leading to the so-called "unfolded protein response" within a cell. When the unfolded protein response is continuously activated owing to unresolved levels of low-grade inflammation, fibroblasts proliferate and produce excess extracellular matrix components. This cascade hardens fascial tissue, leading to fibrosis.

According to Verzella, fibrosis occurs in association with decreased levels of "exclusion zone" water near the surface of collagen. Exclusion zone water has a higher

---

[14]In bone, the interstitium refers to the vascular-lacunar-canalicular network of interstitial-fluid-filled spaces.

viscosity and is more stable than "normal" biological water, and exists near the surfaces of cell membranes and proteins. Verzella suggests that (*a*) the presence of exclusion zone water in fascial tissue could serve as a marker for tissue health, and (*b*) manual therapy (especially indirect manual therapy) could improve the texture and function of fascial tissue by rebalancing levels of exclusion zone water.[15] Verzella also reminds us that exclusion zone water *doesn't only live in fascia*—it is also found in bone, where it stabilizes the triple-helix collagen molecule and collagen-mineral interface. If low-grade inflammation and altered exclusion zone water are markers of nontraumatic fibrosis in fascia, perhaps the same characteristics act as markers for a sort of nontraumatic intraosseous fibrosis in bone. This is an idea worth exploring, I think. Alternately, regarding a traumatic imprint in bone tissue, if the fluid-filled canaliculi and lacunae are impacted or damaged by trauma, restoring fluidic balance within the vascular-lacunar-canalicular network following the traumatic insult would be well indicated.

If these hypotheses hold water (pardon the pun), by entering into a therapeutic dialogue with osseofascial fluid, we can participate in and potentially accelerate the resolution of the "fluid-mediated" formation of both nontraumatic and traumatic osseofascial compactions.

So, it seems that both acute trauma and low-grade inflammation impact osseofascial tissue texture via the same medium: the behavior of interstitial fluid. As Jim Jealous said, "One could reflect on somatic dysfunction as fluid phenomena" (Jealous 2015, 30). For this reason, we cannot fully treat bones—via mobilization, recoils, osteoarticular manipulations, and so on—without first dialoguing with osseofascial fluid first. This is where BST can help.

Vitality and Osseofascial Compactions

What is the difference between an osseofascial compaction and a regular, run-of-the-mill somatic dysfunction? While texture changes are present in both, the loss of vitality is reserved exclusively for osseofascial compactions.

Elasticity and vitality go hand in hand, since elasticity is a hallmark of tissue that is alive. When cells and organisms die, they experience a rapid increase in rigidity, called *rigor mortis*. Compacted osseofascial tissue isn't "dead," of course, but it has lost some of the characteristics that make it vital. In this way, bones resemble other complex organisms that are alive, like birds and blueberries, and as some would argue, computational systems and artificial intelligence.[16]

---

[15]We know that besides hydration levels, other factors may lead to somatic dysfunction in fascia, including dysregulated myofascial contraction, altered myofascial tone and force transmission, altered neuromuscular coordination, autonomic and somatic neural interactions, and fluctuating pH levels, hormonal and metabolic factors, temperature, changes in piezoelectric responses, and breathing patterns (Tozzi 2015b; Bicalho 2020).

[16]Sara Imari Walker and proponents of the assembly theory of the origin of life believe that artificial intelligence is but one component of the technosphere. According to assembly theory, the technosphere has evolved—via natural selection—from our human lineage within the biosphere. Don't worry—while AI shares certain lifelike complexities with living objects, it is not considered to be alive (yet!).

Let's step back from the treatment table for a moment. Referring to computational systems, Chris Langdon, a pioneer in the development of artificial intelligence in the early 1990s, says, "A system can exhibit complex, life-like behavior only if it has just the right balance of stability and fluidity" (quoted in Waldrop 1993, 308). Langdon describes a transition phase between order and disorder called the "edge of chaos." At the edge of chaos, components of a network never quite lock into place, yet never completely descend into turbulence either. These are systems that are stable enough to store information yet fluid enough to transmit it. They are spontaneous, adaptive, and alive. According to Stuart Kaufman, professor of biological sciences at the University of Calgary, "Living systems are actually very close to this edge of chaos phase transition" (quoted in Waldrop 1993, 303). How does this to relate to bone? Well, in bone tissue, just the right balance of stability and fluidity allows healthy bone to be all the remarkable things that it is. Similar to computational systems, too much stability (order) or fluidity (chaos) and the full expression of a bone's life—its vitality— is diminished. In other words, compacted osseofascial tissue sits closer to "rigor mortis" at the extreme "order" end of the order–chaos spectrum. It is my view that by treating osseofascial compactions with BST, we are moving the needle back along the spectrum—closer to that Goldilocks zone just at the optimal edge of chaos. Referring to living organisms, Kaufman says that "evolution always seems to lead to order at the edge of chaos" (quoted in Waldrop 1993, 303). It seems that life (and bone) just prefers it there.

CHAPTER 5

The Pelvic Gather

Marianne was suffering from debilitating bilateral hip pain for years, but imaging ruled out significant pathology. Since our treatments up to that point brought only temporary relief, in June 2023, I tried something new. I had her lie on her back and then placed her legs on a pillow. I brought my hands underneath her pelvis and around each iliac bone, gently hugging her legs with my forearms. I moved my body forward, bringing the pelvis toward the spine and each iliac toward the sacrum, carefully remaining within the fluidic cushion of the tissues. I gathered her pelvis around a quiet stillness at its center. Then I did nothing, and waited. I waited until the stillness spread outward, bringing with it a new kind of symmetry. I waited there, holding space for an ecosystem busy and alive. When the treatment was over, I removed my hands. Marianne got up, feeling very well, and left. When she returned the following month, she had remained pain-free for the first time in three years.

We'll review the pelvic gather technique soon.

CHAPTER 6

A Wilderness of Surprises

At the center of the beholder there must be space for the whole, and this nothing-space is not an empty nothing but a nothing reserved for everything.

—Saul Bellow

We carry inside us our own wildernesses, as particular in their obsessions as they are various in their surprises.

—Carl Phillips

CHAPTER 7

Some Things Happen Only Once

Suzanne developed Parkinson's disease and then ceased coming to see me for treatments. One day in 2014, I felt an urge to check up on her. As I reached for my phone, the call display lit up with her name and phone number. Astonished, Suzanne told me that she had felt a similar unexplained urge to speak with me at that very moment. After our exchange, we wished each other well, and said goodbye. Until our conversation that day, we had not spoken in over four years, and for whatever reason, have never felt the need to speak again.

If something happens only once, is it less or more significant than if it happens multiple times?

CHAPTER 8

Texture, Drive, and Rhythm

Compacted bone and fascia have lost some of the fundamental characteristics that make them bone and fascia. To understand how this happens we'll now discuss the concept of biotensegrity and how (with the help of optimal bone quality and the continuity of the PSE) tensegrity forces are transmitted within and between bones. This section will also introduce and describe two key BST concepts—potency and fulcrum-lever systems. Finally, primary respiration, the three bodies, and Bordoni's three fascias will be explored, to shine even more light on the unique and important combination of texture, drive, and rhythm living within the osseofascial continuum.

BIOTENSEGRITY AND THE OSSEOFASCIAL CONTINUUM

The year 1967 was a busy one. Protests erupted against the Vietnam War, China tested its first hydrogen bomb, Elvis Presley married Priscilla in Las Vegas, a military coup took place in Sierra Leone, the Human Be-In in San Francisco launched the Summer of Love, Louis Leakey discovered *Kenyapithecus africanus*, the Grateful Dead released their first album, a UFO was spotted in the skies above Nova Scotia, Charlie Chaplin appeared in his last film, Muhammad Ali refused military service, a volcano erupted in Antarctica, and in honor of Canada's 100th birthday, Montreal hosted Expo '67.

At the American Pavilion at Expo '67 (now known as the Montreal Biosphere) stands a 250-foot, bubble-shaped, transparent dome made of steel and plexiglass. When my kids were young, we would gaze up at this giant sphere shimmering above us like a hologram. I can almost see it from my kitchen window as I write this. The dome was designed for the Expo by architect R. Buckminster Fuller, and remains his most famous construction. Fuller coined the term *tensegrity*, a combination of the words *tension* and *integrity*, to describe the unique structural relationship between compressive and tensile forces holding the dome up. Architecturally speaking, a tensegrity structure is composed of compression struts that seem to float within a network of tensioned cables. For his sculpture, Fuller subdivided an icosahedron into many smaller icosahedra in a shape large enough to mimic the multidirectional compression resistance of a sphere. He saw structures at every scale as energy systems that harnessed these compressive and tensile forces, and his dome in Montreal was built with these ideas in mind.

The tensegrity principle of *modularity* accounts for how each part or group of parts of a tensegrity structure is integrated, with each module nested within those surrounding it. In Fuller's geodesic dome, any change in any of the struts would impact the next-larger icosahedron-shaped module that it formed. Since each module is inseparable from the next-larger one, each icosahedron at any scale is dependent on the others. The model in figure 8.1 shows three shapes, with each one dependent on the others to complete its own configuration. Here, separate-yet-continuous multiscale modules create a single structure, where any change in one will have repercussions on the others.

Biological systems seem to be governed by similar principles. Tensegrity in living organisms is referred to as *biotensegrity*, and modularity in living organisms (let's call this *biomodularity*) helps explain how any change in one bone or group of bones within the osseofascial continuum leads to changes in the region. Biomodularity also helps explain why we implement both local *and* regional BST treatment: the combination of the two allows us to address smaller osseofascial modules nested within larger, regional ones. In the body, bone A affects bones B and C, and maybe bones B and C eventually impact bones D through G, even maintaining dysfunction back in bone A, potentially creating a network-wide self-perpetuating dysfunctional loop (figure 8.2).

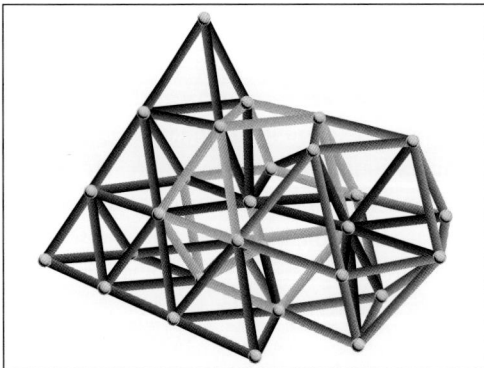

Figure 8.2. Biotensegrity and biomodularity. Dysfunction in bone A could lead to dysfunction in bone B, etc., creating a self-perpetuating dysfunctional loop.

Furthermore, as opposed to a hierarchical organization, where a system is organized from the top down, biotensegrity is powered by a self-organizing, bottom-up, *heterarchal* system, where each component, regardless of size or scale, carries equal importance within the continuum. In the *biodemocracy* (I'm on a bio-roll) of our bodies, no one is in charge because everyone is in charge: the tiniest atom is as crucial as the largest muscle or the longest nerve. Ultimately, it's the actions and reactions at the nanoscale, microscale, and macroscale within our biodemocracy that help determine the shape and behavior of our bodies.[17]

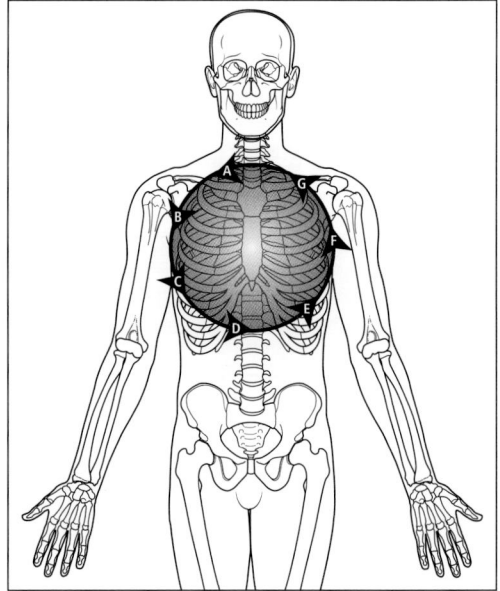

Figure 8.1. Tensegrity modularity. Each of the three shapes is dependent on the others to complete its own configuration. Separate-yet-continuous multiscale modules create a single structure, where any change in one will have repercussions on the others.

[17]In the developing human embryo, Blechschmidt discovered that when shape changes occur at one scale, they also occur at larger and smaller scales, consistent with how heterarchical systems behave. He reasoned that the shape of developing organs and bones is determined not only by genetics but also by the pushes and pulls of neighboring structures. In this way, the human embryo can be viewed as a biotensegrity structure.

Within the osseofascial continuum itself, the same holds true. The pushes and pulls of each phalanx and femur, each rib and zygoma, each bone tiny or large, force each bone to react and then shift back and forth, from compression strut (a part that resists compression) to a tension cable (a part that resists tension) and back again. According to Scarr and Levin, the ability of bones to shift back and forth this way sustains a more cohesive osseofascial biotensegrity. But compromised bone quality has the potential to hinder it.

This shape-shifting idea plays out in everyday activities. Consider jumping up and down on one leg. With normal bone tissue, the femur can balance the compression forces coming from up from the ground with the muscular tensile forces of the quadriceps and hamstrings pulling on the bone to dampen the landing. Healthy bone accomplishes this task without incident—it's rigid yet elastic, like a young tree. But compacted bone may have a harder time here. The ability of the compacted bone to balance compression and tension forces—to shift from compression strut to tension cable—may be compromised. In the case of you jumping up and down, a compacted femur will still do the job, but maybe not as efficiently. If many jumps are performed on the compacted bone day after day, the compromised bone may eventually lead to dysfunction in the muscles and tendons and ligaments attached to it, or in other bones or body systems. For bones to act like bones, bone *quality* matters.

SHARPEY'S FIBERS AND OSSEOFASCIAL TISSUE CONTINUITY

As we learned earlier, Sharpey's fibers are integral to tissue continuity; they expand from soft-tissue attachments and the periosteum, and penetrate deep into the bone matrix (figure 8.3). Via the PSE continuum, Sharpey's fibers connect the periosteum not only to the endosteum but also to all osseous features and compartments in between. Aaron showed how osteoporotic pig bone compromised the quality of the Sharpey's fibers attached to it (figure 8.4), shedding light on the potential impact of bone quality on the connections between structures. As we

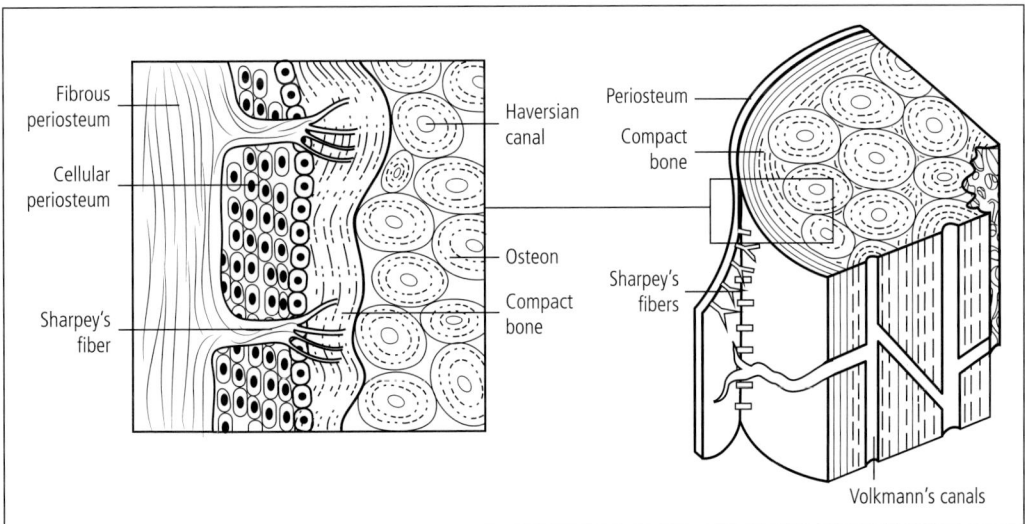

Figure 8.3. Sharpey's fibers expand from the periosteum and penetrate into the bone matrix, connecting bones and parts of bones to each other. Adapted from Aaron 2012.

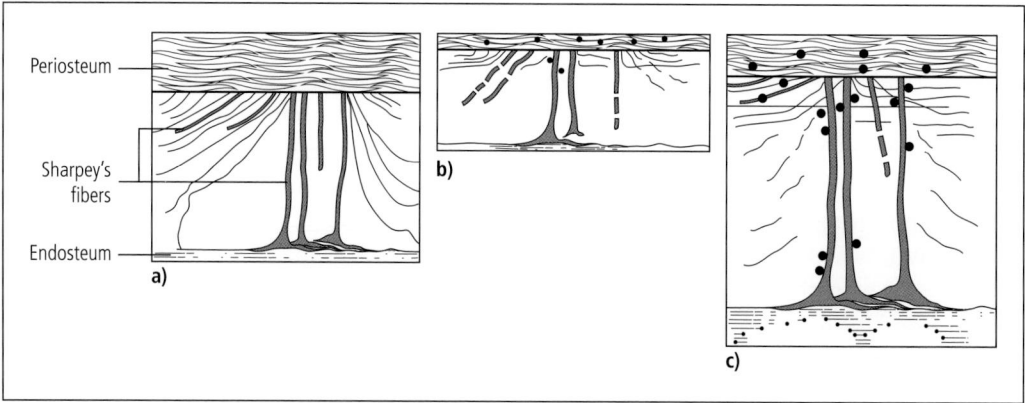

Figure 8.4. The quality of Sharpey's fibers in normal (a) and osteoporotic (b,c) pig bone. Adapted from Aaron 2012.

can see in figure 8.4, in normal pig bone (a) Sharpey's fibers appear healthy; running from the periosteum through the bony matrix reaching the endosteum uninterrupted. The fibers are continuous and unbroken. But as the quality of the bone degrades (b, c), we notice a concurrent degradation in the quality of the Sharpey's fibers. The fibers become thickened and/or disjointed. Here, if bone quality is impaired, so too can be the Sharpey's fibers and the PSE and, by extension, the entire osseofascial continuum.

It's possible—with a capital "P"!—that similar to osteoporotic bone, compacted *nonosteoporotic* bone could also impact the performance of Sharpey's fibers and the PSE continuum—at least temporarily.[18] Then, if the compacted quality of bone tissue can be optimized (again, at least temporarily), the relationship between adjacent structures could be as well. If this were the case, then the

effects of subsequent manual therapies applied to those structures directly after BST could be even more effective, couldn't they? Based on my humble experience, this is what often occurs. Biotensegrity and tissue continuity work together to maintain coherence within and between the structures of the osseofascial continuum, and BST serves as a useful tool to maintain and enhance both.

Now, if we look closer, there's something even more profound going on. Life is buzzing *within* the continuum itself. An ecosystem is alive with rhythm and drive, literally breathing osseofascial tissue from the inside. Along with other tissues and systems, the osseofascial continuum seems to be animated by an enlivened intelligence, an inherent drive toward health and order some have simply called: Potency.

POTENCY

Potency is power. Potency is strength. Potency is the ability to initiate or perform. With his hands cupping the cranium, Sutherland sensed a potency within the cerebrospinal fluid, which he felt made the fluid fluctuate. But the *nature* of Sutherland's potency remains less clear: we really don't know what it is or from where it comes. I think that describing potency in the body

_____

[18]I use the word *temporarily* since we just don't know how long the impact of BST lasts. From my experience, sometimes a bone that I had worked on normalizes itself during the treatment but remains compacted a week, a month, or a year afterward. At some point before the reevaluation, the effect of BST "wore off." Yet, in other instances, the bone will remain normalized. Other scenarios are possible, too.

with words is kind of like describing the color blue or how an apple tastes—it's probably easier to just look up at the sky or bite into a ripe Honeycrisp and call it a day. But before we accept the fact that potency just *is* and move on, let's toss the football around and see if we can find some science in it.

I may have first sensed a version of potency long ago, not within anyone else, but within and around me. When I was five years old, my dad would take me hiking in the Laurentian Mountains in Quebec. We would cross the road and walk up a steep embankment that turned from soft dry sand to damp green moss to taller grasses and shrubs. Multicolored mushroom spores exploded from their caps, blowing upward before returning underground to rot or start over. Tiny plants sprouted, their configurations identical to the taller trees overhead. Perfect miniature replicas, like furniture in a dollhouse. Air currents mixed the scents of daisies with the briny fumes from the lake across the road. Nearly every weekend during those summers, I would be engulfed by this exquisite beauty, by this wilderness of surprises. Each day reminded me of its own painting; colors bleeding into one another, hues and shadow combining and separating again. With eyes closed and with the sun warming my face, I would bask in these sacred moments. On these walks, I felt held and permeated by a larger presence, by a potent life energy living within and around me and between things. What was holding all of it together? Nature? Physics? Chemistry? God?

Perhaps the best place to begin understanding potency is not from how it behaves in and around us, but rather from its behavior in other organisms—like in mold. During your next walk in the woods, look down. If you're lucky, on a damp, rotting tree stump, you may spot an orange or yellow mass of goop staring back up at you. *Physarum polycephalum,* more commonly known as slime mold, is one of the earliest known life forms, and has been oozing around the planet for the last 100 million years or so. Protoplasm is the semifluid substance within cells, and slime mold is basically a blob of protoplasm. But slime mold is far from your average blob.

In his film from the 1930s, botany professor William Seifriz demonstrated that rivulets of liquid protoplasm (protoplasm shifts between liquid and gel states) within slime mold flowed freely until, almost without cause, the liquid reversed flow, pulled by some unknown force in each direction. Seifriz's film also showed slime mold creating a barrier to seal off injected saline, an action that Seifriz interpreted as an attempt to protect the rest of the organism from harm.

At the time of Seifriz's experiments, protoplasm enjoyed special status in biology. Scientists viewed it "as the fundamental stuff of life" (Deitrich 2015) and investigating its behavior was sort of like searching for the meaning of life itself. More recently, it was discovered that the movements within slime mold are powered by the contractile behavior of actin and myosin filaments, a trait shared with human muscle tissue. Other current research demonstrates that slime mold can solve mazes to find food, and how its oscillatory movements relate to mechanisms of learning and movement. Yet, despite these new insights, explaining the *regulator* of the motion in slime mold remains elusive. Could the nature of the slime mold regulator be one that is consistent across all life forms? Could the regulator here be the same potent force—potency itself—that Sutherland sensed in human cerebrospinal fluid?

Sutherland believed that potency was an embodied, intelligent momentum, a life force generated by what he referred to as the "Breath of Life," a term first used in Genesis 2:7. We know that cerebrospinal fluid is clear and colorless and flows within and around the brain and spinal cord. Tiny hairlike cilia on the innermost surfaces of the ventricles beat in coordinated fashion, shuttling the cerebrospinal fluid from one place to another. Along with the vascular pulse and diaphragmatic excursion during respiration, the cilia are at least partially responsible for the fluctuation of cerebrospinal fluid. With the anatomical knowledge of his day, Sutherland surely understood that the cerebrospinal fluid was directed through the ventricles of the brain in these ways, but he still sensed something else at play—a governing force from within.

Referring to potency in the body, Sutherland said: "'Tis the mortar in the space between the bricks that holds the structure together" (quoted in Jealous 2015, 28). In this light, potency can be compared to the spaces between things. For example, the spaces between musical notes hold the notes together, creating a melody. For a song to be a song, it *needs* these spaces. Todd Kepler, researcher at the Santa Fe Institute, describes the curious relationship between negative and positive spaces in Picasso's *Les Demoiselles d'Avignon*, and how the artist gave the spaces between the women and their arms and torsos a peculiar solidity. Here, it's the spaces between shapes that make the painting come alive. Perhaps, then, potency lies in the spaces between biological structures, maintaining the cohesiveness of the organism. Jealous speaks of the space between atoms as a "pure intelligent energy" (Jealous 2015, 29). Like these powerful negative areas, maybe potency is a kind of vital, intelligent (bio)mortar?

But maybe potency resides not only in the spaces between parts, but also in the interactions between them. In the late 1980s,

Aristid Lindenmayer of the University of Utrecht and Prezemyslaw Prusinkiewicz of the University of Regina in Saskatchewan gave a presentation about fake plants. These plants were not made of plastic or cloth— they were grown on a computer screen. The programmers started from a stem and used a handful of simple rules to tell the branches how to grow. The rules said nothing about how the mature plant should eventually look, but only about how the branches should interact. Amazingly, despite having not been given a blueprint of the final outcome, the program was able to produce incredibly realistic computer plants. This seems to occur in living systems, as well. According to Langdon, Lindemayer and Prusinkiewicz's computer plant experiment represented a novel scientific version of vitalism, the idea that life involves an energy or spirit that transcends matter. Langdon argues that, in fact, life *does* transcend matter—not because life is animated by a mysterious energy operating outside the laws of science—but because a system of simple parts following simple rules of interaction can behave in surprisingly complex ways.

So maybe potency is just ingrained in our physical architecture, in the choreographed interactions between our parts, held together by the vital connections between them. If so, this version of potency sounds a lot like the kind of energy transmitted within closed kinematic chains. Closed kinematic chains are a type of architectural powerhouse within tensegrity structures, and have been used in mechanical engineering for a long time. In the body, closed kinematic chains involve a series of linked body segments where the distal end of the chain is fixed or constrained by contact with a stable surface or more stable body part. This configuration allows forces generated in one part of the chain to be transmitted through the entire chain. During a push-up,

for example, force generated into the stable ground leads to forces being transmitted through the body, creating movement.
In response to forces generated though closed kinematic chains, osseofascial tissue shifts into different shapes and arrangements. Scarr explains that forces passing through closed kinematic chains generate a spontaneous reorganization of our architecture into the most efficient configuration possible. Take the hand, an appendage valued by manual therapists. Levin says that there are not enough hand muscles to determine all of the potential combinations of finger positions. To make up for the shortfall, the forces generated by each muscle contraction are processed by the architecture of closed kinematic chains within the osseofascial tissue network of the hand. The network—not the brain!—balances the relative differences in tension, shifting the finger from a straight shape to a bent shape and vice versa. In other words, closed kinematic chains operate outside of neural control. It's the interaction of the parts and the spaces between them that does the thinking.

Another example of this neurally independent architectural intelligence occurs in the womb. The biokinetic view of embryology highlights the importance of kinematic forces in human differentiation. In the 1970s, Blechschmidt discovered that the shape of cells reflects the kinematic forces acting upon them, and that human differentiation begins on the outside of the cell and then proceeds inward. He reasoned that since all cells within the human ovum have the same chromosomes but differentiate in various ways, genetics is influenced by external forces, and not the other way around. That is, besides genetic information, there are *extragenic* kinematic pushes and pulls acting on the cell, driving cellular differentiation. Along with the nature of closed kinematic chains, Blechschmidt's perspectives on embryology nudge us to

consider that an architecturally driven potency exists in our tissues.

So is potency related to a sort of energy pulse distilled from all the pushes and pulls being transmitted through all of our closed kinematic chains? Maybe, but something about this explanation seems too constrained to the musculoskeletal system. No, there has to be more to potency than this.

Besides living within our parts and the spaces between them, potency has been described in all kinds of ways and has been credited with an array of almost metaphysical powers. James Jealous called potency the "silent partner" that guided and augmented his treatments (Jealous 2015). In reference to the Einstein quote "We all dance to a mysterious tune, intoned in the distance by an invisible piper," biodynamic craniosacral teacher Katherine Ukleja sees the Breath of Life as the musician, potency as the music, and primary respiration (to be discussed soon) as the dance (Rieu 2022). McPartland said that potency is related to consciousness, and that our individual consciousness is just a miniature version of the universal consciousness shared by all living things. According to McPartland, protoplasm—the main constituent of slime mold and of our fluid bodies—shares this consciousness, and resonates with the intentions of the universe. Some even say that potency is derived from the very essence of life itself; from the same old-fashioned chemistry that sparked our own misty beginnings.

Roughly 3.5 billion years before Taylor Swift's Eras tour kicked off in Glendale, Arizona, on March 17, 2023, Earth was a very different place, devoid of oxygen, slime mold, TikTok, and any other sign of life. But there was water. And soup! Primordial soup, but soup nonetheless. In fact, contrary to the fiery volcanic hellscape depicted by artists' impressions of the Hadean period, the presence of zircon crystals (which can only form alongside water) indicates a more tranquil, watery world containing more soup than land. Life as we know it emerged from this prehistoric *potage*, but exactly how it did so remains a mystery.

And there are clues from the dawn of human life that may shed light on a possible scientific definition of potency. The idea that life sprung forth from a series of purely random events seems improbable at best. Standard evolutionary theory goes something like this: deoxyribonucleic acid (DNA), ribonucleic acid (RNA), proteins, and polysaccharides were stewing in some warm pond in the presence of amino acids and other molecular building blocks. Over time, these compounds underwent reactions, which grew increasingly complex, eventually including the self-replicating DNA and RNA in their chemical swirl. Once self-replication occurred, natural selection took care of the rest, and billions of years later, you get to take your kids to the Taylor Swift concert (if you can afford tickets).

While contemplating the origin-of-life question, complexity science researcher Stuart Kauffman, who we met earlier, felt something was missing from this scenario. Kauffman reasoned that since most biological molecules are (relatively) enormous, you would have to string together hundreds of amino acid building blocks in just the right way. According to Kauffman, that would be difficult to accomplish in modern laboratories using the most cutting-edge biotechnology. So how could such a thing occur billions of years ago in a scuzzy puddle? Kauffman reminds us that scientists have attempted to calculate the odds of these formations happening and they almost always conclude that, if the connections were truly random, it would take

longer than the *entire lifetime of the universe* to produce a single viable protein molecule, much less all the other stuff needed to make a cell. There had to be something else going on.

According to Kauffman, if the conditions in the pond were just right, each molecule in the network could have catalyzed the formation of other molecules in the network, so that all the molecules in the network would grow more abundant relative to molecules that were not part of the network. In other words, the network would have catalyzed its own formation, accelerating the speed of its evolution. This autocatalysis occurs when the catalyst is both a reactant *and* a product of the reaction, and like elasticity, is a hallmark of living systems. "Beneath our placid exteriors we are a seething mass of autocatalysis" says Rodney Brooks at the Massachusetts Institute of Technology (Brooks 2022).

So, perhaps potency doesn't just live in our architecture but is also a kind of prehistoric "cellular momentum" initiated by autocatalysis, by our built-in chemical drive toward evolution. Maybe autocatalysis is responsible for the "no-name intelligence that [cells] are automatically functioning with," as Rollin Becker saw it (Becker 2023, 20). Maybe Jealous's "silent partner" on the treatment table was just the periodic table doing chemical periodic-table things. Maybe potency lives in our architecture *and* in our chemistry.

At around the same time Sutherland was trying to make sense of his discoveries, physiologist Claude Bernard spoke of a *milieu intérieur*, later clarified in 1926 by Walter Cannon as *homeostasis*. "Homeo," from the Greek word *homoios*, means "similar to," and when combined with *stasis*, the Greek word for "standing still," gives us a term and concept that has become a cornerstone of modern physiology. Homeostasis refers to an innate drive toward a narrow range of balance, despite changing circumstances in the external environment. For homeostasis to work, it requires three things: a defined setpoint range of balance, feedback from what's happening in the body, and the ability to make changes to maintain balance within the setpoint. Luckily for us, the human body has a wide array of control systems to elegantly accomplish these tasks.

Could it be that with their observations and impressions, Sutherland, Becker, Blechschmidt, Jealous, Bernard, Cannon, and others were all referring to the same thing? Perhaps potency is all the things we've mentioned and more. Maybe potency is just the palpable cumulative drive of body systems working to achieve and maintain homeostasis.

Franklyn Sills, a pioneer in the field of craniosacral and biodynamic osteopathy and founder of the Karuna Institute in the United Kingdom, built upon Sutherland's early work to describe how potency manifests not only within the cerebrospinal fluid but within *all* the fluids of the body. As we saw earlier, fluid flow impacts our physiology in all kinds of ways, sloshing through every cell, vessel, organ, and bone. You'll recall that bone is made of roughly 20 percent water, which is enmeshed within the bone matrix at every level. Bone water mediates bone remodeling and fortifies bone composition, making bone tougher and more resistant to fracture. We also discovered how the formation of osseofascial compactions seems to be partly related to altered fluid flow. Again and again, fluidic drive pops up as a fundamental determinant of osseofascial tissue health and behavior. According to Sills, it is through these same

fluids that the action of potency is transmitted to the tissues, creating motility. Sills also reminds us that, similar to how the slime mold sealed off the saline invasion to protect the rest of the organism, potency exerts a comparable protective function in humans by confining impact forces to as small an area as possible—to a muscle, organ, plexus of nerves, or bone.

In May 1962, Rollin Becker had a phone conversation with his son, Donald. In it he described a paper he wrote, in which he discussed his views on potency:

> I called it potency in that paper for the reason that I had to call it something, and talking with a colleague the other day, I made the point that regardless of what terminology we choose to use, the fact is there is something that centers disabilities, traumas, and disease within human anatomicophysiology that carries the power, the authority, the potency for the pattern for that particular problem. Still it's tough to understand. You have to accept it more or less blindly, without too much knowledge of the actual mechanics involved. (Becker 2023, 121)

But accepting something blindly is tough for us to do, Rollin! It takes a rare combination of courage and humility. But maybe we do have to swallow hard and just accept that (*a*) potency exists, (*b*) we can feel it, and (*c*) we can augment its power with our hands. Perhaps, as for the color blue or the taste of a perfect apple, to understand potency doesn't require a scientific explanation based on architecture, chemistry, or fluid dynamics. Maybe to truly understand potency is to just *feel* it, to listen to it, to experience it by putting our hands on our subject or by going for a walk in the woods. I think this would make Rollin Becker proud.

FULCRUMS AND FULCRUM-LEVER SYSTEMS

As we have speculated, potency seems to have been present in the abiotic puddles of primordial soup, in the pulsating goop of slime mold, and in the mysterious Laurentian forests of my youth. It lives within and between every cell and in every bone in Taylor Swift and in you and me, from when we were embryos until right now. And if potency is a drive toward health, a fulcrum is kind of like an *outpost* of that drive. A fulcrum is a point on which a lever balances. It is also a moment and an opportunity. A fulcrum is the eye of a hurricane, an eddy in turbulent water. It is stillness, order within the chaos, a source of organizational power. A fulcrum is like a familiar face in the crowd. It's a dependable friend.

A basic example of a fulcrum is the one under the seesaw in your local park. The fulcrum is the support under the plank that allows the plank to see and saw. Together, the fulcrum (support) and the levers (plank) make up the *fulcrum-lever system* of the seesaw. In the body, there are two types of fulcrum-lever systems: biomechanical and biodynamic.

Biomechanical Fulcrum-Lever Systems

Biomechanical fulcrum-lever systems involve mobility on a macroscale. In these systems, bones act as the levers and the joints between them act as the fulcrums. Three basic types of biomechanical fulcrum-lever systems exist: first, second, and third class.

In a first-class biomechanical fulcrum-lever system, the fulcrum is located between the resistance and the force. The upper cervicals are a first-class fulcrum-lever system. In this case, the weight of the head represents the resistance acting on one side of the fulcrum, at the atlanto-occipital joint, and the muscle action from the trapezius and other posterior muscles attached to the skull represents the force acting on the other side. The base of the occipital bone represents the levers balancing on both sides of the fulcrum.

In a second-class biomechanical fulcrum-lever system, the resistance is located between the fulcrum and the force. When someone stands on their toes, the fulcrum is the metatarsophalangeal joints, the weight of the body is the resistance, and the muscular action of the calf muscles applied to the calcaneus represents the force. The toes and the foot itself are the levers balancing on both sides of the fulcrum.

In a third-class biomechanical fulcrum-lever system, force is applied between the resistance and the fulcrum. A classic example is the elbow joint, where the joint is the fulcrum, the forearm, wrist, and hand represent the resistance, and the muscular action of the biceps provides the force. The bones of the lower and upper arm represent the levers balancing on both sides of the fulcrum.

Biodynamic Fulcrum-Lever Systems

On the other hand, biodynamic fulcrum-lever systems involve motility on a microscale. Here, groups of cells within a structure represent the levers, and a point of stillness represents the fulcrum around which the groups of cells organize. There are three types of biodynamic fulcrum-lever systems: natural, inertial, and external.

In a natural fulcrum-lever system, the fulcrum supports the levers *and* shifts freely as it does so. It has the capacity to react and move to maintain the function and health of the levers it supports. In a way, a natural fulcrum is more fluid (not fluid as in water "fluid," but as in "more free" fluid) in its behavior. If the support for the seesaw were a ball capable of rolling in response to the seeing and sawing and to any translational displacements of the plank, it would be considered a natural fulcrum. Natural fulcrums come in handy! Consider some common anatomical asymmetries: one leg may be an inch shorter than the other, the left foot slightly bigger than the right; there may exist a rotation in a vertebra, or a torsion around a hip, or even all four. Despite these common imperfections, natural fulcrums automatically rebalance us, allowing us to walk in straight lines and stay upright while we brush our teeth or play ping-pong. From a craniosacral perspective, Sutherland's fulcrum at the straight sinus is an example of a natural fulcrum-lever system. The straight sinus is a convergence point within the cranium where the endocranial dural folds meet. These folds connect to the entire reciprocal tension membrane (to be discussed in more detail soon). As the reciprocal tension membrane shifts, so too does the straight sinus, compensating for changing biological circumstances. Both fulcrum (straight sinus) and levers (reciprocal tension membrane) make up this natural fulcrum-lever system.

As opposed to a natural biodynamic fulcrum-lever system, an inertial biodynamic fulcrum-lever system forms in response to trauma, wrapping up the impact forces in a biodynamic hug to protect the rest of the system from harm. When we fall on our butt or get hit by a softball, the forces from the impact are transmitted to our tissues. In a bone, this impact is absorbed by the bone matrix and the fluid-filled cavities within it, potentially impacting fluid flow and bone texture. If the impact is minor, our bodies resolve it without much fanfare. But if the force is substantial and remains unresolved, potency seems to switch into problem-solving mode, engaging those impact forces and creating an inertial fulcrum-lever system

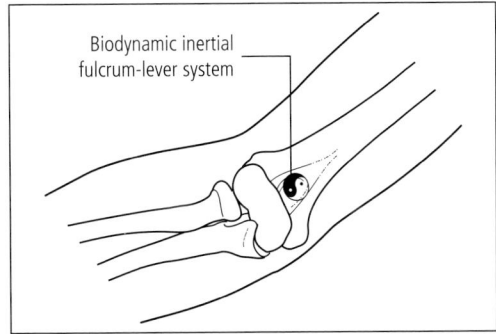

Figure 8.5. An osseofascial compaction is a biodynamic inertial fulcrum-lever system.

to protect the rest of the bone (and body) from harm. Remember how slime mold behaved when it sealed off an invasion of toxins to protect the rest of the organism? This is how human biodynamics seem to behave, as well. Becker: "Your fulcrum point is a neutral point for the staging of the struggle or battle that needs to take place" (Becker 2023, 51). In the body, this "fulcrum point" can appear anywhere—in a bone, in a joint, in an eye socket, in a spleen—and contains both the stillness of potency *and* the traumatized tissue, both engaged in a sort of yin-and-yang, good-versus-evil dance battle.[19] An osseofascial compaction, therefore, is an inertial fulcrum-lever system containing both the stillness of potency (fulcrum) and the compacted osseofascial tissue (levers) (figure 8.5).

---

[19]Often, with good intentions, we are tempted to "fix" an inertial fulcrum-lever system. While noble, this approach is flawed. The duality of the inertial fulcrum-lever system teaches us that perceived dysfunction is not necessarily a problem that needs a solution, but a natural balancing act that should be observed, supported, and appreciated. This light-and-dark equilibrium reminds us to be comfortable engaging with the human system while not always having the answers or even words to explain it. When we place our hands on our subject, a universe of information unfolds. Within that universe is a wisdom—an intelligence—forged over hundreds of millions of years, stratified with layers of breathtaking adaptation that have evolved over time. Let this boundless intelligence be your teacher.

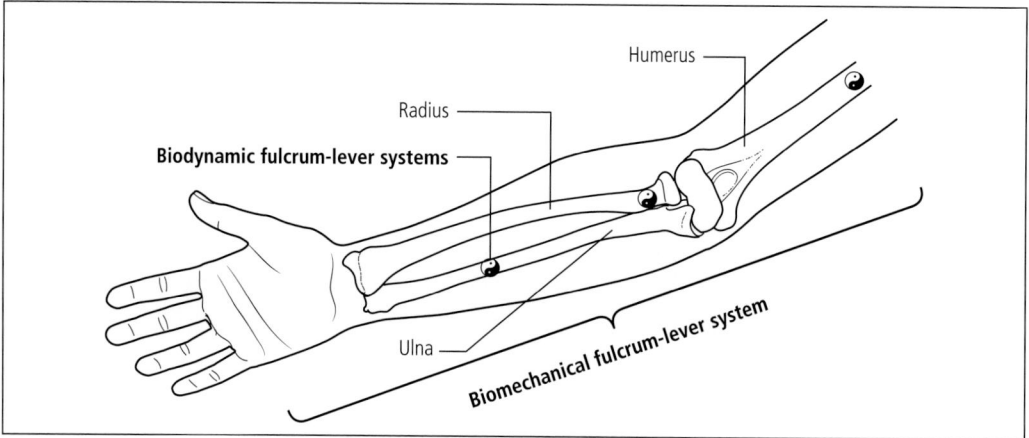

Figure 8.6. Biodynamic fulcrum-lever systems exist within biomechanical fulcrum-lever systems.

One day while out on a run, I was thinking about the interplay between the different types of fulcrums in the body. On that run, it suddenly became clear to me: the biodynamics happen *inside* the biomechanics. In other words, a biodynamic fulcrum-lever system is always found within a biomechanical fulcrum lever-system. In retrospect, this seems strikingly obvious, but bridging the two concepts in such a simple way was revelatory for me. For example, if a (biodynamic) inertial fulcrum-lever system exists in the humerus or ulna or radius, it can impact the texture and quality of that bone, compromising the bone's performance as a lever within the biomechanical fulcrum-lever system around the elbow (figure 8.6).

This example illustrates why it's important to treat both the biodynamics *and* the biomechanics. We use BST to treat the *motility* of the biodynamic inertial fulcrum-lever system *before* working on the *mobility* of the biomechanical fulcrum-lever system.

Remember that the inertial fulcrum within the compaction is an outpost of potency's natural drive toward health, and is linked to the health of our entire system. If our

health were an octopus, the inertial fulcrum within the compaction is the tip of one of its tentacles. Becker considers the inertial fulcrum a vantage point. He explains that "if you could sit at that point, you could evaluate everything that's going on in that tissue. ... [T]he whole picture would unfold from that relative point" (Becker 2023, 140). He also reminds us that "the abnormal ... is only an area that is doing the best it can under the circumstances" (212). In other words, amid the chaos of trauma, health still exists within the fulcrum as a beacon of calm.[20] When treating compactions with BST, we'll first observe and appreciate the dance between trauma and health. Then, we'll engage in the dance by helping potency reanimate the

---

[20]The concept of the inertial fulcrum-lever system blends with ideas from biotensegrity, discussed earlier. The tensegrity icosahedron is a structure whose parts are all spaced equally around a central point, like a sphere. In the body, twisted chains of the tensegrity icosahedrons form the structural basis for collagen-based biological helices and other structures. Scarr stated "The center of the tensegrity-icosahedron is a stress-free zone that allows other things to happen within it" (Scarr 2018, 135). Our bodies contain gazillions of these architecturally shielded stress-free points. In a way, each one of these points is a point of calm, or fulcrum.

levers of the system from within. Ultimately, we'll help an inertial fulcrum-lever system become more like a natural fulcrum-lever system, so it can adapt more easily to the changing biological currents inside of us.

As therapists, resonating with an inertial fulcrum-lever system forces us to appreciate that the dance/struggle occurring within it is not only part of life, but essential to it. The key to treating inertial fulcrum-lever systems is becoming aware of the health balancing the levers from the dynamic stillness within, then helping that health spread throughout the tissue. Becker: "As soon as I am aware of stillness as the mode of power that is in command ... then my hands begin to palpate and feel the shift of the elements of body physiology and their response to this mode of power coming from the stillness" (Becker 2023, 69). If Rollin did it, so can you!

On the topic of you, the third type of biodynamic fulcrum-lever system is an external fulcrum-lever system. That's you (and me), folks! Here, our hands are the external fulcrum upon which the entire (internal) inertial fulcrum-lever system balances (figure 8.7).

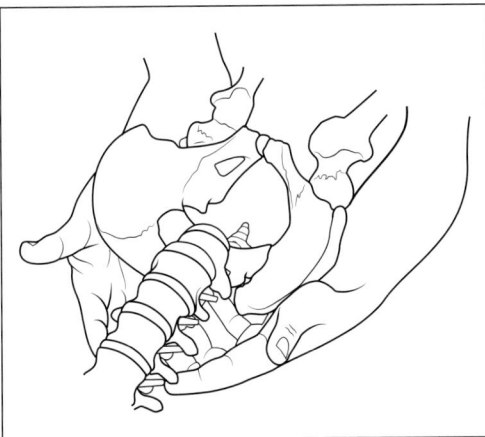

Figure 8.7. An external fulcrum balances the entire inertial fulcrum-lever system from the outside of the body.

For an external fulcrum to be effective, it should possess three qualities. First, it should be *supportive*, to allow the system to lean on it while it changes. Second, it should be *responsive*, to be capable of reacting to the inherent movements of the system. Third, it should be *dynamic*, to physically shift to follow those movements. Allow me to explain.

Treating someone with our hands is kind of like balancing a dowel on a finger. When we balance a dowel, and then shift the arm and body to prevent the dowel from toppling over, we're offering a supportive, responsive, and dynamic external fulcrum to the dowel. Here, our finger is the fulcrum, and the adjustments we make with our arm and body match the amplitude of the dowel's movements. The same phenomenon occurs in a clinical context. By placing our hands on a subject with therapeutic intention, we become the external fulcrum upon which the tissues of the subject can balance.

One of the classic criticisms of manual therapy is that if such subtle intervention could lead to real change within another body, then surely sitting on a chair or sleeping on our backs all night or swimming in a lake would induce similar, if not even more significant, changes. But even if they are significant, such forces exerted on our bodies each day rarely possess those three magic characteristics—supportiveness, responsiveness, and dynamism—that create an effective external fulcrum. A chair is supportive, but neither dynamic nor responsive. For these reasons, sitting on a chair doesn't lead to therapeutic change. While useful, chairs make terrible manual therapists. The good news is that humans are surprisingly good at balancing a dowel on a finger! We were born to offer this very special type of contact. We must respond to the movements of the subject's tissues as we do to the movements of the dowel: being stable enough to support, responsive enough to react, and dynamic enough to move. When our contact is supportive, responsive, and dynamic, we can begin to elicit profound and meaningful change in one another.

To allow us to properly support inertial fulcrum-lever systems from the outside, we must first learn how to dialogue with them. Potency is that fluidic drive toward homeostasis that we discussed earlier, and the inertial fulcrum is an outpost of that drive. Therefore, to communicate with inertial fulcrum-lever systems, we must first learn how to communicate with potency. To communicate with potency, we must understand its language, and the language of potency is called primary respiration.

PRIMARY RESPIRATION

Like English or French or Hindi or Spanish or any other language, primary respiration is the language potency uses to communicate with us. Or, rather, it's the language we must *interpret* in order for us to understand what potency is saying. Primary respiration is its own body system. Alongside the other autonomic body systems like respiration, circulation, and digestion, primary respiration animates our tissues. It expands and contracts, inhaling and exhaling in rhythmic, tidal patterns. These rhythms are neither formless nor imaginary; they are very real, and can be clearly felt with the hands.

The term *primary respiration* was first coined by Sutherland to describe the organizing and healing forces at work within and around us. Almost a century after Sutherland introduced primary respiration to the world, Anne Canarelli interviewed some of the world's most experienced osteopaths, including several of my former teachers.

In her book *Osteopaths: The Philosophy, the Spirit, and the Art of Osteopathy* (2016), the featured practitioners describe how they merely serve as a "facilitators" of the indwelling therapeutics expressed through primary respiration. Colin Dove, director and principal of the British School of Osteopathy from 1962 to 1977, describes the thrill of feeling primary respiration outside the craniosacral system for the first time, and how he "palpated the legs and this is where I finally felt, beyond all reasonable doubt, the so-called cranial rhythm!" (Canarelli 2016, 42). Reuben Bell, near the end of his 40-year osteopathy practice, says that he has been "only a facilitator. Something else did the healing" (13). Bell describes a "subtle tide that animates us from within" (13). Bernard Daraillans, with nearly 50 years of experience as a physiotherapist and osteopath, talks of "surfing on the surface of my subjects' fluid bodies ... breathing of the ocean inside the subjects" (32). Genevieve Forget says that "when the whole reaches a balance point and the acceptance within has agreed, in stillness, the sensation of reinvestment of the [primary respiratory] mechanism was unequivocal" (73).[21] Compelling testimonials from some extraordinary therapists.

To learn the language of potency, we must first learn the words. Here, the words are rhythms, and there are three main rhythms: the cranial rhythmic impulse (CRI), the mid-tide, and the long tide.

---

[21]Forget was one of my teachers at the CEO, and then the lead evaluator during my fifth-year final exam. She had a reputation for having extraordinary palpatory skills and intuition. During the exam she evaluated my cranial and cervical techniques from her hand placed on my patient's foot!

Cranial Rhythmic Impulse

Simply put, the CRI is a *filtered* expression of potency. It is part of the primary respiratory *mechanism*, expressed throughout the craniosacral unit and the rest of the body.

In the early twentieth century, Sutherland described the elements of the primary respiratory mechanism and the features of the CRI for the first time. With his groundbreaking insights, he broadened the realm of manual therapy from a biomechanical model based on structures that move to a biodynamic model based on structures that *possess* movement. A year before he graduated from the American School of Osteopathy in 1900, Sutherland peered at a mounted human skull and thought the beveled cranial sutures looked like fish gills, indicating the potential for motion. Being a rational man of science (and convinced he was wrong), Sutherland tried to disprove this idea but failed. He then spent the next 30 years deciphering a system involving the involuntary movement of the central nervous system and bones of the skull and pelvis, which he called the primary respiratory mechanism. In the foreword to Sutherland's book *Teachings in Osteopathy*, Becker describes Sutherland's vision:

> The primary respiratory mechanism ... produces rhythmic flexion of all midline structures in the body with external rotation of all paired lateral structures, alternating with extension of all midline structures in the body with internal rotation of all paired lateral structures. Every cell and all fluids of the body express this rhythmic, involuntary life and motion throughout life. (Becker, in Sutherland 1990, x)

Since Sutherland's early observations, others have attempted to pinpoint the exact origin of the CRI. After all, there exist a multitude of biological oscillations with numerous sources that vary in scale from seconds, to minutes, to hours. Is primary respiration one of these? Or a combination of them? Sutherland initially proposed that the pulsations of the CRI arose from the motions of the brain, causing a respiratory-like expansion and contraction of the cerebral ventricles, generating a wave of cerebrospinal fluid. In 1976, Harold Magoun expanded upon Sutherland's idea and proposed that it is the choroid plexus that produces cerebrospinal fluid in rhythmic cycles, generating brain motility. In the early 1980s, Upledger and Vredevoogd refined Magoun's hypothesis and named the rhythm the "pressurestat model." In 1997, McPartland and Mein described the CRI as a "harmonic frequency," a summation of several body rhythms, including the cerebrospinal fluid oscillations, cardiac pulse, diaphragmatic respiration, contractile lymphatic vessels, pulsating glial cells, and others.

Regardless of the origin of the CRI (and notwithstanding the fluctuation of cerebrospinal fluid), the primary respiratory mechanism first described by Sutherland was predominantly a biomechanical rope-and-pulley system. But toward the end of Sutherland's life, his philosophy evolved away from the biomechanical principles of the craniosacral unit to focus on the *biodynamic* features of the human form. He shifted his focus from how bones move individually to how bones are moved collectively.[22] In other words, Sutherland began to examine the movement *within* bones, and not just the movement *of* them.

----

[22]Jealous reminds us that by 1953, Sutherland dropped the idea that the reciprocal tension membrane mechanically moved individual bones, calling it "reductionist and linear" (Jealous 2015, 90).

Becker, Jealous, and Sills continued along Sutherland's biodynamic trajectory, becoming more passive in their treatments by doing less and listening more, allowing the movements from within structures to emerge. They expanded and clarified Sutherland's ideas, describing how the CRI is but *one component* of a larger system called primary respiration—a superficial waveform floating on deeper, more stable rhythms.

Sutherland's early description of the CRI within the primary respiratory mechanism had five elements. The five elements work together synchronistically, flexing and extending as a cohesive cranio- (from the cranium) sacral (to the sacrum) unit in a respiratory-type rhythm.

The first element of the primary respiratory mechanism is the fluctuation of the cerebrospinal fluid. Sutherland sensed within the cerebrospinal fluid a "fluid within a fluid" that didn't mix with the cerebrospinal fluid, but had the potency to make it move.

The second element is the mobility of the intracranial and intraspinal membranes and the function of the reciprocal tension membrane. Within the cranium and spinal canal exist tough, inelastic folds of connective tissue, called dura mater, which surround, protect, guide, and limit the movements of the brain and spinal cord. The spinal portion of the dural membrane is continuous with the cranial dura, and descends the length of the spinal column, surrounding the spinal cord. It has several bony attachments along the way, including at the foramen magnum, the upper cervical vertebrae, and at the second sacral segment, before it finally anchors on the coccyx. These membranes maintain a constant level of tension throughout the craniosacral unit.

The third element of the primary respiratory mechanism is the inherent motility of the central nervous system. The central nervous system displays an automatic coiling and uncoiling type of movement, guided by the intracranial and intraspinal membranes and balanced by the reciprocal tension membrane around the natural fulcrum at the straight sinus. This motility powers the primary respiratory mechanism.

The fourth element of the primary respiratory mechanism is the inherent motility and mobility of the cranial bones. When the central nervous system expands during inhalation, the paired bones of the skull externally rotate, and the midline bones flex. As the central nervous system retracts during the exhalation phase, the paired bones internally rotate, and the midline bones extend. The minute movements permitted between cranial bones are enabled by the fibrous sutures that join them, as well as by the viscoelasticity of the bone.[23]

The fifth and final element of the primary respiratory mechanism is the involuntary mobility of the sacrum between the iliac bones. Just as the cranial bones need to move to propagate the pulsations of the brain, the pelvis must allow the sacrum to swivel. During the inhalation phase, the foramen magnum moves superiorly, pulling the base of the sacrum posteriorly. Just as it depends on the mobility of the intracranial and intraspinal membranes, on the function of the reciprocal tension membrane, and on the inherent mobility of the cranial bones, the primary

---

[23]Despite his hypothesis that cranial sutures evolved to permit motion between the bones, Sutherland initially shared the skepticism of the medical community, which collectively agreed that the cranial sutures fused shortly after birth. However, Bordoni et al. (2020a, b) proved Sutherland's hunch to be correct. According to their study, most cranial sutures permit some movement throughout life and even into old age.

respiratory mechanism depends on the mobility of the sacrum.

To summarize, the CRI is but one of the three rhythms of primary respiration produced by the primary respiratory mechanism. During inhalation, the central nervous system expands, flexing and externally rotating the paired and midline bones, respectfully. The foramen magnum moves up, pulling the spinal dural membrane with it, rocking the sacral base posteriorly. During the exhalation phase, these motions are reversed.

The CRI expresses itself through individual bones as internal and external rotations and flexions and extensions (the flexions and extensions generally feel like a rocking-back-and-forth movement). Paired bones, such as the humerus, rotate (figure 8.8). Midline bones, such as vertebrae, flex and extend (figure 8.9).

These movements occur at 5 to 12 full inhalation/exhalation cycles per minute, or one cycle every 5 to 12 seconds. While different authors report different speeds, I usually perceive the CRI at the slower end of the range.

How does the CRI relate to potency? As it does within all tissues in the body, potency

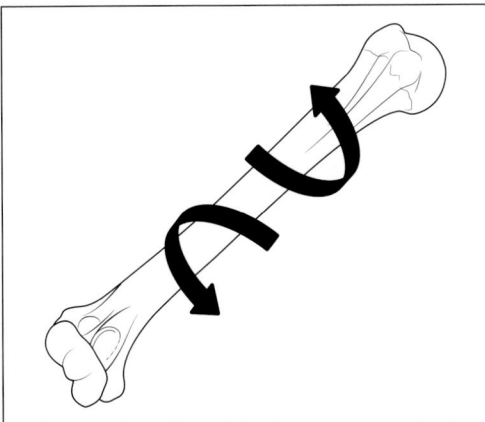

Figure 8.9. Flexions and extensions of the CRI expressed through a vertebra.

animates the fluid within the central nervous system, creating movement within the confines of the skull. Since the skull is a semirigid container, it accommodates the expansion and contraction of the brain. The movements of the cranial bones seem to reverberate through the craniosacral unit and the rest of the body in the form of rotations, flexions, and extensions. Remember that the CRI is a *resultant pattern*—a "lesion phenomenon" (McPartland and Skinner 2005)—reflecting body imbalances. The expression of potency, then, *combined with* the changing physiological patterns of the craniosacral unit and the rest of the body, allows the CRI to give us clues about our underlying health. Its quality and amplitude reflect the changing conditions of the human biosphere. In fact, from within significant dysfunction (like osseofascial compactions), the CRI may not be detectable at all.[24]

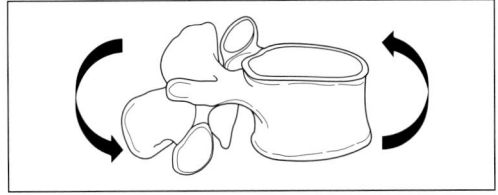

Figure 8.8. Internal and external rotations of the CRI expressed through the humerus.

[24]It is tempting to compare the CRI to the churning of once-calm water moving into and then out of a turbine, reverberating through the rest of the skeleton as patterns that have been filtered and changed. But is this an accurate analogy? This idea contrasts slightly with other perspectives of the CRI occurring *simultaneously* within the craniosacral container and the periphery. Even so, the description of the CRI as a highly variable waveform that changes with the undercurrents of body systems encourages us to consider the turbine analogy. Regardless, whether the peripheral expressions of the CRI occur at a delay or simultaneously does not change how the CRI speaks to us, and for practical purposes, this is what matters most.

Most importantly for us, the presence or absence or diminished amplitude of the CRI within an osseofascial structure gives us clues about the structure's health.

Mid-tide

If the CRI reflects a shaken-and-stirred potency cocktail as it whooshes through the body, the mid-tide reflects a more direct expression of potency. While the CRI as first described by Sutherland includes all kinds of movements reverberating out of the craniosacral unit and throughout the body, several decades later, Franklyn Sills began describing another, slower rhythm called the mid-tide.

Slower and steadier than the CRI, the mid-tide is expressed as a welling-up-and-receding sensation occurring at one to three inhalation/exhalation cycles per minute, or one cycle every 20 to 60 seconds (figure 8.10).

Sills named this rhythm the mid-tide since it reflects a middle ground between potency, fluids, and tissues. According to Sills, when potency acts, fluid is the medium of exchange, bringing potency "into" the cells and tissues. In turn, the cells and tissues pulse. From a

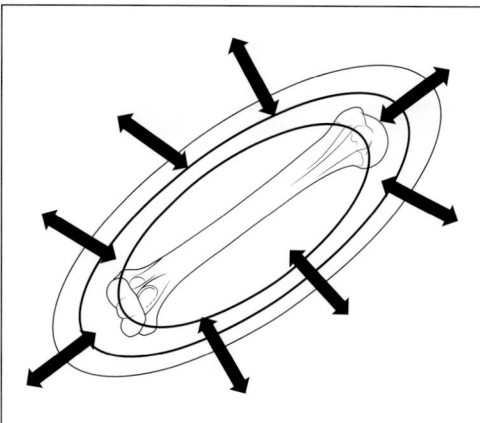

Figure 8.10. Welling up and receding of the mid-tide expressed through the humerus.

biodynamic perspective, this pulse is akin to the motility of our tissues, and is expressed as this welling-up-and-receding sensation that we can feel with our hands. One could even say that the mid-tide *turns into* the CRI once the former passes through the filter of the craniosacral unit and body. With this vision in mind, when palpating the humerus, for example, we feel both the internal and external rotations of the CRI *and* the slower welling-up-and-receding pulsation of the mid-tide within the same bone. Here, we receive two different levels of communication from potency: the CRI, filtered by the changing conditions of the craniosacral mechanism and the rest of the body, and the mid-tide, which has remained relatively unfiltered. Pretty neat, right?

Long Tide

The CRI and the mid-tide are two of the three main rhythms that make up primary respiration, and both of them originate from the long tide. From a biodynamic perspective, the long tide and potency sit atop the primary respiration ecosystem, working together to animate and organize our fluids and cells, from conception and throughout life. The long tide is "part and parcel of the total function within each of us," says Becker, who coined the term in the early 1970s (Becker 2023, 226). According to him, the long tide represents the intrinsic health of the human system. From my humble perspective, the long tide is what life feels like if we could touch it.

Becker graduated from the American School of Osteopathy in 1934 and began his osteopathy practice in Oklahoma, where he worked for a few years before moving to Michigan. In 1944, he met Sutherland, was deeply inspired, and then spent much of his career and life expanding upon

Sutherland's ideas. Becker admits that while the CRI has an explanation, the long tide is harder to describe. When Becker was practicing, sometimes he would not perceive the long tide at all. This statement reflects my own experiences. To Becker, it seemed that only when there were "a lot of general systemic problems—things involving total body physiology" (Becker 2023, 50) did the long tide express itself. According to Becker, it is the *resistance* to the long tide that allows it to be appreciated. This reminds me of something curious Jealous said: "When we can feel anatomy, something is lesioned. Normal soma feels like watery forms and the fascial planes are not palpable" (Jealous 2105, 8). Or as the great Saul Bellow said, the boulders in a stream "show you how fast the water is flying" (Bellow 1976, 327). It seems that we feel the long tide most clearly when it bumps up against dysfunction, illuminating the contrast between the "stream" (where it can express itself fully) and the "boulder" (where it cannot). In other words, only when there is significant resistance to the long tide—like boulders to flowing water—can we sense its true power.

These observations, when considered together, are profound. They show us why treating intraosseous compactions with BST is important. Collectively, these ideas confirm that:

- fluid, tissue texture, and somatic dysfunction are closely related, and
- dysfunction alters the expression of primary respiration by *resisting* it.

These ideas also tie in to what we now know about felt changes in osseofascial tissue. Earlier, we learned that low-grade inflammation or acute trauma can leave their mark on osseofascial tissue, causing fibrosis. This fibrosis seems to "shut the door" on primary respiration. The fibrotic osseofascial tissue becomes "the boulder in the stream." We can feel this interplay with our hands. When we touch an osseofascial compaction, it immediately feels different from normal tissue because primary respiration is absent. Then, once we treat the compaction with BST, the tissue (hopefully) feels normal again. The return to normal is always associated with the return of primary respiration. The boulder is no longer a boulder, and the stream passes right through.

Sills's concepts of the *ordering field* and *ordering matrix* help explain how the long tide governs primary respiration in the body. The ordering field is a term Sills coined to describe a quantum-level energy field established at conception, within which the embryo forms and develops. The ordering field has two aspects: a quantum-level ordering matrix and a bioelectric ordering matrix. The quantum level ordering matrix is laid down at conception and then generates the bioelectric ordering matrix, which is suspended in the tidal body of the long tide. It is within the tidal body of the long tide where potency is "born." Then, via transmutation (a term Sills uses to describe a change of state), potency jumps from the tidal body of the long tide into our fluids and tissues, welling up and receding within the mid-tide. From this perspective, the long tide is a formative field of action—all else derives from it.[25]

According to Becker, compared to the CRI (and thanks to Sills, we can now also compare it to the mid-tide), the long tide is more expansive and stable. Similar to the mid-tide but slower, the long tide expresses a tide-like

---

[25]Michael Shea adds that "the Mid Tide is the total fluid medium of the body and the Long Tide is its brain" (Shea 2006).

"expansion and retraction of the whole being and a gradual receding movement ... followed by another gradual massive expansion and rhythmic interchange within and throughout the total organism" (Becker 2023, 50). Sometimes, it manifests in 100-second inhalation/exhalation cycles as a 50-second inhalation phase moving away from the subject's midline toward the horizon, and as a 50-second exhalation phase moving toward the subject's midline from the horizon (figure 8.11).

The suggestion that the long tide animates us from both the inside *and* the outside hints that the body itself is not a hermetically sealed vessel limited by the boundaries of the skin, but rather semipermeable to the organizational forces of the universe. I like that idea.

When I widen my perspective, the long tide emerges through osseofascial tissue as a slow and stable electric swell. When I hold

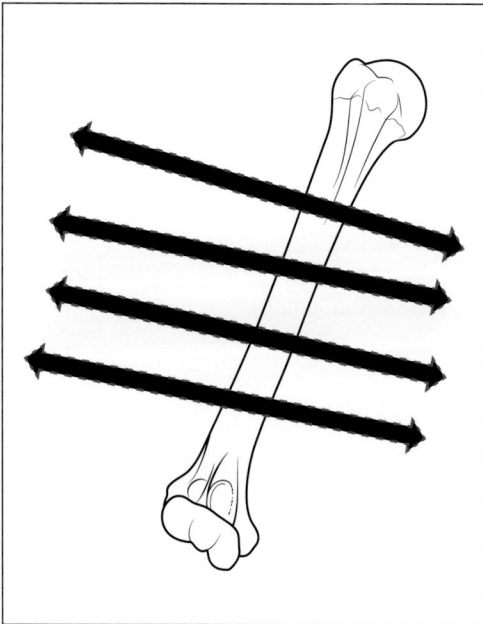

Figure 8.11. The long tide passing through the humerus from the midline to the horizon and then back again.

myself and my subject in a much wider space, trusting in the wisdom of nature, I sense its steady, supportive presence—like a hug.

It has been my experience that during local BST treatment, the long tide plays more of a supporting role. Since we are focused on the "stuff" within bone—the fluidic and physical matter—it is sometimes difficult to perceive the tidal quality of the long tide. For this reason, while treating individual bones, I work mainly with the CRI and mid-tide, while still feeling the support of the long tide, if possible. Like the director of a movie, the long tide is in charge, but during local BST work, often behind the scenes.

In a way, primary respiration is like an ocean inside of us. In nature, gravitational and celestial forces govern the formation of ocean tidal patterns. These forces are always present and stable, unaffected by the conditional forces acting upon them from the ground. In the body, the long tide governs the mid-tide and CRI as potency moves through our bodies and animates our tissues. In the human biodynamic ocean, the mid-tide represents the tidal swells, more stable than the variable waveforms of the CRI. The mid-tide still varies with the intentions of the long tide, but not as much as do the quicker waves of the CRI, which ride atop the larger, more stable swells, changing and reacting to the forces acting underneath them. By perceiving and reading these patterns in compacted osseofascial tissue, we will know when each technique has begun, how it is progressing, and when it ends. Working this way is not complicated or difficult. Feeling and interpreting these phenomena simply requires a calm, receptive state of mind and a little patience. You'll be an expert in no time.

To review, primary respiration contains three rhythms that can be perceived within every healthy cell, structure, and bone. The CRI is expressed as relatively quick rotations and movements at 5 to 12 inhalation/exhalation cycles per minute, or one cycle every 5 to 12 seconds. The mid-tide is expressed as a slower welling-up-and-receding sensation at 1 to 3 cycles per minute, or one every 20 to 60 seconds. Finally, the long tide is the slowest and most stable of the three rhythms, sometimes perceived as an energy wave rising and falling approximately every 100 seconds (table 8.1). If that's a lot of math to remember (it is for me), just think: the CRI is quick, the mid-tide is slower, and the long tide is the slowest. That usually works just fine.

Table 8.1. The three rhythms of primary respiration

Rhythm	Tempo	Cycles/Minute	Seconds/Phase
CRI	Quick	5–12	5–12
Mid-tide	Medium	1–3	10–30
Long tide	Slower	0.6	50

Three Bodies

According to Sills, Jealous developed a concept to help visualize and perceive the rhythms of primary respiration, both separately and together, called the three bodies. The three bodies are fields of action generated by the long tide as the embryo develops, which remain with us throughout life. Sills explains that the fields are suspended in each other, becoming more and more dense.[26] Jealous said that each rhythm of primary respiration manifests in a specific field, or body, and each body has its own unique quality. The three bodies are: tidal, fluid, and physical.

The tidal body is a formative field of action, generated by the long tide, within which the fluid and physical bodies are suspended. It has a windy or electric quality when palpated. It is within the tidal body that the long tide is perceived, and where potency is born.

The fluid body consists of the fluid within and around our cells, and is enlivened by potency. During palpation, the fluid body has (predictably) a watery quality, and it is primarily within the fluid body where the mid-tide manifests.[27]

Finally, the physical body is composed of cells, and it is within the physical body that the CRI expresses itself. The physical body is the densest of the three bodies, and has a dense, earthy quality when palpated.

When palpating osseofascial tissue, visualize the physical body suspended within the wider fluid body, and both the physical and fluid bodies suspended within the even wider tidal body (figure 8.12). This configuration may remind you of the embryo bathing in the amniotic fluid, with both the embryo and the fluid suspended in the "tidal body" of the mother's system (figure 8.13). This is accurate, since according to Blechschmidt, Jealous, and others, biodynamics is within and around us from the very beginning.

When treating osseofascial compactions, visualizing the qualities of the three bodies

---

[26]This progressive densification resonates with scientific findings from Blechschmidt, discussed earlier, who describes a gradual densification of mesenchymal cells as fluid is squeezed out from between them, eventually forming bone.

[27]Jealous describes a state when a patient reaches "neutral." This is when the central nervous system, cerebrospinal fluid, all other fluids and tissues seem to merge into the fluid body.

will allow the three rhythms of primary respiration to jump into our hands more quickly:

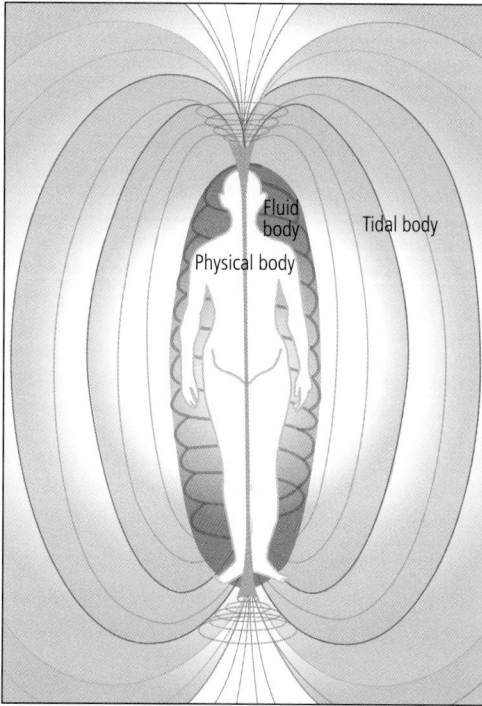

Figure 8.12. The three bodies. Adapted from Sills 2011.

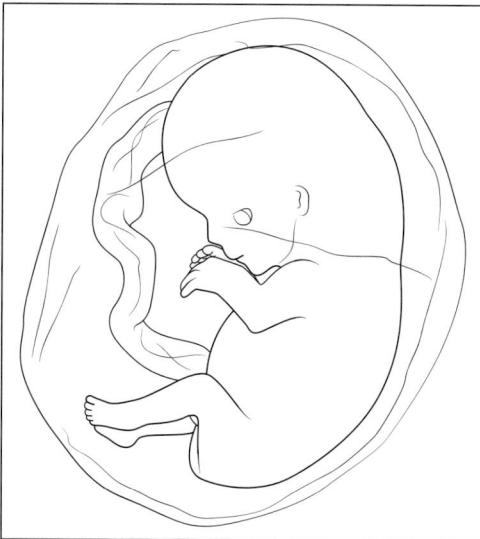

Figure 8.13. The three bodies (in utero).

- To feel the long tide, perceive the windy quality of the tidal body.
- To perceive the mid-tide, sense the watery quality of the fluid body.
- To feel the CRI, visualize the dense, earthy quality of the physical body.

Three Fascias

Curiously, the nesting phenomenon of Jealous's three bodies resonates with work from Italian osteopath and prolific researcher Bruno Bordoni, who discusses three categories of fascia: solid, liquid, and holographic (figure 8.14). As a refresher, here is the definition of fascia, mentioned earlier, put forth by FORCE, Bordoni's work group:

The fascia is any tissue that contains features capable of responding to mechanical stimuli. The fascial continuum is the result of the evolution of the perfect synergy among different tissues, liquids, and solids, capable of supporting, dividing, penetrating, feeding, and connecting all the districts of the body: epidermis, dermis, fat, *blood, lymph, blood and lymphatic vessels,* tissue covering the nervous filaments (endoneurium, perineurium, epineurium), voluntary striated muscle fibers and the tissue covering and permeating it (epimysium, perimysium, endomysium), ligaments, tendons, aponeurosis, cartilage, bones, meninges, involuntary striated musculature and involuntary smooth muscle (all viscera derived from the mesoderm), visceral ligaments, epiploon (small and large), peritoneum, and tongue. The continuum constantly transmits and receives mechano-metabolic information that can influence the shape and function of the entire body. These afferent/efferent

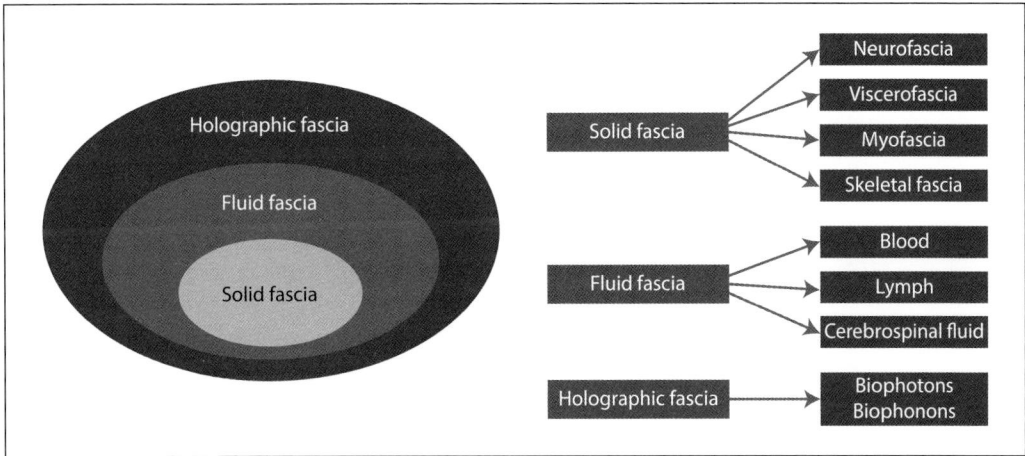

Figure 8.14. Three categories of fascia. Adapted from Bordoni et al. 2022.

impulses come from the fascia and the tissues that are not considered as part of the fascia in a bi-univocal mode. (Bordoni et al. 2022; emphasis added)

Notice how this definition includes blood and lymph, both of which Bordoni groups together as "fluid fascia." His reasoning is compelling, and includes the argument that fluid impacts body shape and function just as much as solid fascia. For this reason, he says, it should be called fluid fascia, and understandably, I think. We know that blood and lymph vessels are snuggled up against other fluidic networks already discussed—Guimberteau's permanently hydrated river of collagen and Bernia's fluid-filled interstitium. Together, these fluidic networks create a body-wide system that permeates every anatomical structure. In this way, fluid does impact body shape and function just as much as other types of fascia.

Holographic fascia completes Bordoni's three-tiered arrangement. Holographic fascia is a term Bordoni uses to describe the fabric of electromagnetic frequencies within and around us.[28] This fabric leads to oscillatory mechanotransduction, similar to Sills's bioelectric ordering matrix, discussed earlier. According to Bordoni, the electromagnetic oscillations of holographic fascia resonate with the oscillations of the DNA within each cell, itself an oscillatory structure. The DNA oscillations are then transmitted to the cellular infrastructure, turning holographic forces into mechanical signals the body can use. Holographic fascia governs the behavior of the fluid and solid fascia, similar to how the long tide governs both the mid-tide and CRI.

When Jealous's and Bordoni's three bodies and three fascias are superimposed (figure 8.15), a beautiful symmetry between osseofascial rhythm and texture emerges.

---

[28]A version of this idea resonates outside the osteopathic community, as well. From his 2018 research into the genome information-procession modes of planaria (little, flat worms with eyes on top of their heads), biologist Mike Levin from Tufts University observed a top-down information distribution system that controls the worms' genome. Levin hypothesized that this system is a "bioelectric code"—a fabric operating outside of the worm's genes.

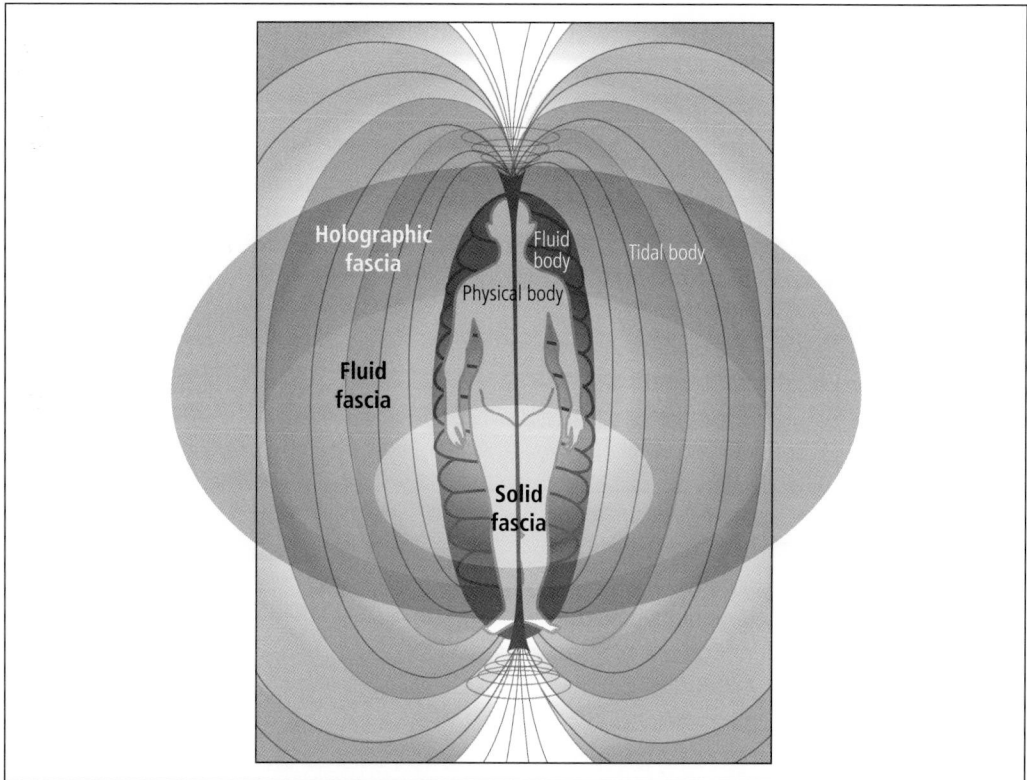

Figure 8.15. Three bodies and three categories of fascia.

Here, solid fascia sits within the physical body, through which the CRI emerges. Fluid fascia blends with the fluid body, through which the mid-tide is expressed. Holographic fascia is immersed in the tidal body, through which the long tide is perceived. Fun fact: in early 2024, when I asked Bordoni if his three fascias were inspired by Jealous's three bodies, he told me that they were not. That makes this juxtaposition even more compelling, I believe.

Holistic Shift

During clinical work, there is sometimes a moment when a shift occurs beneath my hands and within myself at the same time. This shift feels as though the subject's body is telling me that something good has just happened. It's almost as if a "sigh of relief" passes from my patient through my hands. According to Sills, one of Becker's key concepts of biodynamic work is the holistic shift, an idea that has helped put my experiences into context. The holistic shift happens when the practitioner's awareness moves from the variable waveforms of the CRI to the deeper rhythms of primary respiration, and when all three bodies (physical, fluid, and tidal) coalesce (figure 8.16).

When this coalescence arises, the physical, fluid, and tidal bodies have achieved an equilibrium and are sensed to be a unified field manifesting wholeness. When treating osseofascial compactions with BST, the concepts of the three bodies and the holistic shift help give our process context and a framework we can use.

Dialogue:

CRI + mid-tide + long tide = primary respiration

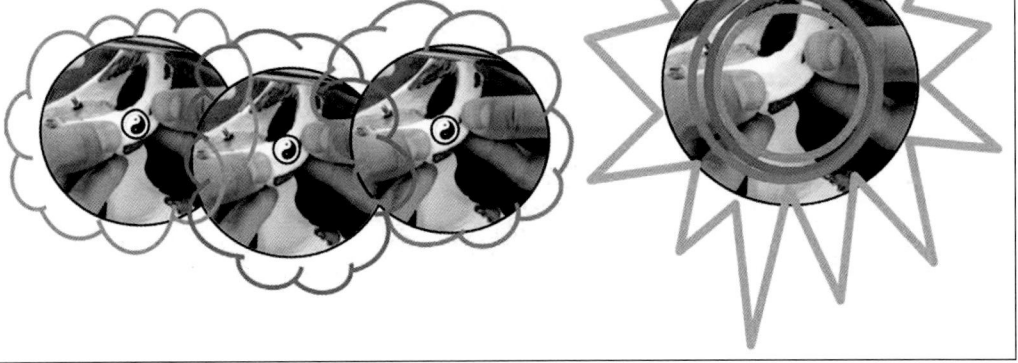

Figure 8.16. The holistic shift is when all three rhythms and all three bodies coalesce into the complete expression of primary respiration.

CHAPTER 9

Doubt

When in doubt, move into deeper water.

—James Jealous

Water

Humans are mostly water.
We melt like wet clay
through fragile fingers,
from a hidden smile,
from a song forgotten,
from things that travel through us like blood,
where they mix and shatter again.
Humans are mostly water,
but also something else
much less strong.

—Scott Sternthal

CHAPTER 11

Biodynamic Skeletal Therapy

Let's now examine how BST emerged from underneath the larger umbrella of craniosacral biodynamics. *Dynamic* is a word used to describe constant change or progress, and *biodynamics* describes dynamics at work in living systems. It appears that biodynamics was first mentioned in reference to the pastures outside any treatment clinic, when in the 1920s, philosopher Rudolf Steiner named a new method of organic farming "biodynamic agriculture," which considers each farm an integrated organism in harmony with the rhythms of the ecosystem. But in relation to the human body, the word was first used in the early 1960s, when Becker used the term *biodynamic potencies* in reference to the teachings of Sutherland.

As we've discussed, Sutherland's approach changed throughout his life. His studies began with bones, progressed to fascial membranes, continued to the cerebrospinal fluid, and then scuba dived into the fluid field. As his experiences deepened, Sutherland began to sense the entire fluid nature of the body as a self-organizing system. His ideas were revolutionary and represented a new take on Still's version of traditional osteopathy. But when Sutherland died, the revolution fizzled,

and osteopathy in the cranial field reverted to the biomechanical model with which he began. Nevertheless, Sutherland's biodynamic "torch" was kept alight by a selection of his students, including Becker, Jealous, Randolph Stone, Sills, and others.

Twenty or so years after Sutherland's death, German embryologist Erich Blechschmidt published *Biokinetics and Biodynamics of Human Differentiation* in 1978, examining the role of fluidic movements in relation to human differentiation. We met Blechschmidt earlier. He proposed that it is the movement of fluid within and around the embryo that kick-starts and then drives human differentiation, bringing genetics along for the ride. Blechschmidt's conclusions profoundly impacted Jealous, who assumed from the former's research that the embryologist must have watched primary respiration at work without actually palpating it.

Inspired by both Sutherland and Blechschmidt, Jealous developed the biodynamic model of osteopathy in the cranial field (BOCF), picking up where Sutherland left off. Jealous's BOCF adheres to the idea that the human embryo serves as a blueprint for our body's ability to heal itself, and that the biodynamic forces of embryogenesis become the biodynamic forces of healing throughout life.

In the late 1970s, at around the same time that Blechschmidt published his findings, Sills came across the work of Stone, and was intrigued by what Stone called "primary energy" and the "neuter essence." In 1986, Sills began sharing his ideas with his students by teaching a biodynamic approach to craniosacral therapy at the Karuna Institute in the United Kingdom. He coined the term *craniosacral biodynamics*, bringing Blechschmidt's, Sutherland's, Becker's, and Jealous's version of biodynamics into craniosacral practice. In 2011, Sills published *Foundations in Craniosacral Biodynamics*, an indispensable resource in the field. Today, biodynamic craniosacral therapy (BCST), a popular synonym for Sills's craniosacral biodynamics, is a growing field, with practitioner organizations developing around the world.

The foundations of BCST lie in a direct orientation to the universal forces of life. The BCST practitioner settles into a receptive state of being, negotiates their relationship to the system of their subject, orients to primary respiration, and creates a wide container within which potency may act. Biodynamic skeletal therapy is not meant to replace BCST—it's meant to complement and enhance it. Biodynamic skeletal therapy shrinks the container of BCST to focus more specifically on the osseofascial continuum. If BCST is the sun, BST is the magnifying glass that harnesses and amplifies the sunlight into a concentrated point, directing the sun's radiance into bone.

In a way, BST began with Sutherland's first observations of the human skull and

continued to develop along with Druelle's methodology at the CEO, which was inspired by other direct descendants of Sutherland. Based on my formal training by Druelle and his teachers at the CEO, on my own experiences as an osteopath, and on my further explorations into the biodynamics of Becker, Blechschmidt, Jealous, Sills, and others, BST was born.

A BRIEF HISTORY OF BIODYNAMIC SKELETAL THERAPY

In 2012, when I was a third-year osteopathy student at the CEO, our teacher Yves Boisvert described what it was like to feel a bone "melt" in his hands, and how it forever altered the lens through which he viewed the human body. It was a fascinating lecture. Curious and excited (and with a healthy dose of skepticism), I began incorporating the treatment principles Boisvert described in class that day, and soon enough, I too sensed strange movements within bone tissue. Astonishingly, these rigid structures began to shift and change, bending and squirming in my hands. Repetitive tidal patterns emerged, pulsating at different rhythms and speeds, expanding and contracting the bone. Where were these rhythms coming from? What did they represent? In my quest for a more thorough understanding of the human system, these and other similar questions remained unanswered.

Soon after that lecture, when I began treating people myself, I boasted hundreds of new techniques in my therapist's toolbox. I had ways to move bones, knead muscles, and dialogue with organs. Furthermore, I could prescribe all sorts of rehabilitative exercises to help my subjects help themselves. I was a one-stop body shop, offering a full suite of therapeutic and rehabilitative care. But as I mentioned in the preface, my toolbox eventually felt too big for the job.

In the fall of 2013, a dear family friend, Ronny Spunt, a family physician, invited me to come work at his medical clinic in Saint-Sauveur, Quebec. He told me to bring my own table and warned me that the room in which I was to work had no windows and was quite small. Ronny also guaranteed (warned?) me that I would be very busy. This was an exciting opportunity for me. I had not yet even finished osteo school, and was eager to gain real-life experience. At the time, I had already started treating patients at my own clinic in Montreal,[29] but since I had just started practicing, I had only a few appointments booked each day. Despite the one-hour commute from Montreal, a full day of work at Ronny's clinic would be well worth the drive.

On that first cold Thursday morning in October, I loaded my cat-scratched treatment table into the trunk of my car and drove north along Highway 15. Upon my arrival at the clinic, a single sheet of white paper lay unassumingly on my desk. It had many names written on it. I stared at my patient list with adrenalized horror. I was scheduled to see 11 patients that day! Not only was that number double or triple my normal daily patient load, but the duration of each treatment was shorter than I was accustomed to. I needed to readjust my approach on the fly.

The first item I changed that day was my evaluation protocol. Normally, my evaluation routine took 15 to 20 minutes, but since my treatments here would be shorter, I needed to condense the procedure. Thinking quickly,

[29]In Quebec, we were allowed to issue receipts for osteopathic treatment once we had completed our third year of osteopathy school.

I focused on finding "big things," problems that jumped out at me in an obvious way. I began by quickly scanning patients for these big things, and what lit up right away was extra-rigid bone tissue; bone that felt more like concrete than like normal bone. So, I treated these zones the way I knew how: with a combination of compression and tension. I finished the interventions with simple mobilizations, adjustments, or recoils.

I ended that first day exhausted, but exhilarated. I felt proud, but I had doubts. Did my adapted approach yield results? Did my patients like me? Did they feel better? Was that first day so busy because there had simply been a backlog of people who needed to be treated?

My worries were assuaged the following week, when my schedule was full again, this time with a waiting list of names scratched into the side-margins of the page. Something I did that first day worked.

The take-away message from those early years was that I didn't need all of my techniques. All I required was a sound principle. This principle was finding and treating compacted osseofascial tissue *first*. Treating the biodynamics *before* the biomechanics. Addressing motility *before* mobility. Enhancing the texture of the osseofascial tissue *before* enhancing its connections. Today, more firmly than ever, this principle forms the foundation of my practice.

Fast forward to a mid-COVID-pandemic evening in late 2021. As I was washing dishes, a strange and wonderful feeling came over me. The sensation was so clear and so pure that I became almost giddy with joy. Over the past few years, beginning with my experiences in Saint-Sauveur and leading up to that very night pre-rinsing Tupperware lids, my osteopathy practice had evolved tremendously. Patients were feeling much better after seeing me. They were referring their friends and siblings, their kids and cousins. My waiting list was expanding. Yes, something I was doing seemed to be working quite well. My revelation that evening emerged from this one thought: I was ready to share my experiences with the world, and I would do it through a book. So here we are. Thank you for joining me.

I was drawn to biodynamics and BST through the back door, like a home buyer to a house with an apple pie in the oven. I was led there—pulled by some unseen but undeniable force. Once I arrived, I sat down at the table with a big piece of that pie and never left. In *Harry Potter and the Sorcerer's ('Philosopher's' outside of the US) Stone*, Ollivander says to Harry, "The wand chooses the wizard, Mr. Potter." In a way, like Harry Potter's wand, BST chose me.

Just as the mid-tide is a middle ground between the long tide and the CRI, BST is a kind of middle ground between biodynamics and biomechanics—it combines the best of both, making each one work better.

I'll say it again because I like the way it sounds: like a magnifying glass harnessing the sun's light, BST captures the brilliance of BCST and focuses it on bones. The beauty of BST is that it is as powerful as it is simple. While using BST requires a kind of presence and dialogue, with some practice, you'll master it.

THE PRINCIPLES OF BIODYNAMIC SKELETAL THERAPY

The goal of BST is to reanimate osseofascial compactions in order to restore and enhance function. To synthesize what we have already discussed (and we have discussed a lot) here are the main principles of the approach.

Osseofascial compactions are a high-priority type of somatic dysfunction.
Osseofascial compactions lack elasticity and vitality and can negatively impact the cohesiveness of the osseofascial continuum. This makes osseofascial compactions a high-priority type of somatic dysfunction. Therefore, they should (generally) be treated before other, less disruptive somatic dysfunctions.

Fluid behavior seems to be involved in the formation *and* reanimation of osseofascial compactions.
Fluid behavior seems to be associated with osseofascial tissue texture. Very low intensities of compressive and tensile force applied to osseofascial tissue impact these same fluids, helping us reanimate osseofascial compactions from within.

Potency exists in all fluids and tissues, is palpable, and is augmentable.
Potency is a fluidic drive toward homeostasis and exists in all fluids and tissues. In the body, it manifests within the fluids and animates both the fluid and physical bodies with an organizational intelligence. Potency is also palpable, and through our therapeutic dialogue, we can help augment its power.

Primary respiration is the language of potency.
Potency has a voice, and it speaks to us via the rhythms of primary respiration. Based on the amplitude of these rhythms, we can follow the progress of potency as it works, taking cues from it about how and when to begin, continue, or finish a technique. In short, primary respiration helps guide our treatments.

Osseofascial compactions are inertial fulcrum-lever systems.

Potency is a natural drive toward order, and an inertial fulcrum is an outpost of that drive. Together, potency and compacted bone tissue form an inertial fulcrum-lever system, which expresses lower amplitudes of primary respiration compared with healthy osseofascial tissue. The lower amplitude of primary respiration is associated with compromised tissue texture, and by extension, tissue quality.

Osseofascial tissue quality impacts adjacent structures.

Osteoporotic bone has been shown to negatively affect the quality of Sharpey's fibers. In this book, I suggest that osseofascial compactions also lower tissue quality, and may also impact Sharpey's fibers in similar ways. This remains unproven.

The relationship between adjacent structures impacts mobility.

If the connections between adjacent bones are compromised owing to compromised Sharpey's fibers, the mobility between those bones may be, as well.

Mobility impacts function.

Finally, decreased mobility between bones limits function.

SIX STAGES OF BIODYNAMIC SKELETAL THERAPY TREATMENT

The six stages of BST treatment form the backbone (ahem) of the approach. In fact, their description and design were the main objectives of this book. For this reason, I want to spend ample time discussing and describing each one of them. Understanding each stage as well as possible puts the odds of success in our favor. Again, this may serve as more of a review for some of you. For others, it may be brand new. Review *or* new, take your time here—it will be well worth it once we start practicing.

Permit me to go back in time, again. People have been giving and receiving manual treatment for centuries. In Greek and Roman times, Aëtius of Amida, a physician, used massage for headaches, vertigo, and epilepsy. Based on hieroglyphic records, Egyptians used manual therapy to treat various ailments and injuries. Healers and shamans from these and other civilizations have claimed for thousands of years that healing forces can pass from practitioner to patient.

In the nineteenth century, "bonesetters" in England offered medical care for people who could not afford to see a doctor. Bonesetters soon began to attract the attention of the mainstream medical community. Sir James Paget, a physician, noted that bonesetters seemed to help patients who didn't respond to traditional medical care. Eventually, bonesetters settled in the United States. The Sweet family practiced bonesetting in Connecticut and Rhode Island for nearly two centuries, and were likely among the earliest influencers of a visionary young medical doctor living in the southern United States named Andrew Taylor Still.

Still, whose ears must be ringing in the great beyond since we've been talking about him so much, is widely considered the founder of osteopathic manipulative therapy. After carrying out autopsies on cadavers retrieved from exhumed graves, as well as performing adjustments and other manual therapies on humans (both dead and living), Still was convinced that human anatomical structure was linked to health. A staunch opponent of pharmacology and wary of the medical doctors of his day with their often-barbaric interventions, Still believed that by nonsurgically manipulating body structure with the hands, function could be restored. As the first medical doctor known to have combined manipulative therapy with traditional medicine, Still believed that if a bone was precariously positioned, it could impact the function of the blood, lymph, and nerves. For instance, discussing ailments of the foot, Still said:

> A partial dislocation of one side of the spine would produce a twist which would throw one muscle on to another and another, straining ligaments, producing congestion and inflammation, or some irritation that would lead to a suspension of the fluids necessary to the harmonious vitality of the foot. (Still 2004, 32)

Still famously never wrote a technique book, but his teachings have influenced much of modern-day manual therapy. His approach (now called the Still technique) has two parts: indirect and direct. The indirect part of the Still technique allows the myofascial structures to release. Then, the direct part improves range of motion by challenging the extensibility of the connective tissue.[30]

---

[30]More specifically, the Still technique involves passively moving the joint and tissue into a position of ease, and then exaggerating the position slightly to increase the relaxation of the connective tissue. A compression or traction force is then applied for a few seconds parallel to the structure being used as a lever (for example, an arm) to further relax the tissues. While maintaining the traction/compression force, the structure is then brought back into the restriction and through the barrier.

Fast-forward to right now. With its multistage approach, BST reflects Still's biphasic direct-indirect techniques. Instead of just two phases, BST has six, and they are:

1. Cocooning
2. Compression
3. Dialogue
4. Augmentation
5. Spreading
6. Integration

Stage 1: Cocooning

Cocooning is the first stage. To begin BST treatment, we surround the inertial tissue with our hands and fingers, providing a contained arena for potency to do its work. Becker referenced this:

> I don't impose any channels I want it to go in, but I give it a nice tight fit so it will keep going where there is work to do. I don't let it just dissipate blindly, but I give it room to play in. I'm there to hold the stuff into focus so the work can be accomplished. (Becker 2023, 51)

Becker's idea of giving the inertial zone a "nice tight fit" and giving potency "room to play" resonates nicely with BST. In a way, cocooning a compaction is like capturing fireflies in a jar. It's a way of temporarily containing a kind of potent luminescence.

I mentioned before that, in nature, wind and water currents are invisible, but we still feel them. A similar phenomenon applies here. An osseofascial compaction is invisible, but we can still palpate it. During the cocooning stage, we surround the area of compacted tissue with the hands and fingers until we have the entirety of the compaction within our grasp. The compaction could be an entire bone, a dime-sized zone within a bone, or a sliver of connective tissue between two bones. If the compaction is within one part of a bone, we cocoon that specific area. If the compaction feels more diffuse throughout the entire bone, we cocoon it by grasping the bone at each end. If the compaction exists between two bones, we cocoon it from all sides.

Remember that the rhythms of primary respiration express themselves fully only through tissue that is *healthy*. At this very early stage, the compacted tissue is still "less healthy," so some or all of the rhythms may be absent or weak.

Stage 2: Compression

Compression is the second stage. Compression exaggerates the compaction by compacting it even more, making it the main indirect portion of BST treatment. But even though we are squeezing the tissue, compression is also a way to create *more* space. This is counterintuitive, I know. But when applied with just the right amount of force and at just the right angle, compression "opens the door" for potency to enter the compaction and act. Like the frayed shoelace from earlier, axial compression— compression applied from the ends of and parallel to the collagen substrands—may create more micro-space between the strands. Of course, working this way with osseofascial tissue is not an exact science— we can't see the actual collagen substrings to know if we are applying our compression exactly parallel to them. But this is where our orientation of compression becomes key. More on this soon.

Sutherland and Becker were fans of using compression, Jealous not so much. I certainly am. Sharon Wheeler, founder of the BoneWork

approach, uses compression with both hands to create a "field of pressure" around compacted bone tissue, helping reanimate the traumatized tissue. Druelle and our teachers at the CEO were pro-compression, as well.

Becker believed that compression was a way of balancing the energy within inertial tissue. When he applied compression from the periphery toward the center—from the levers toward the fulcrum—the strain patterns would unwind, and he would achieve better results. "The compression is going toward the point out of which energy comes," he explained (Becker 2023, 57). The key to therapeutic compression, according to Becker, is to apply just enough compressive force so that the energy applied from the *outside* matches the energy coming from *within*. By doing this, a kind of compressive "neutral point" is established, akin to two people pushing their hands together but remaining still. It's at this moment of neutrality that the levers reorganize themselves, unwinding from a disordered state to an ordered one. This is exactly what we are aiming for during this stage. Below, Becker references Sutherland's approach, discussing the latter's accumulation of parameters with a compression toward the fulcrum.

> The corrective principle in physiological biodynamics is more than mere exaggeration, direct action, opposing physiological action, etc. It is as Will Sutherland suggested when he was asked what to do with a convulsive case in a convulsive state: lock them up. Bring all the contributing factors present into the fulcrum, from the ends of all the levers, into physiological biodynamic focus or balance. This is the point of physiological and pathophysiological efficiency. This is

the point at which entropy can modify its dynamic. (Becker 2023, 249)

While Sutherland and Becker used compression to unwind strain patterns, Jealous considered compression unnecessary and potentially detrimental to the cause. He reasoned that since all lesions still contain motion, why would we add compression and potentially stifle it? To this, I would argue that, indeed, too much compression applied too quickly and in the wrong direction *can* stifle it, but just the right amount of compression at the just the right speed and angle opens it.

Several kinds of manual therapy use indirect approaches, of course. Myofascial release techniques incorporate indirect work. In the Still technique, discussed earlier, the first part of the maneuver is the indirect exaggeration of the position of dysfunction to relax the myofascial elements. Counterstrain, a myofascial therapeutic approach developed by Lawrence Jones in the 1950s, uses compression to further shorten painful already-shortened tender points within muscles and tendons. These and other indirect manual approaches often impact the reflex loops between proprioceptive organs and the central nervous system. But Golgi tendon organs and muscle spindles are absent in bone. Could other mechanisms explain the impact of therapeutic compression on bone tissue? Well, as we well know, injuring a bone hurts. And when there is pain, the central nervous system can become sensitized, causing the pain to linger long after the acute injury has healed. This is aptly referred to as *sensitization*. This may seem obvious, but I think it's worth saying anyway: the fact that we feel pain and experience sensitization is proof that the central nervous system is involved in bone pain. But during BST, we're definitely not hurting anyone—the forces

are just too small—and less is known about how *nonpainful* stimuli in bone are linked to the central nervous system. It seems that either (*a*) our impact on bony compactions is not mediated by the central nervous system, or (*b*) we just haven't figured out how non-painful stimuli in bone are linked to the central nervous system. So what else is going on here?

But we do understand quite a bit about how bones respond to load. We know that, via fluid flow, osteocytes detect mechanical load and initiate bone remodeling. While BST doesn't lead to bone remodeling in the classic sense (at least not in the duration of one or several sessions), perhaps the melting sensations we feel result from us temporarily altering the behavior of bone water. Another possible explanation for the changes we feel could involve electricity. Through compression, collagen emits an electrical charge, which leads to changes in its structure. We know from earlier that our bodies and cells contain bioelectricity, and that a bioelectric fabric may even govern our genome and evolution. We also learned how crystalline materials within collagen generate piezoelectricity when compressed or stretched, and how this electric charge contributes to mechanotransduction. It has been shown that electric impulses lead to changes in tissue sensitivity, symmetry, motion, and texture. Maybe our impact is fluidic *and* bioelectric.

A third possibility is that our therapeutic compression acts on the twisty nature of collagen itself, counterwinding it like a twisted rope. Once the rope is unwound (think of the frayed shoelace), more space is created within the compaction for potency to enter and act. My very-unproven-yet-plausible twisted rope theory may help illustrate this.

Scott's very-unproven-yet-plausible twisted rope theory

We covered the basics of collagen structure earlier. Remember that collagen is mainly responsible for the viscoelastic properties of bone and fascia, and the ability of collagen fibers in osseofascial tissue to ease under compression allows us to enter into a special therapeutic dialogue with the osseofascial continuum. We saw how the hierarchical structure of the collagen fibril makes it similar to a twisted nanoscale rope, and due to structural imperfections in the collagen triple helix molecule, the twisted rope is flexible. Similar to actual ropes or cables, collagen fibrils are naturally loaded with tension and are prone to buckling when compressed. Like multistrand ropes when they are compressed or counterwound, Bozec demonstrated that pure collagen displays "birdcaging," a separation of individual substrands. Notice how *more* (not less) space is created between some of the strands (figures 11.1 and 11.2).

This idea helps explain how *pure* collagen behaves, but what about collagen in bone? Is the same birdcaging phenomenon present? It kind of feels that way, doesn't it? Due to the staggered arrangements of hydroxyapatite crystals within the collagen fibrils, there is much less room for collagen in bone to buckle than it would on its own. After all, if the crystals didn't resist compressive load, bone

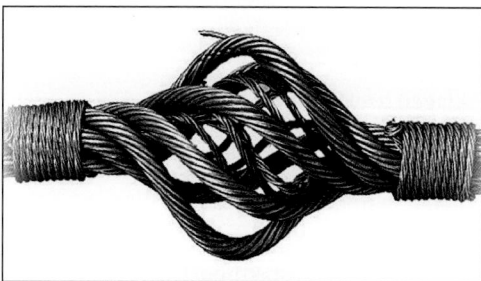

Figure 11.2. Birdcaging in collagen fibrils. Also see, figure 4.5. Adapted from Bozec, van der Heijden, and Horton 2007.

just wouldn't be bone. But Stock showed us that some collagen distortion in bone is not only present but necessary for optimal load transfer to occur. This tells us that there is still room for collagen in bone to *act like pure collagen*. Even though bone is rigid, under just the right amount of compressive force at just the right angles, an unmistakable softening occurs. And when we fine-tune the compression—making microadjustments in the amount and angles of force—we seem to enhance the release even more.

We can now envision an invisible yet palpable scar-like bony imprint composed of tiny, twisted collagen molecules arranged into disorganized tangles of larger, bunched-up collagen fibrils, all of which are bungled up in a frazzled, scar-like mess. Then, under just the right amount of compression and at just the right angles, the disorganized pattern of collagen "slackens" (at least temporarily), creating more space between

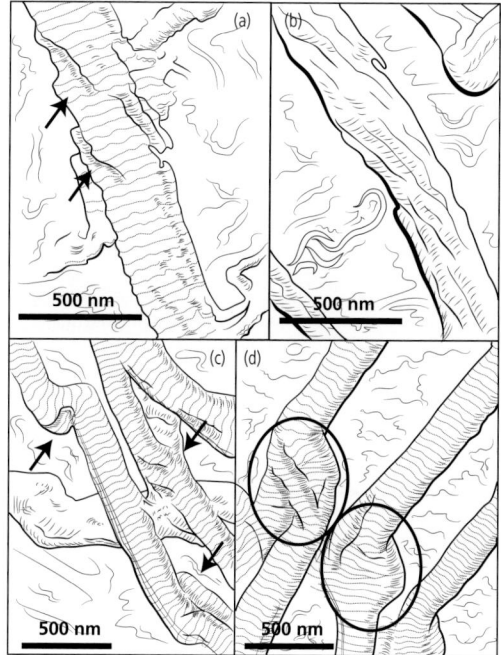

Figure 11.1. Birdcaging in actual twisted rope.

(some of) the individual twists of collagen. More research is needed to substantiate this, but I think that the twisted rope theory is compelling. Combined with picturing the squishy viscoelastic cushion of the collagen "accordion" described earlier, the image of unwinding the twisted rope may serve as a helpful visualization. It does for me.

Okay, enough chit chat—back to our subject waiting patiently on the table! We've already cocooned the compaction. Now, we need to figure out how to apply that tricky axial compression that will open the system. I have found that the best way to do this is ... well, there is no best way, actually. Our best bet, I think, is to find where the compaction feels most rigid in tension, and then compress the bone directly back into that line of rigidity, twisting a bit here and a bit there, fine-tuning our contact. We may have to play that mini-accordion (described above) to find the best angle. If we use too much compressive force, the spring of the collagen bottoms out. But, if we carefully remain within the fluidic cushion of the bone, collapsing the twists and tensions, counterwinding the collagen like a twisted rope or shoelace, we seem to create more space for potency to enter and act. Again, this is far from an exact science. As in all the stages of treatment, listening to the tissues in our hands is paramount. The tissues tell us what to do.

If the compaction is within one part of a bone, compress that specific area. If the compaction feels more diffuse throughout the entire bone, compress it from each end. If the compaction exists between two bones, compress it from all sides.

Stage 3: Dialogue

The third stage of BST treatment is dialogue, and is very much about listening. This is when we begin to feel (listen to) and decipher the rhythms of primary respiration as they emerge from osseofascial tissue. In my opinion, manual dialogue should unfold like verbal dialogue between two people. Through verbal dialogue, we listen to words and observe other nonverbal cues to understand how we can help. During manual dialogue, we listen and observe with our hands. We interpret tactile sensations to understand how to best offer support. During a verbal conversation, nonjudgmental listening is sometimes enough for a patient or friend to find a solution for themselves. Listening on its own provides an empowering opportunity for self-healing. Through manual dialogue, when we listen using a similar nonjudgmental presence, we offer the body a chance to lean on us so it can change. Both verbal and manual listening can be profoundly therapeutic, since they invite meaningful change to occur from within.

During this stage of BST, as we continue to maintain the compressive dialogue from earlier, the inertial fulcrum itself may come into focus. The inertial fulcrum feels like stillness—a calm, vital presence—within the somewhat chaotic inertial fulcrum-lever system of the compaction. We are not only dialoguing with the levers, here, but also with the fulcrum. The fulcrum is hard at work, balancing the disorganized patterns of osseofascial tissue swirling around it. As we dialogue in compression, creating and holding space for potency to enter and act, primary respiration should begin emerging from the bone, manifesting more strongly from within the compaction. It manifests more strongly because the tissue is getting "healthier" in our hands. We may begin to feel the rotations and movements of the CRI, then the welling up and receding of the mid-tide, and finally the steady presence of the long tide. Remember, if the long tide is hard to perceive, focus on the CRI and mid-tide. Eventually, we may sense a shift when the rhythms coalesce, inhaling and exhaling the bone in one resultant rhythm.

During the dialogue stage, we remain active yet nonjudgmental listeners—volunteering support when necessary, making subtle suggestions here and there, offering encouragement when needed. Our role here is to keep the levers of bone tissue in contact with the fulcrum, bathing them in stillness. As we hold the entire ocean of primary respiration in our hands as the tissue continues to unwind, we fine-tune the pressure to encourage it even more. Like a dependable friend, we reassure the tissue that it can lean on us while it changes.

If the compaction is within one part of a bone, dialogue with that specific area. If the compaction feels more diffuse throughout the entire bone, dialogue with the whole bone from each end. If the compaction exists between two bones, dialogue with it from all sides.

Stage 4: Augmentation

Augmentation is the fourth stage of BST treatment. Like a proud parent running beside their child learning to ride a bike, or like a drama teacher mouthing the words as their student recites them during the school play, the augmentation stage of treatment is when we support the phenomena unfolding before us. We're not interfering, but we're still right there, offering encouragement.

Now that primary respiration is breathing the bone beneath our hands, we should be able to recognize the maximum amplitudes of the phases. At the height of the inhalation phase, a natural disengagement of the bone tissue occurs. Here, it's as if the compaction is expanding, stretching its wings, creating more

space for itself as it shifts to a more natural state. We remain in contact with the tissue as it does so and until primary respiration has reached a maximum amplitude for a few complete cycles.

If the compaction is within one part of a bone, augment primary respiration from within that specific area. If the compaction feels more diffuse throughout the entire bone, augment primary respiration within the entire bone from each end. If the compaction exists between two bones, augment primary respiration within it from all sides.

Stage 5: Spreading

The spreading stage is the fifth stage and is the *direct* part of BST treatment. Once potency has unwound and expanded the inertial bone tissue as much as it can on its own, and the expression of primary respiration is robust, spreading the bone will encourage the tissue to expand a little bit more. As we saw earlier, the expansion occurs within the relaxation phase of the collagen tensile stress/strain curve. Our role here becomes more active again, reversing the direction of our compressive force by applying a spreading action directly against the most rigid torsional shape or pattern of compaction. Here, the term *spreading* is used instead of *stretching* or *tension*, since the idea is to slowly spread the bone as if it were made of taffy. The "taffy" image is another visualization that works quite well. Remember, the spreading stage is slow, gentle work.

Earlier, we learned that in pure collagen, very low tensile loads lead to an unkinking of the collagen molecules. The unkinking leads to a kind of re-jigging of the collagen-water relationship, or a molecular hydroplaning within the tropocollagen, causing a "relaxation" of the collagen. If the tensile force continues to increase, the higher load shifts from the viscosity of the collagen-water relationship to the elasticity of the solid collagenous matrix. **Since we're interested in engaging the same fluids responsible for the formation of the dysfunction, we use very low tensile forces.** I've put this in bold type because it is important. During BST treatment, it helps to view bone tissue as a fluidic medium. Regardless of the stage of treatment, we are always working within the fluid body of osseofascial tissue. Also, remember that viscosity is rate dependent, so the effectiveness of this stage depends not only on the amount of force applied but also on the rate at which it's applied. If we spread too hard and too quickly, we'll bypass the fluidic cushion of the bone, and the taffy will resist. It is worth repeating that this is slow, gentle work.

A helpful way to avoid applying too much spreading force is to simply *imagine* spreading the bone, and wait for a very subtle relaxation to manifest from deep within the bone matrix. We're not "lengthening" bones here. Rather, we are waiting for quiet "sigh of relief" texture change from deep within the tissue. When we're at the right level, sometimes it feels as though two conflicting things are happening at once: the collagen relaxes while the crystal reinforcements hold. So, with our fingers and hands, we cover as much of the surface area of the tissue as we can, and then we just imagine spreading the bone like cold honey on toast.

During the spreading stage, primary respiration sometimes fades temporarily. Once it reemerges, we remain in contact with the tissue for a few complete cycles.

If the compaction is within one part of a bone, spread that specific area. If the compaction feels more diffuse throughout the entire bone, spread the entire bone from each end.

If the compaction exists between two bones, spread it from all sides.

Stage 6: Integration

Once the spreading stage is complete and primary respiration is being more robustly expressed from the once-inertial site, we integrate our local work into the global human system. Here, we remain in contact with the once-inertial tissue, expanding our perception to include the entire body and sensing primary respiration breathing within it. We wait for this larger ocean of primary respiration to recognize the local mini-ocean in our hands and then carry it away with its tide. We stay with this sensation for a few complete cycles of primary respiration until the local structures become almost indiscernible from the rest of the body. Once this occurs, we remove our hands or transition to other modalities, if necessary.

SENSING PRIMARY RESPIRATION

Before finding and treating actual osseofascial compactions, I suggest practicing perceiving the three rhythms (CRI, mid-tide, and long tide) within the three bodies (physical, fluid, and tidal) in *normal* bone tissue. This way, you'll develop a sense for the normal expression of primary respiration and be able to compare it to compromised expression in compacted tissue.

For each of the three rhythms, we'll practice from the sacrum and from one location on the periphery. You can either practice listening to one rhythm from each hold before moving on to the next hold, or practice sensing all three rhythms from the same hold before switching.

I've listed the exercises in an order that I feel is appropriate to follow, especially for beginners. Feel free to jump from one exercise to another based on your expertise and preference.

If some of the descriptions contain sections that seem repetitive, forgive me. My intention is to provide as complete instructions as possible for each section of each exercise to accommodate those who choose to review one or several of the exercises outside the order listed. Feel free to skim over these repetitive sections if needed.

Sensing Your Primary Respiration I

This exercise is the first part of a two-part series (see also page 258).

Before sensing primary respiration in someone else, start by sensing it in yourself. Sensing your own primary respiration can be a useful learning and centering exercise to perform before the first treatment of the day, or before a treatment that you anticipate being more challenging. It will also prime your awareness to better sense the rhythms of primary respiration in your subject. I suggest performing this exercise lying supine with your eyes closed. Allow your mind to settle. Visualize the midline of your body, from the top of your head down to your coccyx, as an ever-present shaft of calm, liquid light.

Begin with the CRI. See if you can feel the CRI expressed through the internal and external rotations of the arms and legs. Stay grounded within your midline while you perceive the three-to-six-second inhalation phase of external rotation and then the three-to-six-second exhalation phase of internal rotation of the limbs. Once you've identified the CRI within the limbs, see if you can extend your awareness to the structures closer to your midline, such as the pelvis and rib cage. You'll notice that the CRI doesn't always rotate structures,

but moves them in other ways, too. This is normal. Regardless of how they're moving, the movements should all roughly express the same cadence. If you have difficulty here, it may help to resonate more intently with the earthy quality of your physical body. Imagine that you are made of earth—of physical matter. You may also sense that the symmetry of the CRI changes from one area of your body to the next, or is absent in one part or another. That's also normal. For now, just stay with the CRI for a few complete cycles, observing and appreciating it without too much analysis.

Now, move to the mid-tide. Remember that the mid-tide is slower than the CRI, and instead of rotational movements in individual structures, it is expressed as a slower welling-up-and-receding sensation, rising and falling one to three times per minute. Remain grounded in your midline. Begin by sensing the 10-to-30-second inhalation phase of the mid-tide ascending inferior to superior and from the midline outward as your cranium and body well up. Then, feel the 10-to-30-second exhalation phase descending superior to inferior and from outward toward the midline as your cranium and body empty. If at first you have difficulty sensing the mid-tide, it may be helpful to resonate with the watery quality of your fluid body. Imagine yourself as a person-shaped water balloon. As you may have noticed with the CRI, you may sense that the amplitude or symmetry of the mid-tide differs from one area of your body to the next. For now, just observe it. Settle into your awareness of the inhalation and exhalation of the mid-tide for a few complete cycles.

Move from the mid-tide to the long tide. The long tide is the slowest and most stable of the three rhythms. It's also inconsistent, so you may not sense it at all. Sometimes, it's helpful to begin with the long tide, then proceed to the

CRI and mid-tide, and return to the long tide again. However you choose to sense it, stay grounded within your midline. For the long tide, I find it useful to not only resonate with the electric wind-like texture of the tidal body right away but also to extend my awareness to the room around me and out to the horizon, and even further. Simply visualize yourself in a much larger space. See if you can feel a steady 50-second inhalation phase moving away from your midline toward the horizon, followed by a 50-second exhalation phase moving from the horizon back to the midline. Observe the long tide for a few complete cycles.

Once you have sensed the rhythms separately, see if you can now feel them together, like words coming together to form sentences, and then paragraphs, and then a story. If you were only able to feel one or two of the rhythms, that's okay. Stay with primary respiration for a few complete cycles. Feel how the rhythms coalesce. Take a few more moments to bask in the ocean of primary respiration animating you from within.

Sensing CRI

Now that you've felt primary respiration within yourself, it's time to feel it in your patient. Sit at the head of the treatment table, with your feet flat on the floor, hips moved to the back of the chair, shoulders relaxed. Allow your mind to settle. Visualize the midline of your body, from the top of your head down to your coccyx, as an ever-present shaft of liquid light. Become a responsive, dynamic, and supportive external fulcrum on which your subject can depend while potency acts.

From the sacrum

With the subject lying prone, stand or sit by their pelvis and gently place your hands on the sacrum (figure 11.3).

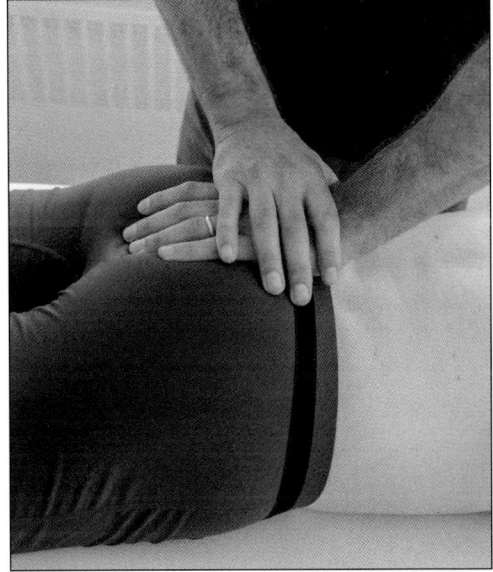

Figure 11.3. Sacral listening hold.

Since the CRI manifests within the physical body, focus on the physical characteristics of the sacrum. Appreciate the texture and vitality of the bone. Begin by sensing a subtle three-to-six-second inhalation, rocking the base of the sacrum posteriorly (toward the ceiling), then feel the three-to-six-second exhalation, rocking the base of the sacrum anteriorly (toward the table). The CRI may be expressed more noticeably in different areas of the sacrum, the rocking may seem asymmetrical, or the movement may be absent. All of these are possible. Remember, if there's a compaction within the sacrum, the expression of primary respiration will be limited. Settle into your awareness of the inhalation and exhalation of the CRI, in whichever pattern or amplitude it brings, for a few complete cycles.

From the femur

Remove your hands from the sacrum and have the subject return to the supine position. Sit or stand by their left thigh. Envelop the thigh with both hands (figure 11.4).

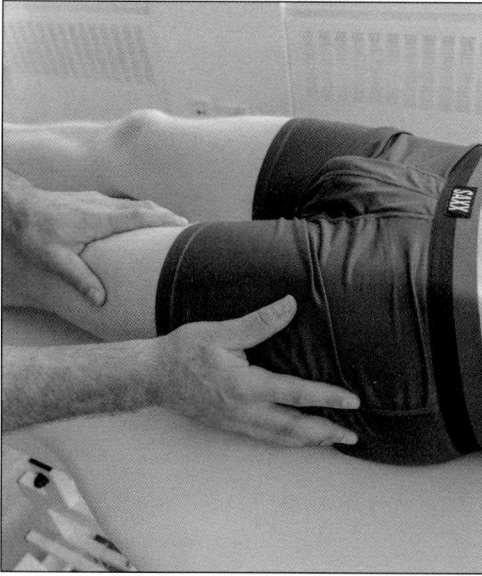

Figure 11.4. Sensing CRI from the femur.

Without physically applying more pressure, slowly bring your awareness deeper into the musculature of the thigh until you visualize and sense the femur. Feel the gradual change in density as you descend through the skin, adipose tissue, muscle, then on to the bone. When contacting the femur, focus on the physical characteristics and movements of the bone. Sense the CRI as it expresses a three-to-six-second inhalation, rotating the femur externally, and then the three-to-six-second exhalation, rotating the femur internally. As always, the CRI may be expressed more noticeably in different areas of the bone. Settle into your awareness of the inhalation and exhalation of CRI for a few complete cycles. Sensing primary respiration from peripheral holds sometimes takes more practice than it does to sense primary respiration from the craniosacral positions, so be patient here.

Sensing Mid-tide

Sit at the head of the treatment table, with your feet flat on the floor, hips moved to the back of the chair, shoulders relaxed. Allow your mind to settle. Visualize the midline of your body, from the top of your head down to your coccyx, as an ever-present shaft of liquid light. Become a responsive, dynamic, and stable external fulcrum on which your subject can depend while potency acts.

From the sacrum

We'll use the sacral listening hold demonstrated in figure 11.3. Here, switch your perception from the physical characteristics of the CRI to a more fluidic awareness. Imagine the sacrum becoming a sacrum-shaped water balloon, and your hands becoming hand-shaped water balloons, each with very delicate balloon containers so that any excess pressure could pop either of the balloons. Begin by sensing a subtle 10-to-30-second inhalation and filling of the sacrum, and then feel the 10-to-30-second exhalation and emptying of the sacrum. You may notice the CRI rocking the sacrum. If so, don't engage it, just appreciate it, and continue to resonate with the mid-tide. The filling and emptying should feel as if the sacrum-shaped water balloon is literally filling up with water and then emptying. The mid-tide may be expressed more noticeably in different areas of the sacrum, or the filling and emptying may seem asymmetrical. Remember, if there is a compaction within the sacrum, the expression of primary respiration will be limited. Settle into your awareness of the inhalation and exhalation of the mid-tide for a few complete cycles.

From the humerus

Remove your hands from the sacrum and have the subject return to the supine position. Sit or stand by their left humerus and envelop the upper arm with both hands, with one hand on either end of the bone. Compress your hands together ever so slightly to engage the tissue (figure 11.5).

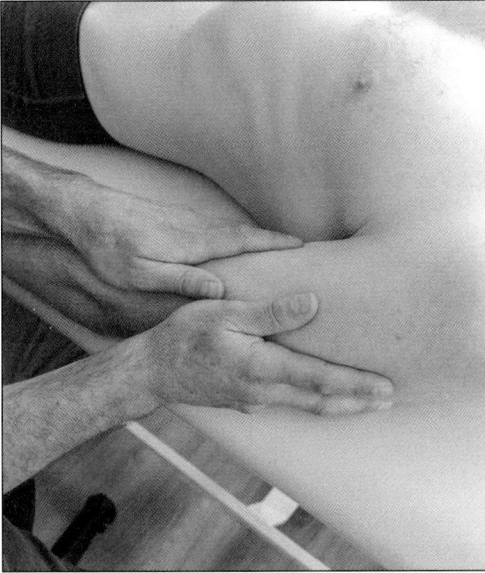

Figure 11.5. Sensing mid-tide from the humerus.

Without applying more physical pressure, slowly bring your awareness deeper into the upper arm, feeling the change in density as you descend from the soft tissues to the bone itself. Switch your perception from the physical characteristics you visualized when sensing the CRI to a more fluidic awareness. Imagine the humerus becoming a humerus-shaped water balloon, and your hands becoming hand-shaped water balloons. Sense the 10-to-30-second inhalation filling the humerus, and then the 10-to-30-second exhalation emptying the humerus. You may notice the CRI manifesting via internal and external rotations of the humerus. Don't engage these movements, just notice them. It should feel as if the humerus-shaped water balloon is literally filling up with water and then emptying. The mid-tide may be expressed more noticeably in different areas of the humerus, or the filling and emptying may seem asymmetrical. Settle into your awareness of the inhalation and exhalation of the mid-tide for a few complete cycles.

Sensing Long Tide

As always, sit at the head of the treatment table, with your feet flat on the floor, hips moved to the back of the chair, shoulders relaxed. Allow your mind to settle. Visualize the midline of your body, from the top of your head down to your coccyx, as an ever-present shaft of liquid light. Become a responsive, dynamic, and stable external fulcrum on which your subject can depend while potency acts.

From the sacrum

Remove your hands and have your subject turn over so they are now lying prone on the table. Stand or sit by their pelvis and gently place your hands on the sacrum as described above (figure 11.3). When sensing the CRI, you focused on the physical characteristics of the structures beneath your fingers. When sensing the mid-tide, you focused on the fluidic quality of those structures. Since the long tide manifests within the wider tidal body in and around the subject's body, imagine that your hands are translucent, and both you and your subject are immersed in a very wide-open space. You may notice the CRI manifesting via rocking of the sacrum or the welling-up-and-receding tidal motion of the mid-tide. For the moment, do not engage these rhythms, just appreciate them.

Now, widen your perception to fill the room, then move it out toward the horizon while staying in contact with the sacrum. Hold the sacrum in this much wider perception. You may start to notice a 50-second-inhalation tidal motion moving away from the midline through the sacrum toward the periphery, followed by a 50-second-exhalation tidal motion moving back from the periphery through the sacrum toward the midline. Some people may also sense an endless expansive force or a dynamic stillness within and around the subject's body. This is all possible, since the long tide can assume different shapes and currents. The long tide is also inconsistent, so you may not feel it at all. Settle into your awareness of the inhalation and exhalation of the long tide for a few complete cycles.

From the left radius

Remove your hands from the sacrum and have your subject return to the supine position. Sit or stand by their left arm. Grasp the proximal head of the radius with your right hand and the distal end with your left hand (figure 11.6).

Visualize the bone. Gently approximate your hands to better appreciate its texture. When sensing the CRI, you focused on the physical characteristics of the bone. When sensing the mid-tide, you focused on the fluidic quality of the bone. Since the long tide manifests within the wider tidal body in and around the subject's body, imagine that your hands are

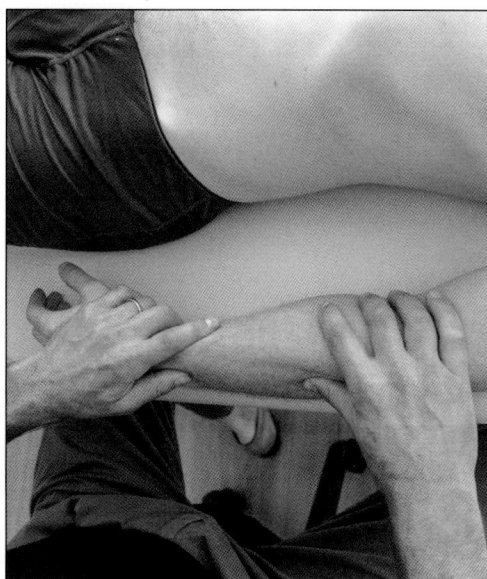

Figure 11.6. Sensing long tide from the radius.

translucent, and both you and your subject are immersed in a much wider space.

You may notice the CRI manifesting via external and internal rotations of the bone or the welling-up-and-receding tidal motion of the mid-tide. Don't engage these rhythms, just watch them. Move your perception out toward the horizon while maintaining contact with the radius. Let your mind hold the radius in this much wider perception. You may start to notice a 50-second-inhalation tidal motion moving away from the midline and through the radius toward the periphery, and the 50-second-exhalation tidal motion moving back from the periphery through the radius toward the midline. Some people may also sense an endless expansive force or a dynamic stillness within and around the subject's body. The long tide is also inconsistent, so you may not feel it at all. This is all normal and possible. Settle into your awareness of the inhalation and exhalation of the long tide for a few complete cycles.

Sensing the Holistic Shift

The holistic shift happens when the practitioner's awareness shifts from the variable waveforms of the CRI to the deeper rhythms of primary respiration. You've already practiced sensing all three rhythms within all three bodies separately. Now, you'll practice experiencing and resonating with all three rhythms and all three bodies as they coalesce as the total expression of primary respiration.

From the sacrum

Have the subject lying prone on the table. Stand or sit by their pelvis, and gently place your hands on the sacrum as described above (figure 11.3).

First, notice the variable waveforms of the CRI manifesting within the physical body of the sacrum in 3-to-6-second inhalations and 3-to-6-second exhalations. Now, switch your perception to a more fluidic awareness. Imagine the sacrum becoming a sacrum-shaped water balloon and imagine your hands becoming hand-shaped water balloons. Now, sense the mid-tide with its subtle 10-to-30-second inhalation and filling of the sacrum, and 10-to-30-second exhalation and emptying of the sacrum. Then, imagine your hands becoming translucent. Widen your awareness even more to include the tidal body that fills the room and extends to the horizon, and see if you can feel the long tide as a 50-second inhalation moving away from the midline through the sacrum toward the periphery and a 50-second exhalation moving back from the periphery through the sacrum toward the midline.

Try to remain aware of the individual textures of the three bodies (physical, fluid, and tidal) and the cadence of each of the three rhythms (CRI, mid-tide, and long tide) blending into one resultant texture and rhythm. Settle into this awareness for a few complete cycles.

From the left clavicle

Remove your hands from the sacrum and have the subject return to the supine position. Sit or stand by their left shoulder. Grasp the left clavicle by gently pinching the medial end with the fingers of your left hand, with your left thumb tucked gently into the subclavicular space, and by gently pinching the lateral end of the clavicle with the fingers of your right hand, with your right thumb tucked gently into the subclavicular space (figure 11.7).

Gently approximate your hands to better appreciate the texture and quality of the bone. First, notice the CRI manifesting within the physical body of the clavicle in 3-to-6-second inhalations and 3-to-6-second exhalations. This may feel like anterior and posterior rotations of the bone. Now, switch your

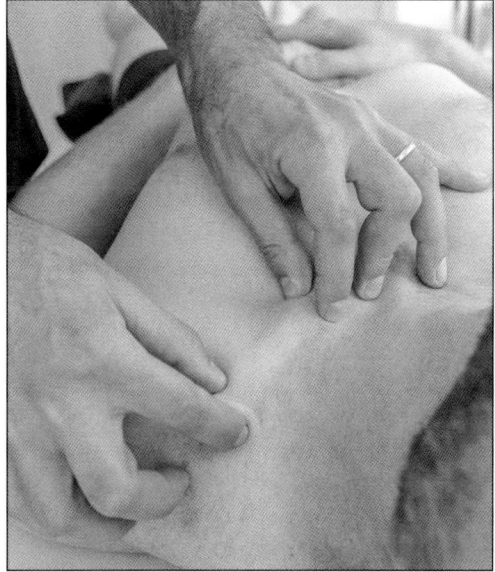

Figure 11.7. Sensing the holistic shift from the clavicle.

perception from the physical characteristics of the CRI to a more fluidic awareness. Imagine the clavicle becoming a clavicle-shaped water balloon and your hands becoming hand-shaped water balloons. Feel the mid-tide with its subtle 10-to-30-second inhalation filling the clavicle, and 10-to-30-second exhalation emptying the clavicle. Now, imagine your hands becoming translucent, and see if you can feel the long tide as a 50-second inhalation moving away from the midline through the clavicle toward the periphery and a 50-second exhalation moving back from the periphery through the clavicle toward the midline.

Try to remain aware of the individual textures of the three bodies (physical, fluid, and tidal) and the cadence of each of the three rhythms (CRI, mid-tide, and long tide) blending into one resultant texture and rhythm. Settle into this awareness for a few complete cycles.

Practice these exercises as many times as needed, and feel free to return to them from time to time to tune up your palpation and perception skills.

Trust

The difference between you and the greatest therapist who ever lived is not trust or knowledge.

The difference between you and the greatest therapist who ever lived is trusting your knowledge.

Steven's Jaw

Steven walked into my office. He was in a bad mood. "How are you feeling?" I asked. "Terrible," Steven replied, "and I'm not telling you why. Figure it out." Intrigued, I asked him to lie on his back. I started at his feet and moved up his body, touching each bone. When I arrived at the right side of Steven's face, I noticed that the texture of the mandible and temporal bone was different. The bones had less elasticity. They felt less alive. When I finished my evaluation, which took a few minutes, I asked Steven if the right side of his face and neck were involved in his symptoms. He sat straight up on the table in disbelief, nodding his head. He explained that he had been having debilitating right-sided facial and jaw pain with cervical radiculopathy down his right arm. In this case, I didn't need to test the movement of the bones, only the movement within them. After I had treated him, Steven left my office in less pain and in a (slightly) better mood.

CHAPTER 14

How to Test and Treat Bones

Now comes the fun part: testing and treating bones with BST. Like reintroducing a rehabilitated bird back into its flock, we'll find bone tissue that needs help, bring it back to health, and set it free. Before getting into specifics about testing and treating bone, this section explains the general approach of how to put what we've learned into practice. This chapter will introduce *touch-testing*, the evaluation protocol used in BST. We'll also discuss the differences between local and regional BST treatment, and how each relates to the other. Other items will be unpacked here, including tips on palpation, how much force to use, and how long each BST technique should last. To end the chapter, and before diving into actual practice, we'll answer some frequently asked questions.

TOUCH-TESTING

Before we treat compactions, we need to find them! In my practice, sometimes I find compactions while I'm working on something else. For example, I could be mobilizing the scapulae and detect an extra-rigid section of the bone around the acromion process. Or I could be releasing the cervical fascia and feel that the second cervical vertebra (C2) is compacted. I also find compactions by deliberately scanning the body for them, a procedure I call touch-testing.

Touch-testing is like a treasure hunt for bony compactions, and it involves what the name implies: touching a bone to test it. Every bone? Well, yes. This may seem cumbersome within the confines of a single treatment, but with a little practice, you'll be able to scan the entire body in minutes.

Touch-testing involves more than a simple touch, but less than a full mobility test, and accomplishes two things at once. First, contacting a bone for only a second or two allows us to quickly appreciate its texture and quality. Does it feel like wood or concrete? Wood is normal; concrete is not.

Second, touch-testing allows us to appreciate the *micromobility* of a bone in relation to its neighbors. Is there at least some micromovement between that bone and the bone to which it is connected? Some movement is normal; no movement is not. Some may suggest that the only way to test the mobility of a bone is to mobilize it through its full range of motion around a joint, including rotations, glides, and translations. True—touch-testing does *not* test the full range of motion. However, since we're concerned with finding compacted bone(s), testing the micromobility of a bone is all we need. If a compaction is present between two bones, there'll be virtually no discernible mobility in any direction or of any amplitude.

Trusting First Impressions

Trusting first impressions is important since we have the tendency to second-guess ourselves, especially while learning. In 2018, I took a postgraduate class at the CEO called "The Evaluation and Treatment of the Osseous Head." The teacher of the course was Eric Prat, one of the cofounders of the osteopathic mechanical link (OML), a fascinating approach to osteopathic manual therapy that he developed with his teacher Paul Chauffour in the 1970s.

The OML approach involves evaluating a strictly defined series of points before making decisions about where to begin treatment. The points of the series are preselected according to their significance, so the series never changes. The tests are done quickly, relying on first impressions of tissue elasticity to determine the health of a structure.

When I watched Prat work, I was astounded at how fluidly he contacted and assessed dozens of points, especially around the face and skull. It was as if he wasn't even touching the points, but gliding over them, perceiving them. Using more classical methods of cranial evaluation—evaluating each cranial and facial bone for mobility—could take up to an hour to complete. Using the OML system, Prat achieved this in about a minute.

Impressed, I immediately began using his protocol for my cranial evaluations. The first time I did the OML cranial series, it took 15 minutes—just for the head! But the more I practiced, the more efficient I became. Even more surprising to me was that the quicker I moved from one point to the next, relying on my first impressions, the more accurate the tests became.

Test Quickly, Treat Slowly

With OML and BST, we test a bone *quickly*. This is important for two reasons. First, a quick touch forces us to trust our first impressions (which are usually correct). Second, since bone is a viscoelastic material, its deformation is rate dependent. Therefore, the more quickly we touch a bone, the less chance there is of it changing (even if this change is infinitesimal) before we make a decision.[31] Remember that viscoelasticity is the combination of the gooiness of a liquid and the elasticity of a solid, and it plays out in all kinds of neat ways across a wide range of materials. A shear-thickening fluid, for example, exhibits an abrupt increase in viscosity with an increasing shear rate. Oobleck, that weird combination of cornstarch and water, behaves this way. If you rest a spoon on the surface of a bowl of Oobleck, the utensil slowly sinks to the bottom. But if you tap the surface of the Oobleck with the same spoon, the spoon bounces off. Other viscoelastic materials include Silly Putty, taffy, thick honey, and your kids' homemade

---

[31] The quick/slow duality resonates with the idea discussed earlier about how the absolute solidity of many biomaterials is questionable. To adequately transfer force throughout the biotensegrity structure of the body, materials like bones must shape-shift between compression strut and tension cable, sometimes acting more like soft-matter gels than solid structures.

slime concoctions made with borax. In all these materials, when force is applied suddenly, they feel solid. When force is applied slowly or removed altogether, they ooze. The bone-as-Oobleck visualization seems to work here.

The Two Phases of Biodynamic Skeletal Therapy Touch-Testing

There are two phases of the touch-test: phase 1 and phase 2. Phase 1 is an initial touch-test to determine if a compaction exists, and phase 2 is a more specific "spread-and-twist" test to determine the orientation of the torsional pattern of the compaction.

During phase 1, touch-test each point for no more than a few seconds (figure 14.1). The touch may be combined with a spread or a squeeze or a wiggle or a push. For some of the smaller bones of the hands and feet, squashing the bone will "spread" it from the center outward. Use your fingers, the palm of your hand, or your thumb. The specifics are unimportant. What's crucial here is getting the information you need from making quick contact.

For phase 2 (and only once you've identified the presence of a compaction in phase 1), identify the torsional pattern of the compacted tissue. Retest the bone(s) by applying tension and torsion, spreading and twisting the tissue (figure 14.2).

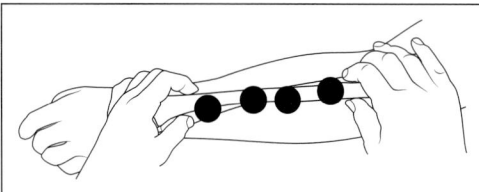

Figure 14.1. Example of phase 1 of touch-testing. A series of quick points of pressure.

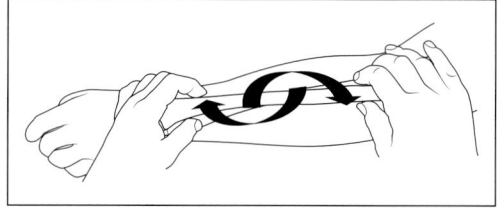

Figure 14.2. Example of phase 2 of touch-testing. A spreading and twisting of the bone.

TWO PHASES OF BIODYNAMIC SKELETAL THERAPY TREATMENT: LOCAL AND REGIONAL

There are also two phases of BST treatment: local and regional. Local treatment usually precedes regional treatment and addresses osseofascial compactions within a bone or between two bones. Regional treatment addresses the regional strain patterns within groups of bones. For example, we may first treat the local compaction within the fibula (figure 14.3), followed by the regional strain pattern within the entire lower extremity (figure 14.4). In this case, local treatment precedes regional treatment.

We discussed biotensegrity and modularity earlier. Combining local and regional treatment allows us to address the modularity of the osseofascial continuum. With this

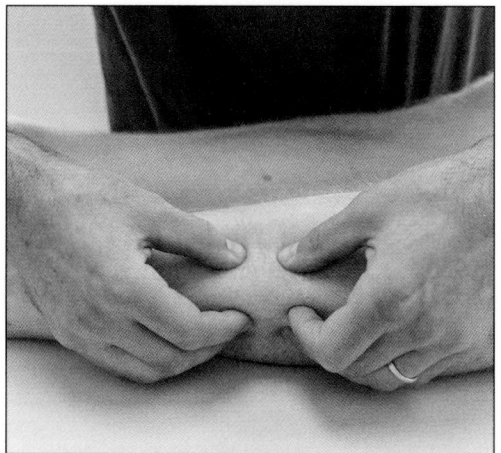

Figure 14.3. Local treatment of the fibula.

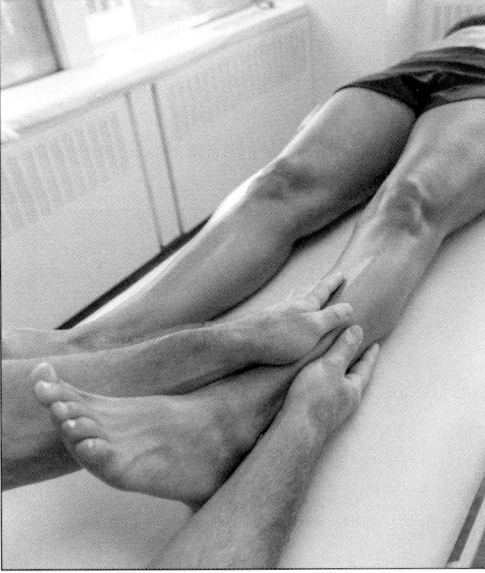

Figure 14.4. Regional treatment of the lower extremity.

local-regional approach, we can treat smaller, local modules of one or two bones nested within larger, regional modules of other bones, addressing the biotensegrity of the entire region.

Palpation

To be proficient at both local and regional BST treatment, our palpatory skills must be sharp. Akin to snowflakes melting in the sun, each interaction between two people is unique and temporary, and only happens once. BST is a way to participate in and enhance the magic of that moment. But in order not to miss the moment, reliable palpation is key. Our hands must become more like hand-ears so they can listen to potency at work.

Our fingers and hands are miraculous instruments, and our palpation is astonishingly sensitive. If we remain attentive and present, a universe of information will unfold. But like any skill worth acquiring, palpating primary respiration in bone tissue requires practice, and can take years to

perfect. Becker: "It took four solid years from 1945 to 1949, for my stupid palpatory sensory cells to wake up and feel the things that I was supposed to be picking up" (Becker 2023, 42). I admire Becker's humility.

Palpation is often easier to talk about than to do. After all, humans are complex. When we touch another person with therapeutic intention, two complex systems merge, and the outcome is hard to predict. Consider the difference between a rock and bird. If you were to toss a rock into the air, it would trace a nice even curve in the air. The rock goes up and then comes down. The rock is a simple structure that can only make a simple response to the forces acting upon it. But if you were to release a pigeon into the air, the bird would act very differently from the rock. Despite being subjected to the same atmospheric forces, the pigeon may swoop and drop or fly back up into a tree or to the top of a building. The bird is strong and light. It can counterbalance the force of gravity. It is dynamic and agile, so it can change direction and altitude. The bird may even use the wind currents to its advantage, accelerating more quickly or climbing higher than it could on its own. Unlike the rock, the bird possesses intelligence and agency. Compared to the rock, the bird is complex.

But is the rock really that boring and predictable? It depends on who you ask. To most of us, a rock is just a rock. But if you were a geologist, the number of different ways you could interact with the rock would increase. A geologist could scan it, radiometrically date it, analyze it, or test it for hardness and density. From a geologist's vantage point, the rock is a much more complex system.

To some, bone tissue seems and acts much like that rock being tossed into the air: inert and rigid with predictable behavior. But to us BST'ers, bone is complex. As we have seen, bone contains a sort of architectural intelligence. It shape-shifts in our hands. It can surprise us with its reactions to the forces acting upon it. To us, bone and osseofascial tissue are more like the bird than the rock.

Like the concepts of beauty and truth, complexity resides as much in the eye of the observer as it does in the behavior of the system itself. The neat thing about BST is that if we trust our palpation, we can let the interplay between two complex systems unfold naturally, so we don't have to predict the outcome of the interaction. So while you practice, let bone surprise you. Follow it. Encourage it. Don't over-analyze or stifle it. From my experience, this attitude makes our work more effective (and more fun). Thomas Walker, Certified Advanced Rolfer®, calls this type of presence "inclusive attention," which involves keeping a neutral state of mind with no preference to outcome (T. Walker 2014). From my experience, operating with inclusive attention allows great things to happen.

I was a beginner once, too. In my first year of osteopathy school, our teacher at the time, Stephanie L'Espérance, was guiding us through an exercise examining the excursion of the thoracic diaphragm. She had us place our hands on the abdomen of a fellow student, with our thumbs tucked under the rib cage. As the subject took a few breaths, L'Espérance asked us to compare the movements of the right side of the diaphragm to those on the left side. After a few moments I said, "They're equal ... I guess?" She looked at me with one raised eyebrow, placed her hands gently on mine, made sure I was on the right level, and within seconds, I could feel how unequal the movements really were. It was a humbling moment and one of many I had as I was developing my skills. A year or so later, I had my hands on the

cranium of one of my classmates, desperately trying to perform a correction of a side-bending rotation lesion of the sphenobasilar symphysis. Seeing I was having difficulty, our perceptive teacher, Jeannine van Vliet, came up behind me and put her hands on mine. She told me to soften my grip and wait for the fluids to shift under my fingers. Under her guidance, I felt a surge of fluid move from one side of the cranium to the other. As I followed the movement, it became so clear that now I couldn't *not* feel it. I was stunned and inspired to learn (and feel) more.

The way we first touch our subjects is important. It sets the tone of the entire therapeutic relationship. I read an excerpt from a conversation between Peter Armitage from the European School of Osteopathy and Steven Sanet in Sanet's book *Talking with Healers in Osteopathy*. Armitage says:

> I saw a picture once of a crocodile on a muddy bank of a lake or a river going into the water, you know I think it'd seen prey or something. And it went down the bank and into the water and there wasn't even a ripple and I thought "Ah, that's how to put your hands on the body." And if you could do that, without a ripple, you would also have honored that "need" to perceive everything and not put your own color on it, as you've said. Undisturbed physiology reporting itself in full to you. (Sanet 2020)

Crocodiles do make great first impressions, don't they? When you first contact your client, be that crocodile on the riverbank. Even before touching the skin, feel the thin air cushion between the subject's body and your hands. Take a moment to perceive the silence of that space. Feel how the temperature of the air cushion is different from the surrounding air. Then, let your hands land softly on the skin, without a ripple. Sutherland said,

"Let your hands be like the bird lighting on the branch of a tree, quietly touching and then settling down over the area" (Sutherland 1990, 151). Let the information come to you without trying to interpret it right away. Remain quiet and receptive.

Next, visualize the structure being palpated. I can't emphasize enough how important this is. If your hands are on the parietal bone of the skull, see that parietal completely. See the color, the shape, the ridges and protrusions. While practicing, having an anatomy book or plastic model close by could be helpful. Look at the structure on the page, study it, and then place your hands on the subject. This routine has helped me considerably over the years.

Also, while you are in dialogue, imagine bathing the levers of compacted bone in the dynamic stillness of the fulcrum. Stillness is nourishing, and our job is to amplify and propagate it. Becker talks about "palpating the interchange between the stillness and the problem" (Becker 2023, 69). Bathing the levers (problem) in the inertial fulcrum (stillness) enhances the interchange between the compacted tissue and health.

Force

Biodynamic skeletal therapy is slow, gentle work. We saw earlier how during very low intensities of compressive force, pure collagen seems to unwind like a watery, counterwound, twisted rope. During very low tensile force, the viscosity of the tropocollagen molecule undergoes a kind of watery reorganization and subsequent relaxation. In bone, it feels as if collagen acts the same way, and has just enough wiggle room between the hydroxyapatite reinforcements to do so. But our window here is small. In both compression and tension, if we exert too much force into the bone

too quickly, we surpass the fluidic "cushion" where we can elicit real change.

So how much force is too much or not enough? Instead of using finite measurements to guide our work,[32] the cushion test, discussed next, is a simple and practical way to orient to the right amount of force to use within any given bone.

The cushion test

The test is simple. Once you find the bone to treat, grasp it at each end or at the limits of the compacted tissue. Gently compress the bone until you reach the end of the springiness of the tissue (figure 14.5). Once there, slowly release the compressive force, letting the natural rebound of the bone separate your hands again. As the compression lessens, you'll sense a moment where the bone starts to dance or squirm. If you release too much tension, the squirminess will stop again. Return to the squirminess and stay there. This is the sweet spot or cushion of compression where the magic happens. Now, spread the bone, applying increasing amounts of tension until the system blocks again (figure 14.6). As you did with compression, slowly back off the tensile force, allowing the natural recoil of the bone to bring your hands closer together. As you do this, wait for the bone dance to start again. The dance means that you're back in the right place. The space between the compression and tension limits (figure 14.7) is our cushion. This is where BST happens.

Another very unscientific force gauge I use was inspired by a wise man named James,

---

[32]During a typical massage, pressures of three to five pounds per square inch are used, and this general range would probably apply to our work, as well. I like the cushion test better, since it is more specific to each bone and involves less math.

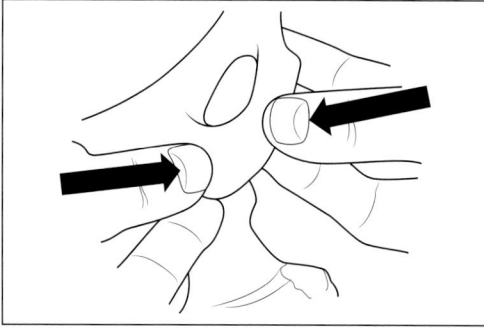

Figure 14.5. Compressive cushion test.

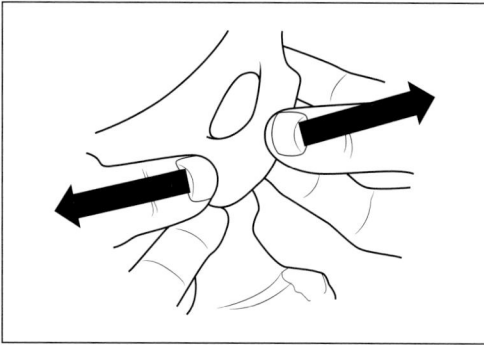

Figure 14.6. Tensile cushion test.

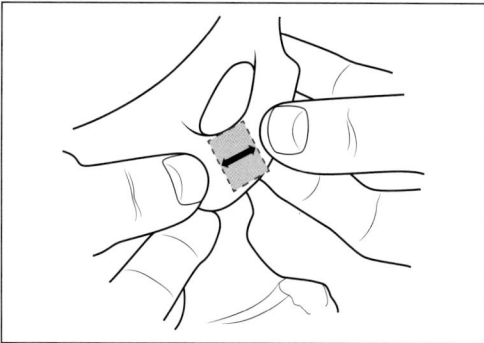

Figure 14.7. Cushion between compression and tension dialogue limits (gray rectangle).

my driving instructor when I was 16 years old. During one of my lessons, when we were merging onto the Decarie Expressway in Montreal, James whispered into my ear like a mystical sage: "Just *imagine* changing lanes, and the car will follow." Somehow, this was all the force the steering wheel needed, and it always seemed to work. Especially during

the spreading stage, remember James and his wise advice: just *imagine* spreading the tissue, and the bone will follow.

Duration

Different therapeutic modalities require varying amounts of time. For example, an osteoarticular adjustment takes a split second. A counterstrain technique lasts 2 minutes. According to Becker, his "corrections" took approximately 10 minutes. From my experience, each BST technique takes between 4 and 16 minutes, with the dialogue and spreading stages usually requiring the most time. Here's a very general breakdown by stage:

- Cocooning: 10 to 30 seconds
- Compression: 10 to 30 seconds
- Dialogue: 60 to 300 seconds
- Augmentation: 30 to 180 seconds
- Spreading: 60 to 300 seconds
- Integration: 20 to 60 seconds

What is more difficult to predict is how long the *impact* of BST lasts. In other words, once we reanimate the inertial tissue, we really don't know the duration of the reanimation (at least I don't, yet). For this reason, if post-BST manual therapies like adjustments, recoils, mobilizations, or myofascial work are planned, it's best to incorporate these as soon as the BST work is complete and within the same treatment session.

Contraindications

While BST is extremely gentle and safe, there are a few contraindications to consider.

Fractures

Do not use BST on a fractured bone that is not yet healed. Bones take between 8 and 10 weeks to heal. Wait until the 10-week post-fracture mark, or until imaging confirms that the fracture has completely healed.

Bone disease

Proceed with caution when treating patients with bone diseases or conditions that cause bone fragility, such as bone cancers, osteogenesis imperfecta, Paget's disease, osteomalacia, hyperparathyroidism, or advanced osteoporosis. Regarding bone cancer, there is some conflicting evidence that manual therapies applied directly to malignant bone tumors can increase the prevalence of metastasis. If in doubt, please speak to the client's doctor before proceeding.

Age

One of the questions I get asked the most is "Can BST be used on kids?" The answer is yes. I've used BST on children of all ages without any issues. If in doubt, speak to the child's pediatrician before proceeding, or defer to another professional with more experience in pediatrics. On the other side of the age spectrum, BST is not only safe but beneficial for the geriatric population, especially on those clients or patients who are too fragile for more vigorous therapies.

FREQUENTLY ASKED QUESTIONS

Can BST be used on kids?
As mentioned above, yes. For newborns and infants whose fontanelles have not yet closed, refrain from using BST on the cranium. If in doubt, speak to the child's pediatrician before proceeding.

Is an extra-rigid bone necessarily a compacted bone?
Bone tissue is rigid, but still full of life. When touch-testing osseofascial tissue for compactions, true compactions will jump out. They will be obvious. Compacted bone

feels more like concrete than like wood. If in doubt, the bone is probably not compacted, so move on to the next point.

When I find more than one compaction, which one do I treat first?
Some practitioners use comparative inhibition to prioritize dysfunction, and this can be applied here, too. By touching a few compactions, the one that releases or "melts" last is the most compacted and gets treated first. For example, if you found compactions within the right greater trochanter of the femur, the right clavicle, and the left temporal, you could rank these by comparing them. First, touch the greater trochanter with one hand and touch the right clavicle with the other. Within seconds, one will appear to change or soften. In this example, if the femur softens first, the clavicle is a higher treatment priority than the femur. Next, contact the clavicle and the temporal. If the clavicle softens first, the temporal takes the lead and should be treated first. Since it has already been established that the clavicle was higher priority than the femur, the three compactions can now be arranged by treatment priority as follows: (1) temporal, (2) clavicle, then (3) femur. Use the comparative inhibition test if you have numerous compactions to treat. This will help save time by addressing the most important lesions first.

Patient energy level may also help you decide how many points to treat in a given session. Some therapists, including Gerald Lamb, co-developer of the specific adjustment technique with his teacher Tom Dummer, prefers to treat only one lesion per session. When I asked Lamb about this, he explained that the body has limited energy to devote to any given task. By performing only one key adjustment, the body will have the best chance of resolving the issue. I generally agree and prefer to treat no more than one or two true compactions per session.

Of course, time is always a factor. Even though the touch-test of a point may take only seconds, the local and regional treatment of each point will take much longer. Whether your allotted treatment time is 20, 40, or 90 minutes, treatment duration will affect how many points to treat per session.

Why is nothing happening during the compression or spreading stage?

There are two reasons this may occur. First, you may be using either too much or too little force. If you suspect that this may be the case, retest the bone using the cushion test. This should help reorient you to the correct amount of force to use in both the compression and spreading phases. Once you're in the cushion, the bone tissue should come back alive. This cushion is where our therapeutic dialogue occurs and where great things happen. Second, you may not have oriented your compression and spreading with the specific torsional pattern of the compaction. Even with practice, you may find this difficult. Make sure you're working within the most rigid line of compaction and in accordance with its most rigid torsional pattern. If the tissue is still not responding, it may be that it just needs more time to react. If you have time to spare, experiment with a few extra-long applications of either compression or tension and evaluate the results. Remember, we're all still exploring this together, which makes this work exciting. If you're still struggling, come to one of our workshops—I'll be happy to help if I can!

During the dialogue stage, why do I only feel one or two of the three rhythms of primary respiration?

Primary respiration is the language of potency, and it is composed of rhythms.

Three of these rhythms have been called the long tide, mid-tide, and CRI. Like dark clouds temporarily hiding the sun, compacted tissue temporarily "hides" the expression of primary respiration. If only one or two of these rhythms emerge during the dialogue stage, that's fine. Remember that the long tide is inconsistent: sometimes we can feel it, sometimes we cannot. Even if it is there, it is often difficult to sense the tidal quality of the long tide while also being focused on the fluid and physical qualities of osseofascial tissue. If you're having difficulty sensing the long tide, work with the CRI and mid-tide, remaining aware of the supportive presence of the long tide in the background. Work with the rhythms that you feel. Even if you cannot identify all three rhythms, wait until a general coherence within the bone develops. Wait for the bone to soften and breathe in a steady, stable pattern. During the dialogue stage, once you feel that potency has done all it can on its own, regardless of whether all three rhythms are present, move on to the augmentation and spreading stages.

Is it okay to use BST *after* other modalities during the same treatment?

Yes. BST is best used as a primer coat for the osseofascial continuum *before* moving on to other manual therapies, but it can also be applied during or after other modalities. If you happen to find a compaction while doing myofascial work, for example, perform the six stages of BST treatment, then return to the work you were doing.

I have never worked as a manual therapist before. Can I start with BST?

Yes. BST is a simple, safe, and powerful way to begin learning about the skeleton and osseofascial continuum through touch. It will undoubtedly reveal opportunities for further development as a manual therapist.

As always, make sure that your manual therapy practice adheres to the regulations set forth by your certifications, associations, or organizations. If in doubt, best to double-check if BST fits within the scope of your profession or practice.

Can BST be the whole treatment?

Yes, but remember that BST addresses *biodynamic* fulcrum-lever systems embedded within *biomechanical* fulcrum-lever systems. Once the biodynamic fulcrum-lever system has been treated, other modalities are often required to optimize the range of motion within the biomechanical fulcrum-lever system. For this reason, BST is best used in combination with other manual therapies.

Can I skip some of the stages and still get results?

Yes. But experience has shown me that progressing through all six stages leads to a more profound dialogue with the subject, and possibly to longer-lasting and faster results.

Process and Results

If we focus on the results, the process is hard.
If we focus on the process, the results are easy.

Jerry's Shoulder

Some years ago, Jerry had a sore shoulder. He was told by a friend of a mysterious healer working out of a hotel in Montreal. Desperate for help, Jerry made an appointment. When he arrived at the hotel, Jerry was greeted by a receptionist and directed toward the treatment room. The room was subdivided into several cubicles. In each cubicle, there was a table, and on each table, a person. Jerry was not asked any questions about his complaint, nor did he volunteer any information. Instead, he was simply instructed to lie face down on the table and wait. After a few moments, Jerry sensed the presence of another person circumnavigating the table. Moments later, Jerry's shoulder began to burn ferociously. He turned his head and saw a man standing there, his hand inches from Jerry's burning arm. "How did you know my shoulder hurt?" Jerry asked. "It was easy," the man said; "there was yellow light emanating from it." Sometime later, when Jerry called the hotel to make another appointment, he was told that the man had left without notice, his whereabouts unknown.

CHAPTER 17

Bones and Regions

Before we dive into actual BST practice, here are a few notes:

- I've divided the body (and the next part of this chapter) into 11 body regions:
  1. Forefoot
  2. Midfoot
  3. Hindfoot
  4. Lower extremity
  5. Pelvis
  6. Lumbar spine
  7. Thorax
  8. Hand and wrist
  9. Upper extremity
  10. Cervical spine
  11. Cranium

  Each section includes a description of each bone in the region and information on how to find, test, and treat it. Regional treatments are described in a separate section.
- We discussed the six stages of BST treatment earlier. As a refresher, I've included a "Quick Guide to the Six Stages of BST Treatment," which you can refer to when treating each bone. Any additions or modifications to this master list are included with each bone.
- Notwithstanding a few exceptions, the descriptions of bones and regions generally flow from distal to proximal, but feel free to start anywhere you like and proceed in the order of your choice.

- I've confined the descriptions in this section to the aspects of osteology that concern us most: bones and parts of bones that we can find, feel, test, and treat. There's more detail provided about the posterior surface of the sacrum than for the anterior surface, for example, since it's only the posterior surface that can be accessed. The same applies to some of the bones of the face, which can only be reached from the mouth. As my dad used to teach me when I was learning to catch a football: "If you can't touch it, you can't catch it." Here, if you can't touch it, you can't treat it (with BST, at least).
- For palpation, testing, and treatment, I generally offer guidelines with the subject in supine or prone position, since this is how I prefer to work. A few exceptions to this rule include the fibula, innominates, ribs, and scapulae, where some side-lying options are discussed. If you prefer or if needed, feel free to work with your subject in these positions or any others that feel most comfortable for both of you.
- I usually suggest the two phases of touch-testing. Remember that touch-testing should happen *quickly*. Like how a photocopier lamp lights up sections of the page as it passes, phase 1 of testing is meant to quickly illuminate the presence of compactions in the osseofascial

continuum. Once identified, the spreading and twisting of phase 2 gives us more information about the torsional patterns of the compaction. While there are a few exceptions, this general two-phase routine often saves us time. But sometimes you may decide to combine the two phases into one step. It really is up to you. As you become more proficient at touch-testing, you can adjust the routine accordingly.

- In the descriptions of the local treatment for any given bone, and for the sake of practicality, I only describe the steps and provide images for the treatment compactions *within* a bone. If the compaction exists between a bone and a neighbor (within the softer osseofascial tissue—i.e., the ligaments), apply the same six stages of treatment but from either side of the joint and into the connective tissue.
- Finally, since this book is mainly about bones, I avoid naming all of the ligaments, tendons, and muscles, usually just referring to them as "connections." This will spare us from too much anatomical jargon.

QUICK GUIDE TO THE SIX STAGES OF BIODYNAMIC SKELETAL THERAPY TREATMENT

Here's a quick guide to the six stages of BST treatment. As you progress through the bones and regions, refer to this list as needed.

1. **Cocooning:** Start by cocooning the pattern or shape of the compaction by surrounding it with the hands and fingers. Be as precise as you can with finger placement. Surround the compacted zone within the bone or the entire bone itself with a nice, tight perimeter.
2. **Compression:** If necessary, perform the cushion test to orient to the compressive viscoelastic cushion of the bone. Gently compress the osseofascial tissue,

unwinding *into the ease* of its torsional pattern, counterwinding it like a rope. Exaggerate the compaction by compressing it even more. Stay within the fluidic cushion of the tissue. If the bone feels solid, you may have compressed it too much. If this is the case, let the natural recoil of the tissue move you back into the fluidity.

3. **Dialogue:** Begin to identify and dialogue with the rhythms of primary respiration. If possible, sense the CRI emerging from the physical body of the bone. Next, sense the mid-tide emerging from the fluid body of the tissue. Imagine your hands as hand-shaped water balloons and the bone as a bone-shaped water balloon. Then, if possible, sense the long tide passing through the bone from the midline of the body toward the periphery and then back through the bone from the periphery toward the midline. This occurs within the tidal body, and may have more of a breezy or electric quality. If the long tide is absent or more difficult to detect, focus on the CRI and the mid-tide. You may also want to begin with the long tide, then progress to the mid-tide, and then to the CRI. See if you can sense the inertial fulcrum around which some or all these rhythms are organizing. If so, bring the levers of bone tissue in toward the fulcrum, bathing them in stillness. Stay within your compressive dialogue as the health from the fulcrum spreads outward, reanimating and unwinding the compacted tissue. Wait until the rhythms coalesce, steadily breathing the bone with a new resultant oscillation.
4. **Augmentation:** Maintain your compressive dialogue but shift to a slightly more passive contact, allowing your fingers to inhale and exhale with the bone for a few complete cycles of primary respiration. Again, if the expression of the long tide is less clear, focus on the CRI and mid-tide.

5. **Spreading:** If necessary, adjust your finger positions to accommodate a more efficient spreading action. Reestablish contact with the bone tissue from the new hand position, and if necessary. Perform the cushion test to orient to the tensile viscoelastic cushion of the bone. Make sure you apply enough pressure to penetrate the *whole* section of bone, and not just the surface. Sense the tissue as it is, and then without applying too much more force, imagine spreading the bone directly against the most rigid torsional pattern of compaction. Here you are directly reversing the compressive force used in stage 2. Feel the bone begin to slowly spread from a place deep inside itself. As you did during the compression stage, stay within the fluidity of the bone. If it feels too solid, or if it feels as though nothing is happening or as if the dialogue stops, you may be using too much force. If this is the case, let the natural recoil of the bone bring you back to the fluidity. Often, the rhythms of primary respiration temporarily fade during the spreading

stage. If so, wait for them to re-emerge from the tissue for a few more complete cycles before moving to the next stage. If the expression of the long tide is less clear, focus on the CRI and mid-tide.

6. **Integration:** Finally, imagine the primary respiration of the whole body, acknowledging and accepting the primary respiration under your hands. Let your local work integrate into the whole. Once this occurs, remove the hands and/or proceed to regional BST treatment or other modalities.

FOREFOOT

There are 19 bones in each forefoot: 14 phalanges and 5 metatarsals (figure 17.1). The phalanges are the small bones of the toes. Due to their small size, testing and treatment is rather straightforward. For the sake of practicality, I only describe the testing of the connections between neighboring bones once. For example, when I discuss the first proximal phalanx, I only describe testing the connection between it and the metatarsal, since its connection with the first distal

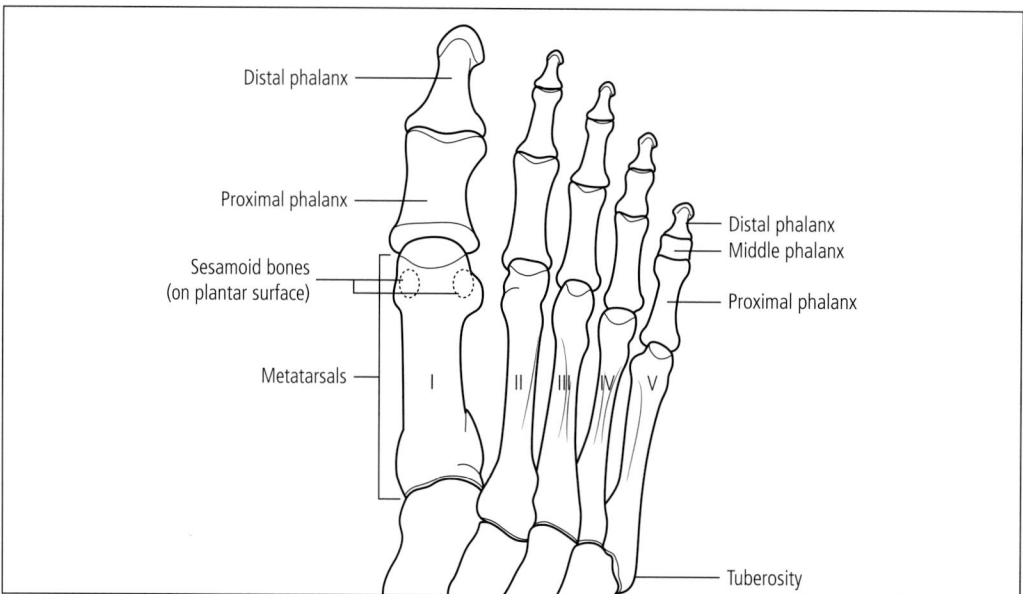

Figure 17.1. Forefoot.

phalanx has already been discussed in the "First distal phalanx" section.

Phalanges

The big (first) toe has two phalanges, a distal phalanx and a proximal phalanx. The other four toes each have three phalanges: distal, middle, and proximal. Due to their similarities, the second through fifth phalanges are described together but in three categories: distal, medial, and proximal.

First distal phalanx

Neighbor

First proximal phalanx

Palpation

The first distal phalanx is the tip of the big toe, home of the toenail (figure 17.2). If you slide your fingers proximally over the toe until you feel a bump just proximal to the base of the nail, you have reached the interphalangeal joint, the articulation between the first distal phalanx and the first proximal phalanx.

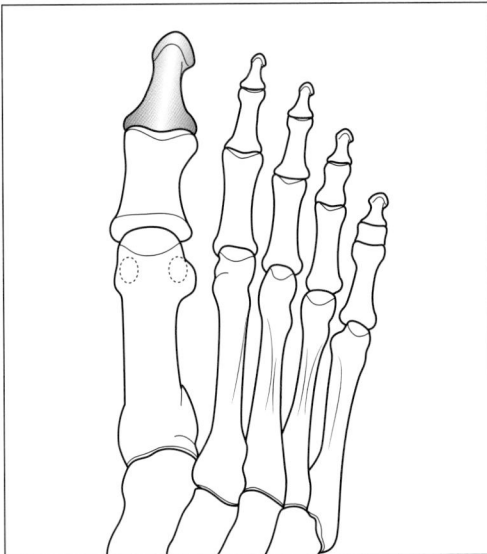

Figure 17.2. First distal phalanx.

Testing

Phase 1: Pinch and spread the distal phalanx between your thumb and finger, as if squeezing a gumdrop, squashing the bone from the center (figure 17.3). Does the bone feel more like wood or like concrete?

Now, test the connection between the first distal and first proximal phalanges by squeezing and spreading the joint line (figure 17.4). Does the connective tissue between the bones feel compliant or fibrotic?

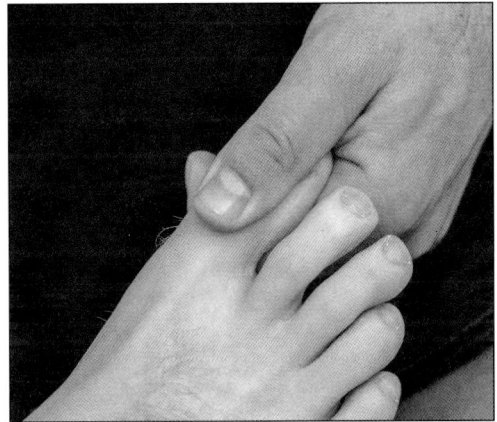

Figure 17.3. Phase 1: Testing the first distal phalanx by pinching and spreading the bone from the center.

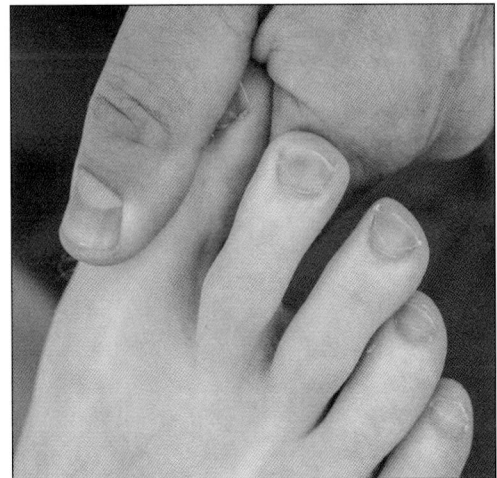

Figure 17.4. Phase 1: Testing the connection between the first distal and first proximal phalanges by squeezing and spreading the joint line.

If both the bone and the connections possess some bounce, move to the next bone to be tested. If the bone feels more like concrete or the connective tissue between the bones feels fibrotic, move to phase 2.

Phase 2: Spread and twist the bones in different directions to determine the most rigid pattern within (figure 17.5) and between them (figure 17.6).

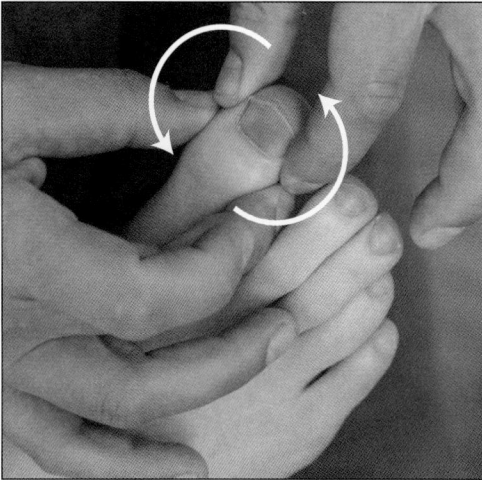

Figure 17.5. Phase 2: Spreading and twisting the first distal phalanx to determine the most rigid torsional pattern of compaction.

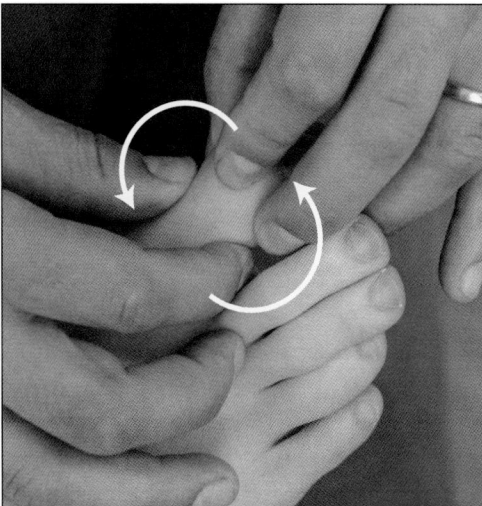

Figure 17.6. Phase 2: Spreading and twisting the connection between the first distal and first proximal phalanx.

Local treatment

An example of a hand position for treatment is shown in figure 17.7. Grasp the bone in a comfortable way and proceed with the six stages of BST treatment (see "Quick Guide to the Six Stages of BST Treatment").

Regional treatment

Integrate the local treatment of the first distal phalanx into the region by using the forefoot gather technique (see "Regional Treatment").

First proximal phalanx

Neighbors

First distal phalanx
First metatarsal

Palpation

The first proximal phalanx is located between the first metatarsal and first distal phalanx (figure 17.8). If you slide your fingers proximally from the distal phalanx over the bump just proximal to the base of the toenail, you will be on the first proximal phalanx.

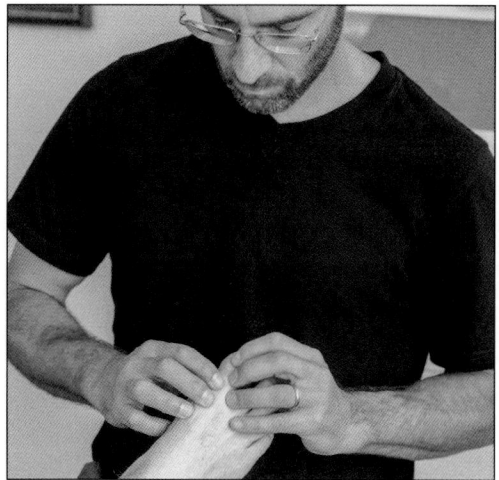

Figure 17.7. Local treatment of the first distal phalanx using the thumbs (plantar surface) and the index and middle fingers.

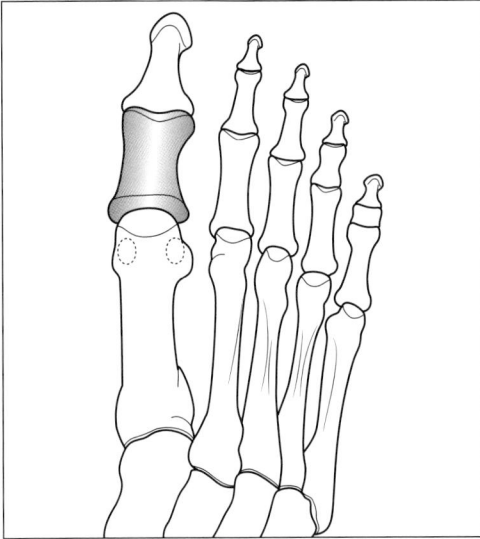

Figure 17.8. First proximal phalanx.

If you keep moving proximally until you reach the large knuckle, you will have reached the metatarsophalangeal joint, the proximal end of the bone.

Testing

Phase 1: Grasp the first proximal phalanx (figure 17.9). Pinch and spread the bone between your thumb and fingers, squashing the bone from the center. Does it feel more like wood or like concrete?

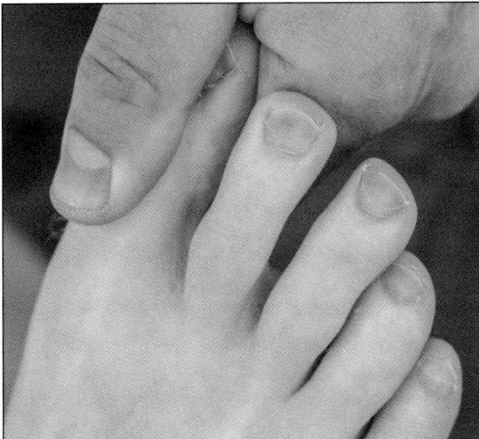

Figure 17.9. Phase 1: Testing the first proximal phalanx by pinching and spreading the bone from the center.

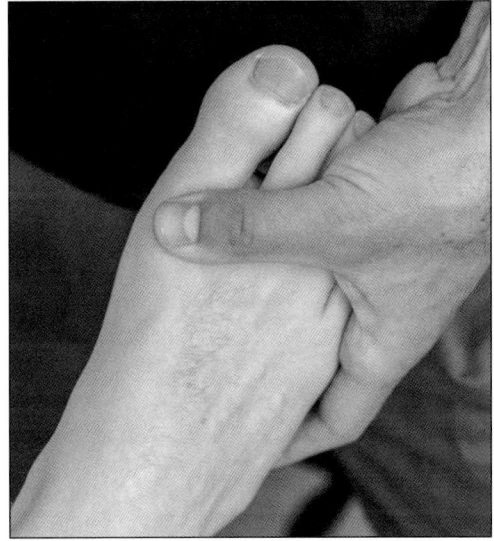

Figure 17.10. Phase 1: Testing the connection between the first proximal phalanx and the first metatarsal by pinching and spreading the joint line with the thumb and fingers (plantar surface).

Now, adjust your fingers if necessary and test the micromobility between the bone and the first metatarsal by squeezing and spreading the joint line (figure 17.10). Does the connective tissue between the bones feel compliant or fibrotic?

If both the bone and the connections possess some bounce, move to the next bone to be tested. If the bone feels more like concrete or the connective tissue between the bones feels fibrotic, move to phase 2.

Phase 2: Spread and twist the bones in different directions to determine the most rigid torsional pattern within (figure 17.11) and between them (figure 17.12).

Local treatment

An example of a hand position for treatment is shown in figure 17.13. Grasp the bone in a comfortable way and proceed with the six stages of BST treatment (see "Quick Guide to the Six Stages of BST Treatment").

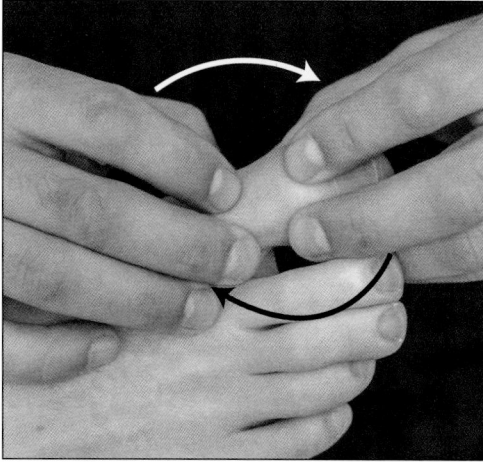

Figure 17.11. Phase 2: Spreading and twisting the proximal phalanx using the thumbs (plantar surface) and the index and middle fingers.

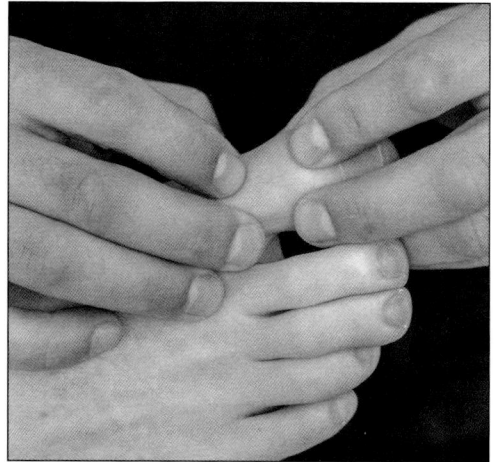

Figure 17.13. Hand position for treatment of the first proximal phalanx using the thumbs (plantar surface) and the index and middle fingers.

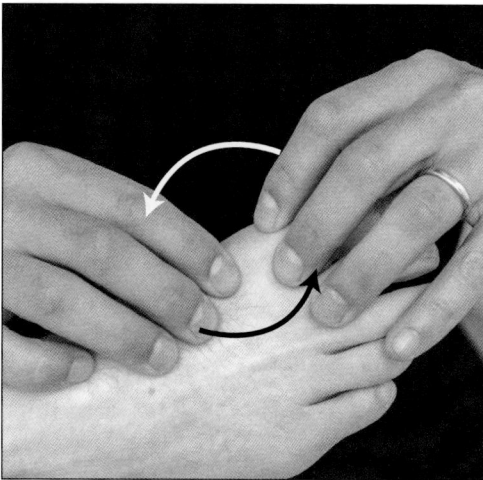

Figure 17.12. Phase 2: Spreading and twisting the connection between the first proximal phalanx and first metatarsal using the thumbs (plantar surface) and the index and middle fingers.

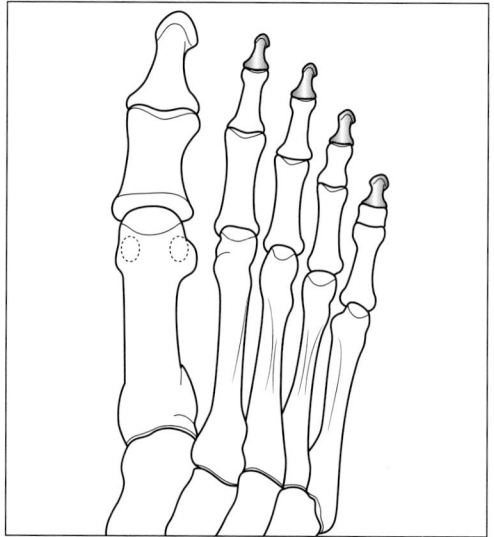

Figure 17.14. Second to fifth distal phalanges.

Regional treatment

Integrate the local treatment of the first proximal phalanx into the region by using the forefoot gather technique (see "Regional Treatment").

Second to fifth distal phalanges

A similar protocol is used for the second to fifth distal phalanges (figure 17.14),

so they will be grouped together here. We'll use the fourth distal phalanx as an example.

Neighbors

Second to fifth middle phalanges

Palpation

The second to fifth distal phalanges are the tips of the other four toes. If you slide your

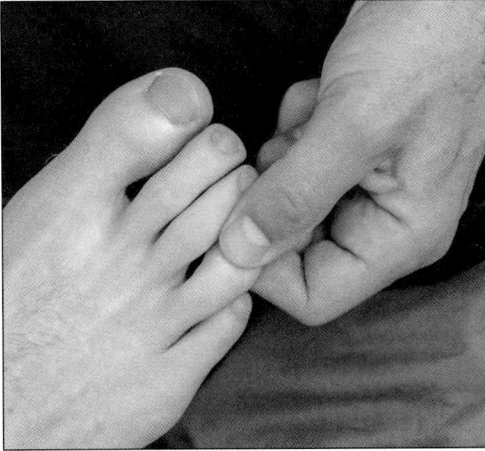

Figure 17.15. Phase 1: Testing the fourth distal phalanx by pinching and spreading the bone from the center.

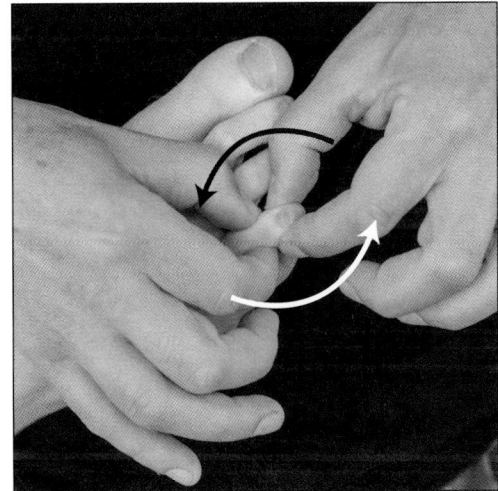

Figure 17.16. Phase 1: Testing the connection between the fourth distal and middle phalanges by squeezing and spreading the joint line with the thumb and index finger (plantar surface).

fingers proximally over the toe until you feel a bump just proximal to the base of the nail, you have reached the distal interphalangeal joint, which joins the distal phalanx to the middle phalanx.

Testing

Phase 1: Pinch and spread the distal phalanx, as if squeezing a gumdrop, squashing the bone from the center (figure 17.15).

Now, adjust your fingers if necessary and test the micromobility between the bone and the fourth middle phalanx by squeezing and spreading the joint line (figure 17.16).

If both the bone and the connections possess elasticity, move to the next bone to be tested. If the bone itself feels like concrete or the connective tissue between the bones feels fibrotic, move to phase 2 for further testing.

Phase 2: Spread and twist the bones in different directions to determine the most rigid torsional pattern within (figure 17.17) or between them (figure 17.18).

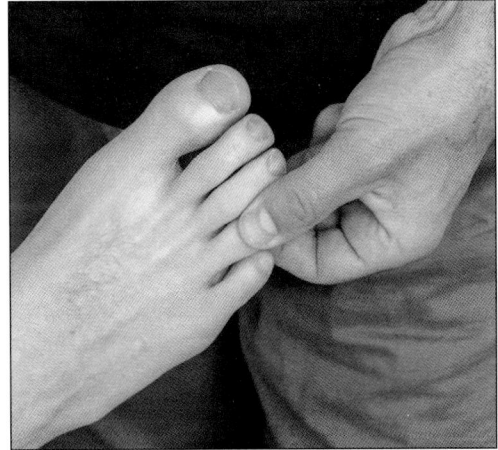

Figure 17.17. Phase 2: Spreading and twisting the fourth distal phalanx.

Local treatment

An example of a hand position for treatment is shown in figure 17.19. Grasp the bone in a comfortable way and proceed with the six stages of BST treatment (see "Quick Guide to the Six Stages of BST Treatment").

Regional treatment

Integrate the local treatment of the second to fifth distal phalanges into the region by using

105

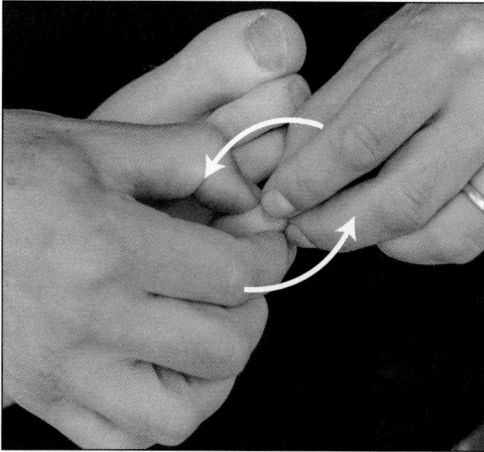

Figure 17.18. Phase 2: Spreading and twisting the connection between the fourth distal and middle phalanges.

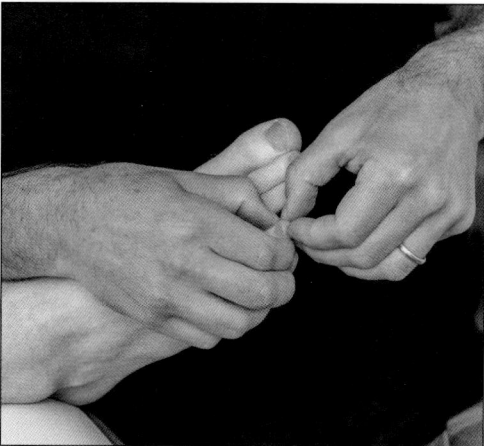

Figure 17.19. Hand position for the local treatment of the fourth distal phalanx.

the forefoot gather technique (see "Regional Treatment").

Second to fifth middle phalanges

Once again, a similar protocol is used for the second to fifth middle phalanges (figure 17.20), so they will be grouped together. We'll use the third middle phalanx as an example.

Neighbors

Second to fifth distal phalanges
Second to fifth proximal phalanges

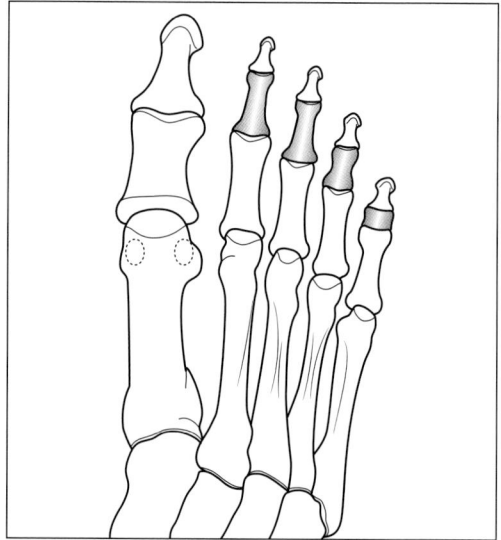

Figure 17.20. Second to fifth middle phalanges.

Palpation

The second to fifth middle phalanges are located between the corresponding distal and proximal phalanges. If you slide your fingers proximally from the distal interphalangeal joint to the next eminence on the toe, you will have reached the proximal interphalangeal joint, which joins the middle phalanx to the proximal phalanx.

Testing

Phase 1: Pinch and spread the middle phalanx between your thumb and fingers, as if squeezing a gumdrop, squashing the bone from the center (figure 17.21). Does it feel like wood or like concrete?

Now, adjust your fingers if necessary and test the micromobility between the middle and proximal phalanges by squeezing and spreading the joint line (figure 17.22).

If both the bone and the connections possess elasticity, move to the next bone to be tested. If the bone itself feels like concrete or the connective tissue between the bones feels fibrotic, move to phase 2 for further testing.

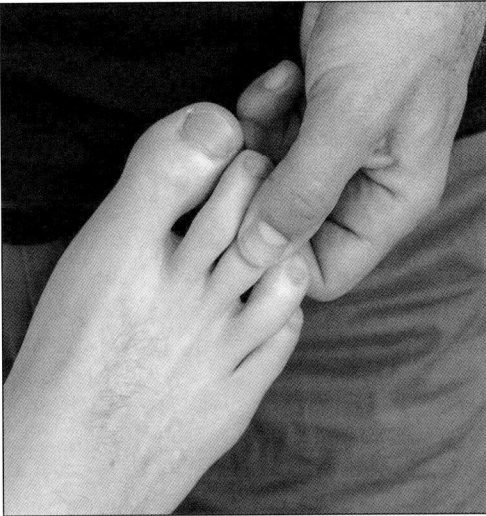

Figure 17.21. Phase 1: Testing the third middle phalanx by pinching and spreading the bone from the center with the thumb and index finger (plantar surface).

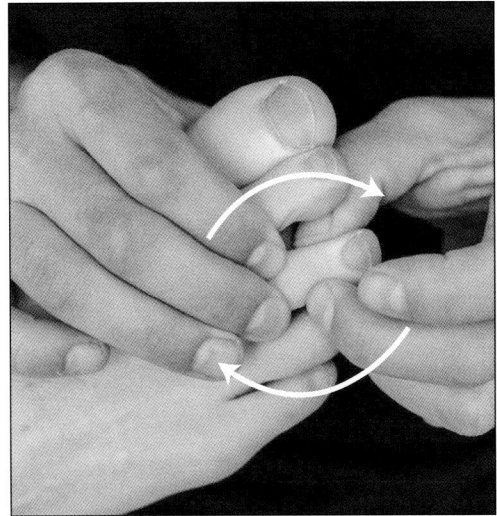

Figure 17.23. Phase 2: Spreading and twisting the third middle phalanx.

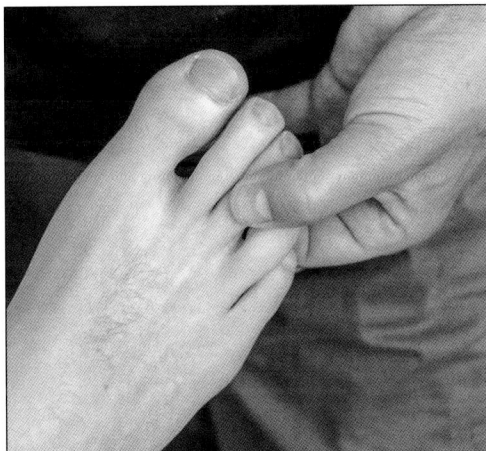

Figure 17.22. Phase 1: Testing the connection between the third middle and proximal phalanges by squeezing and spreading the joint line with the thumb and index finger (plantar surface).

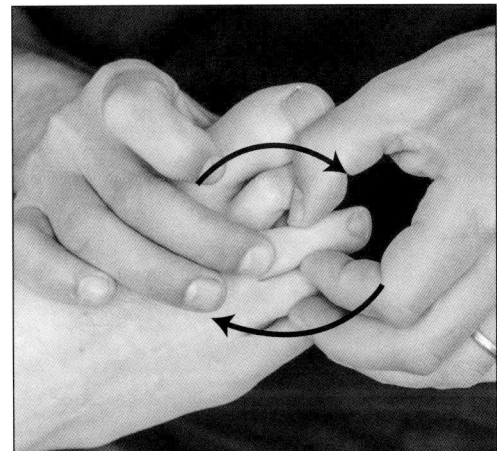

Figure 17.24. Phase 2: Spreading and twisting the connection between the third middle and third proximal phalanges using the thumbs and index and middle fingers.

Phase 2: Spread and twist the bones in different directions to determine the most rigid pattern within (figure 17.23) or between them (figure 17.24).

Local treatment

An example of a hand position for treatment is shown in figure 17.25. Grasp the bone in a comfortable way and proceed with the six stages of BST treatment (see "Quick Guide to the Six Stages of BST Treatment").

Regional treatment

Integrate the local treatment of the second to fifth middle phalanges into the region by using the forefoot gather technique (see "Regional Treatment").

107

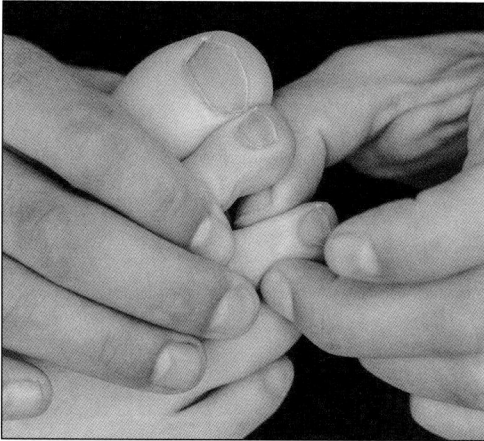

Figure 17.25. Hand position for the local treatment of the third middle phalanx.

Second to fifth proximal phalanges

Once again, a similar protocol is used for the second to fifth proximal phalanges (figure 17.26), so they will be grouped together. We'll use the fifth proximal phalanx as an example.

Neighbors

Second to fifth middle phalanges
Second to fifth metatarsals

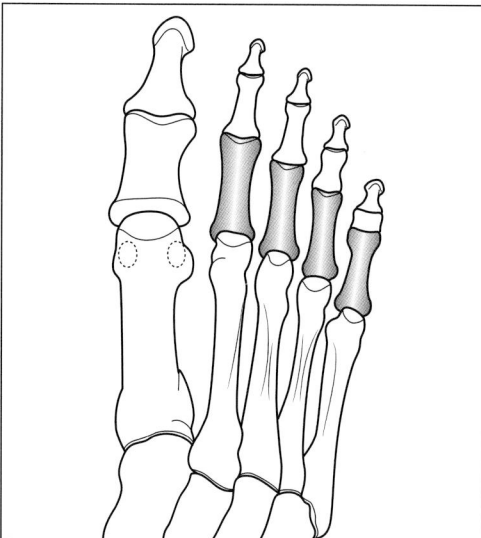

Figure 17.26. Second to fifth proximal phalanges.

Palpation

The second to fifth proximal phalanges are located between the corresponding middle phalanges and metatarsals. If you slide your fingers proximally along the phalanx from the proximal interphalangeal joint to the next eminence between the toe and the foot, you will have reached the metatarsophalangeal joint, which joins the proximal phalanx to the metatarsal.

Testing

Phase 1: Pinch and spread the proximal phalanx between your thumb and fingers, squashing the bone from the center (figure 17.27). Does it feel like wood or concrete?

Now, adjust your fingers and test the micromobility between the proximal phalanx and the corresponding metatarsal by squeezing and spreading the joint line (figure 17.28).

If both the bone and the connection with its neighbor possess elasticity, move to the next bone to be tested. If the bone feels like

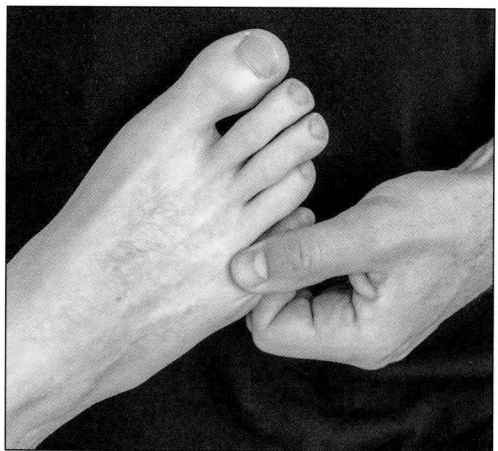

Figure 17.27. Phase 1: Testing the fifth proximal phalanx by pinching and spreading the bone from the center with the thumb and index finger (plantar surface).

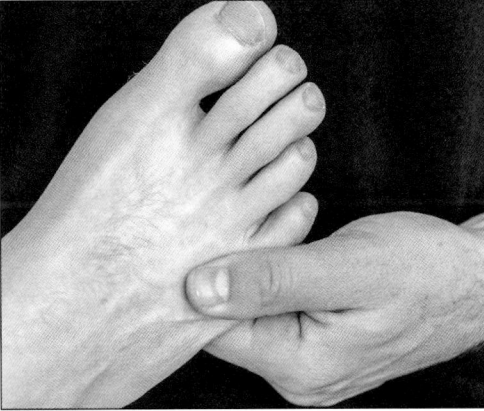

Figure 17.28. Phase 1: Testing the connection between the fifth proximal phalanx and the fifth metatarsal by squeezing and spreading the joint line with the thumb and fingers.

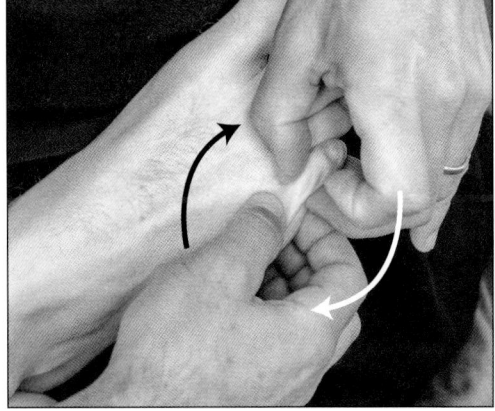

Figure 17.29. Phase 2: Spreading and twisting the fifth proximal phalanx.

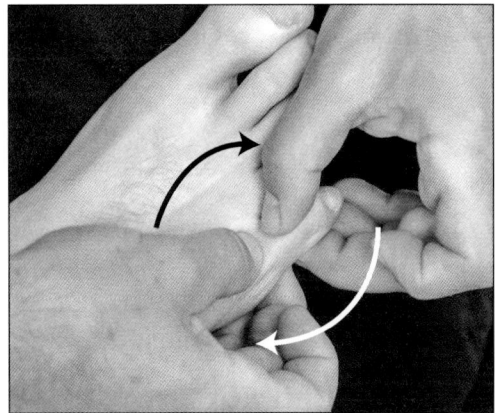

Figure 17.30. Phase 2: Spreading and twisting the connection between the fifth proximal phalanx and the fifth metatarsal.

concrete or the connective tissue between the bones feels fibrotic, move to phase 2.

Phase 2: Spread and twist the bones in different directions to determine the most rigid torsional pattern within (figure 17.29) or between them (figure 17.30).

Local treatment

An example of a hand position for treatment is shown in figure 17.31. Grasp the bone in a comfortable way and proceed with the six stages of BST treatment (see "Quick Guide to the Six Stages of BST Treatment").

Regional treatment

Integrate the local treatment of the second to fifth proximal phalanges into the region by using the forefoot gather technique (see "Regional Treatment").

Metatarsals

Since the five metatarsals are similar in shape but have varied proximal articulations, there are a few palpatory quirks that deserve separate descriptions. So we'll review each

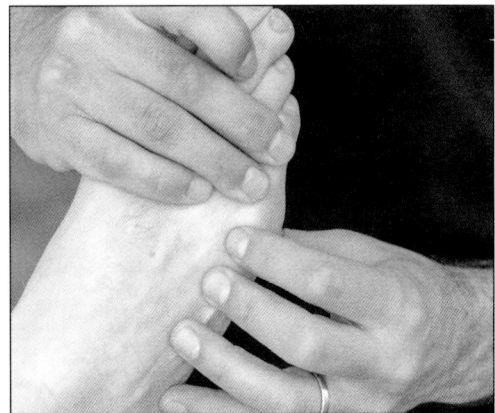

Figure 17.31. Hand position for the local treatment of the fifth proximal phalanx using the thumbs (plantar surface) and the index and middle fingers.

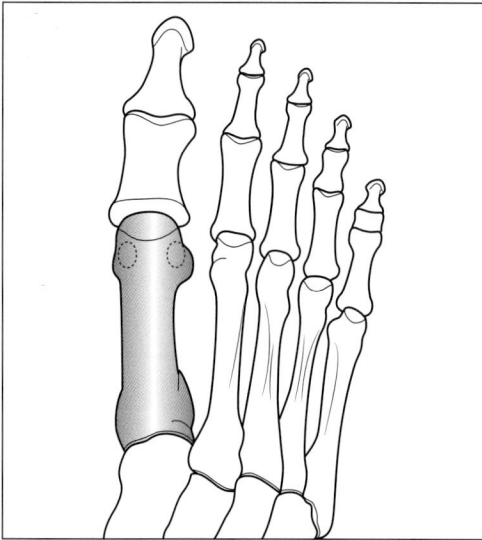

Figure 17.32. First metatarsal.

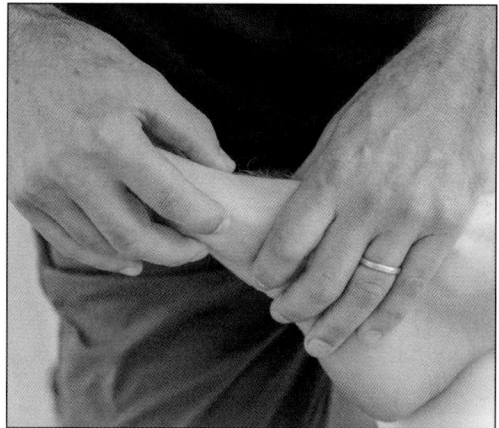

Figure 17.33. Locating the base of the first metatarsal. In this configuration, your index finger should naturally sit on the base of the bone.

metatarsal individually. Here we'll get to know the "wiggle test," a useful exercise for palpating the metatarsals and their neighbors.

First metatarsal

The first metatarsal is the thickest and shortest of the five and forms the medial aspect of the midfoot (figure 17.32). On the plantar surface of the head there are two small facets, over which glide the sesamoid bones.

Neighbors

First proximal phalanx
First cuneiform
Base of second metatarsal

Palpation

When you move your fingers proximally from the first metatarsophalangeal joint, you will be on the distal end, or head, of the first metatarsal. The proximal end of the first metatarsal joins the first cuneiform at the first tarsometatarsal joint. The first metatarsal also connects to the medial aspect of the base of the second metatarsal. A neat trick for finding

the base of the first metatarsal is to place your hand on the medial aspect of the foot, with your little finger on the talus, ring finger on the navicular, and middle finger on the first cuneiform (figure 17.33). In this configuration, your index finger should naturally sit on the base of the first metatarsal. Hold the bone in both hands and wiggle it. The wiggle test will delineate the first metatarsal from the first cuneiform and second metatarsal, since neither of the latter will move during the test.

Testing

Phase 1: Simultaneously squash the bone and spread it with your fingers (figure 17.34). Does it feel like wood or concrete?

Now, adjust your fingers and test the micromobility between the base of the first metatarsal and its neighbors by squeezing and spreading the joint lines (figures 17.35 and 17.36).

If both the bone and the connections possess elasticity, move to the next bone to be tested. If the bone feels like concrete or the connective tissue between it and any of its neighbors feels fibrotic, move to phase 2.

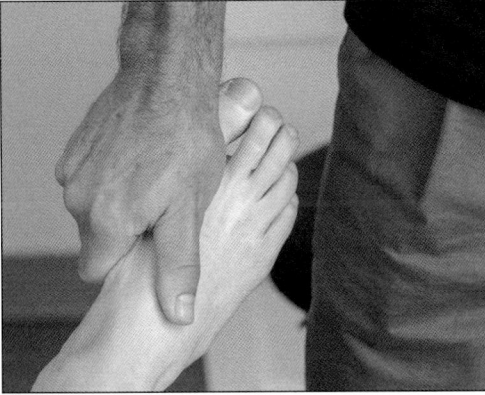

Figure 17.34. Phase 1: Testing the first metatarsal by squeezing and spreading the bone with the thenar eminence and fingers (plantar surface).

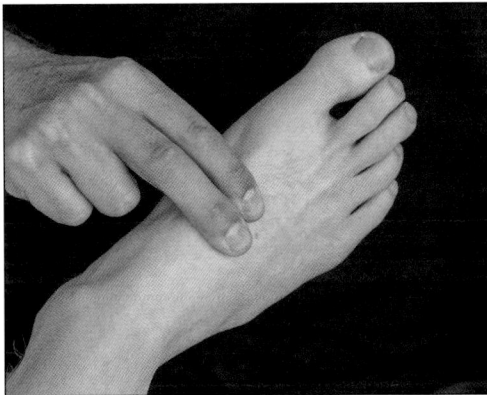

Figure 17.35. Phase 1: Testing the connection between the first metatarsal and the first cuneiform by squeezing and spreading the joint line with the thumb (plantar surface) and index and middle fingers.

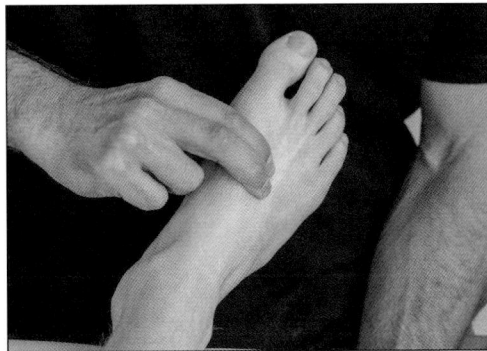

Figure 17.36. Phase 1: Testing the connection between the first metatarsal and the base of the second metatarsal by squeezing and spreading the joint line with the thumb (plantar surface) and index and middle fingers.

Phase 2: Spread and twist the bone(s) in different directions to determine the most rigid torsional pattern within (figure 17.37) or between them (figures 17.38 and 17.39).

Local treatment

An example of a hand position for treatment is shown in figure 17.40. Grasp the bone in a comfortable way and proceed with the six stages of BST treatment (see "Quick Guide to the Six Stages of BST Treatment").

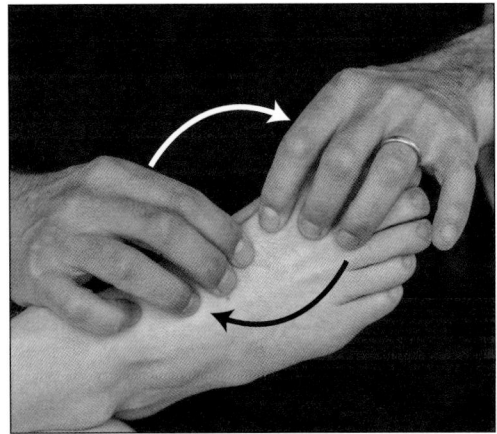

Figure 17.37. Phase 2: Spreading and twisting the first metatarsal using the thumbs (plantar surface) and index fingers.

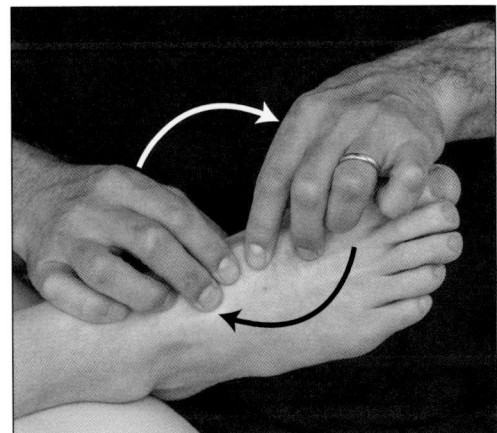

Figure 17.38. Phase 2: Spreading and twisting the connection between the first metatarsal and the first cuneiform using the thumbs (plantar surface) and index and middle fingers.

111

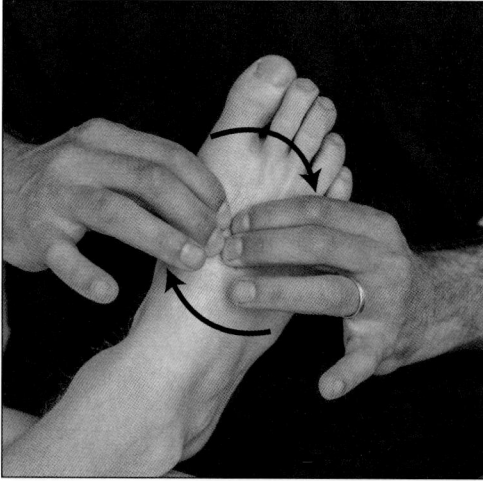

Figure 17.39. Phase 2: Spreading and twisting the connection between the first metatarsal and the base of the second metatarsal using the thumbs (plantar surface) and index and middle fingers.

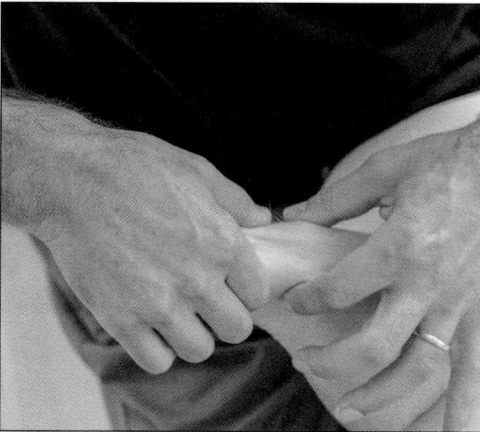

Figure 17.40. Hand position for the local treatment of the first metatarsal with the therapist standing on the lateral side of the foot.

Regional treatment

Integrate the local treatment of the first metatarsal into the region by using the forefoot gather technique (see "Regional Treatment").

Second metatarsal

The second metatarsal is the longest of the five metatarsal bones (figure 17.41).

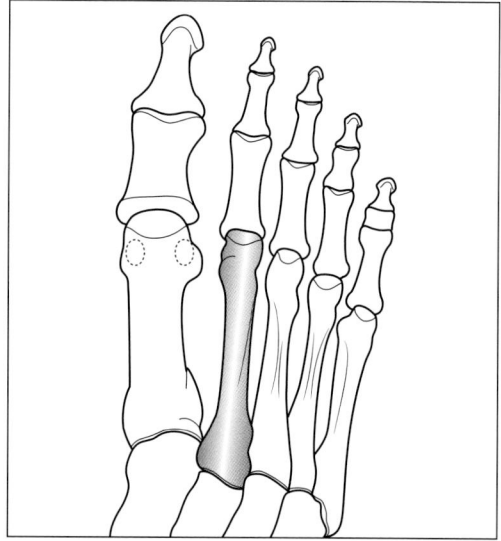

Figure 17.41. Second metatarsal.

It has multiple neighbors, articulating distally with the second proximal phalanx, proximally with the three cuneiform bones and the base of both the first and third metatarsals.

Neighbors

Second proximal phalanx
First, second, and third cuneiforms
Base of the first and third metatarsals

Palpation

When you move your fingers proximally from the second proximal phalanx over the second metatarsophalangeal joint, you will be on the head of the second metatarsal. Pinch the head of the metatarsal with one hand and wiggle the bone. At the same time, slide your other hand proximally down the shaft toward the tarsometatarsal joint line, monitoring the movement. If you bypass the base of the bone and land on the second cuneiform or any of the other neighbors, the wiggling will cease. Move back into the wiggling and you'll be back on the second metatarsal.

Testing

Phase 1: Pinch the second metatarsal between your thumb and fingers, squashing and spreading the bone (figure 17.42). Does it feel like wood or concrete?

Now, adjust your fingers and test the micromobility between the base of the second metatarsal and its neighbors by squeezing and spreading the joint lines (figures 17.43 and 17.44).

If both the bone and the connections possess elasticity, move to the next bone to be tested. If the bone feels like concrete or the connective tissue between it and any of its neighbors feels fibrotic, move to phase 2.

Phase 2: Spread and twist the bone(s) in different directions to determine the most rigid torsional pattern of compaction within (figure 17.45) or between them (figures 17.46 and 17.47).

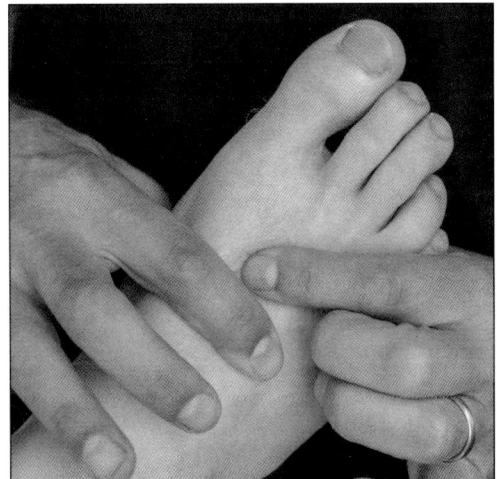

Figure 17.42. Phase 1: Testing the second metatarsal by squeezing and spreading the bone with the thumb and fingers (plantar surface).

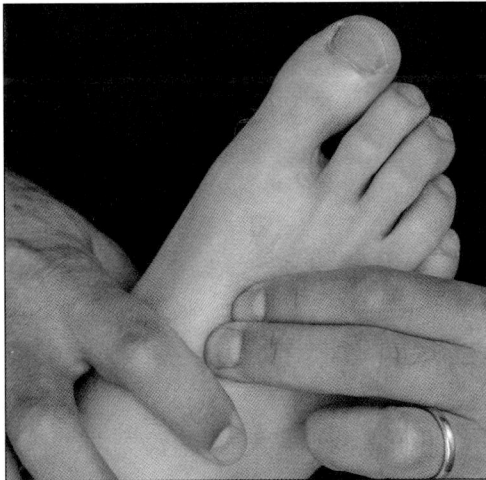

Figure 17.44. Phase 1: Testing the connection between the second metatarsal and the base of the first and third metatarsals by squeezing and spreading the joint lines with the thumbs (plantar surface) and index fingers.

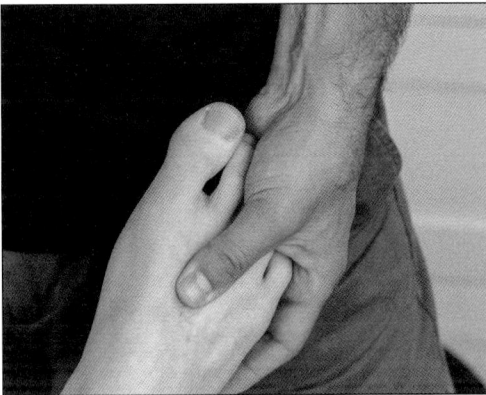

Figure 17.43. Phase 1: Testing the connection between the second metatarsal and the first, second, and third cuneiforms by squeezing and spreading the joint lines with the thumbs (plantar surface) and index and middle fingers.

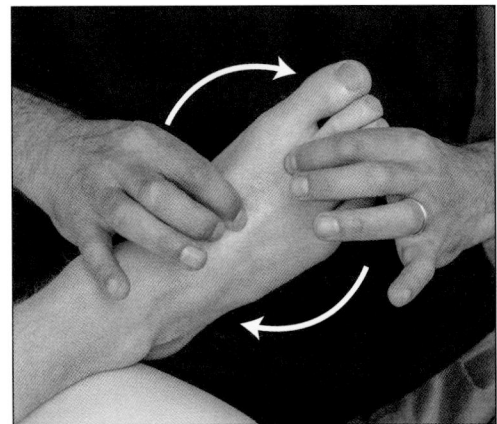

Figure 17.45. Phase 2: Spreading and twisting the second metatarsal with the thumbs (plantar surface) and index fingers.

113

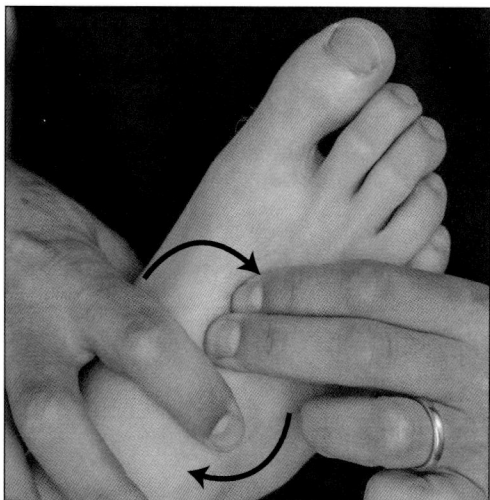

Figure 17.46. Phase 2: Spreading and twisting the connections between the second metatarsal and the three cuneiforms with the thumbs (plantar surface), index, and middle fingers.

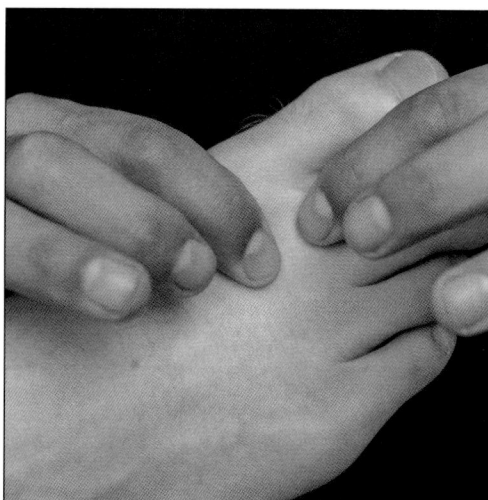

Figure 17.48. Hand position for the local treatment of a section of the shaft of the second metatarsal with the thumbs (plantar surface) and index fingers.

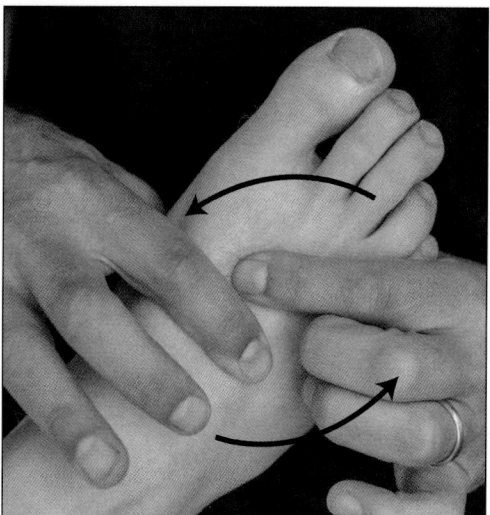

Figure 17.47. Phase 2: Spreading and twisting the connections between the second metatarsal and the bases of the first and third metatarsals with the thumbs (plantar surface) and index fingers.

Local treatment

An example of a hand position for treatment is shown in figure 17.48. Grasp the bone in a comfortable way and proceed with the six stages of BST treatment (see "Quick Guide to the Six Stages of BST Treatment").

Regional treatment

Integrate the local treatment of the second metatarsal into the region by using the forefoot gather technique (see "Regional Treatment").

Third metatarsal

The head of the third metatarsal joins the third proximal phalanx, and the base of the third metatarsal articulates with the third cuneiform and the bases of both the second and fourth metatarsals (figure 17.49).

Neighbors

Third proximal phalanx
Third cuneiform
Bases of the second and fourth metatarsals

Palpation

When you move your fingers proximally from the phalanx over the third metatarsophalangeal joint, you will be on the head of the third metatarsal. As you did with the first two, pinch the head of the third metatarsal with one hand and wiggle the bone. At the same time, pinch the bone with

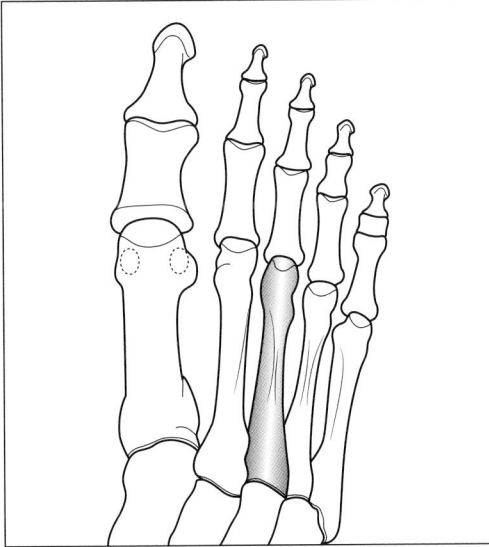

Figure 17.49. Third metatarsal.

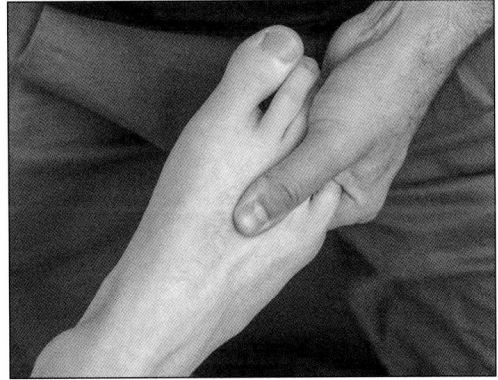

Figure 17.50. Phase 1: Testing the third metatarsal by squeezing and spreading the bone with the thumb and fingers (plantar surface).

your other hand, sliding it proximally down the shaft toward the tarsometatarsal joint line, monitoring the movement. If you bypass the base of the bone and land on the third cuneiform or any of the other neighbors, the wiggling will cease.

Testing

Phase 1: Pinch the third metatarsal between your thumb and fingers, squashing and spreading the bone (figure 17.50). Does it feel like wood or concrete?

Now, adjust your fingers and test the micromobility between the base of the third metatarsal and its neighbors (figures 17.51 and 17.52) by squeezing and spreading the joint lines. If both the bone and the connections possess elasticity, move to the next bone(s) to be tested. However, if the bone feels like concrete or the connective tissue between it and any of its neighbors feels fibrotic, move to phase 2.

Phase 2: Spread and twist the bone(s) in different directions to determine

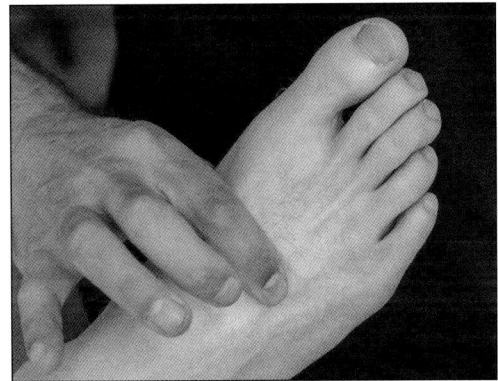

Figure 17.51. Phase 1: Testing the connection between the third metatarsal and the third cuneiform by squeezing and spreading the joint line with the thumb (plantar surface) and index finger.

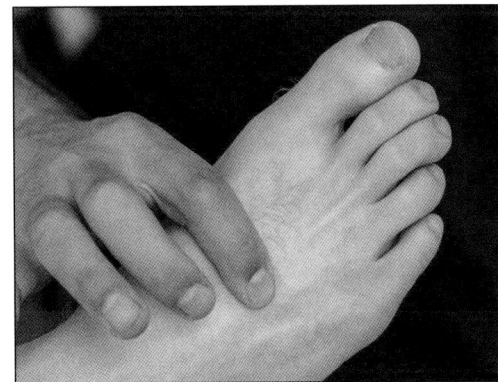

Figure 17.52. Phase 1: Testing the connection between the third metatarsal and the bases of the second and fourth metatarsals by squeezing and spreading the joint lines with the thumb (plantar surface) and index finger.

the most rigid torsional pattern within (figure 17.53) or between them (figures 17.54 and 17.55).

Local treatment

An example of a hand position for treatment is shown in figure 17.56. Grasp the bone in a comfortable way and proceed with the six stages of BST treatment

(see "Quick Guide to the Six Stages of BST Treatment").

Regional treatment

Integrate the local treatment of the third metatarsal into the region by using the forefoot gather technique (see "Regional Treatment").

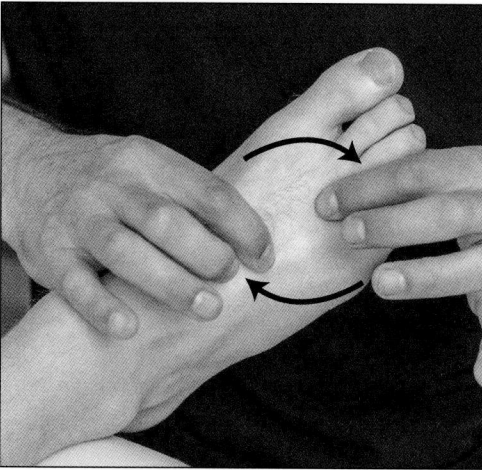

Figure 17.53. Phase 2: Spreading and twisting the third metatarsal with the thumbs (plantar surface) and index fingers.

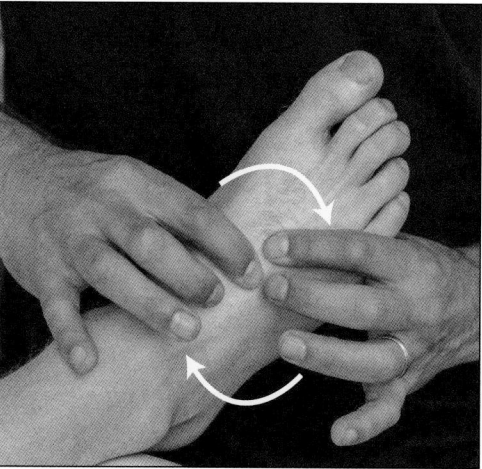

Figure 17.55. Phase 2: Spreading and twisting the connection between the third metatarsal and the bases of the second and fourth metatarsals with the thumbs (plantar surface) and index fingers.

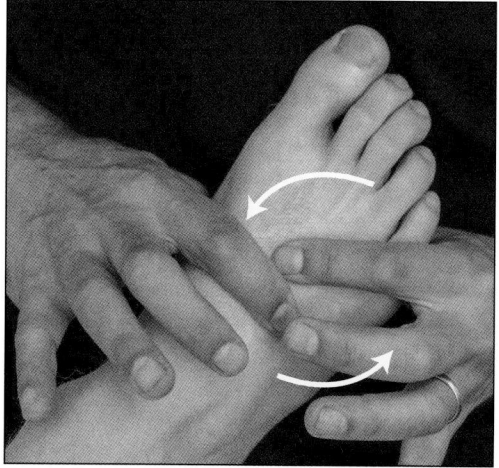

Figure 17.54. Phase 2: Spreading and twisting the connection between the third metatarsal and the third cuneiform with the thumbs (plantar surface) and index fingers.

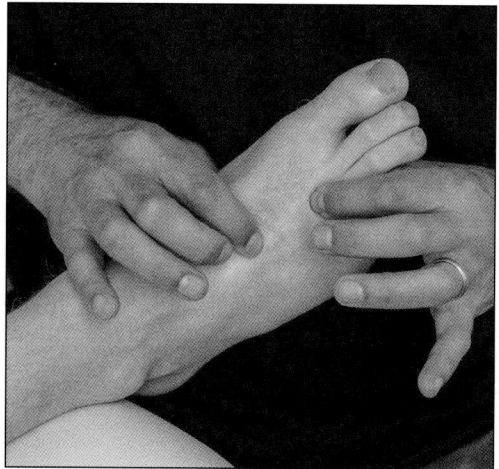

Figure 17.56. Hand position for the local treatment of the third metatarsal with the thumbs (plantar surface) and index fingers.

Fourth metatarsal

The head of the fourth metatarsal joins the fourth proximal phalanx, and the base of the fourth metatarsal articulates with the cuboid and the bases of both the third and fifth metatarsals (figure 17.57).

Neighbors

Fourth proximal phalanx
Cuboid
Bases of third and fifth metatarsals

Palpation

When you move your fingers proximally from the phalanx over the fourth metatarsophalangeal joint, you will be on the head of the fourth metatarsal. Pinch the head of the metatarsal with one hand and wiggle the bone. At the same time, pinch the bone with your other hand, sliding it proximally down the shaft toward the cuboid, monitoring the movement. If you bypass the base of the fourth metatarsal and land on the cuboid or any of the other neighbors, the wiggling will cease.

Testing

Phase 1: Pinch the fourth metatarsal between your thumb and fingers, squashing and spreading the bone (figure 17.58). Does it feel like wood or concrete?

Now, adjust your fingers and test the micromobility between the base of the fourth metatarsal and its neighbors by squeezing and spreading the joint lines (figures 17.59 and 17.60). If both the bone and the connections possess elasticity, move to the next bone to be tested. If the bone feels like concrete or the connective tissue between it and any of its neighbors feels fibrotic, move to phase 2.

Phase 2: Spread and twist the bone(s) in different directions to determine the most rigid torsional pattern within (figure 17.61) or between them (figures 17.62 and 17.63).

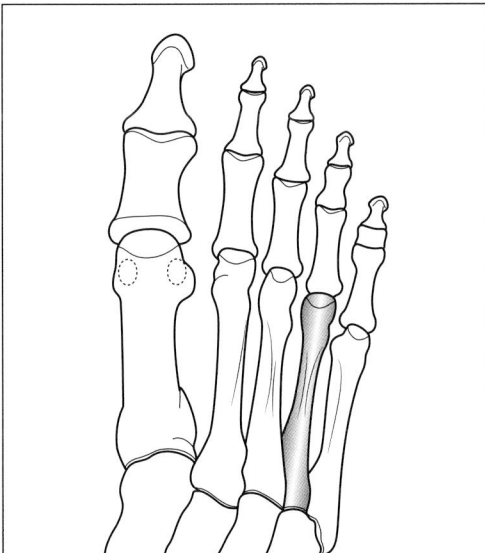

Figure 17.57. Fourth metatarsal.

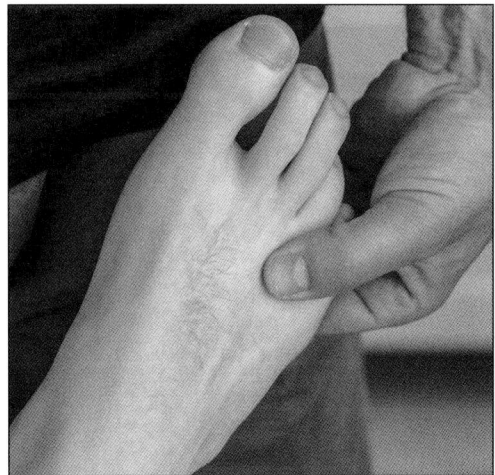

Figure 17.58. Phase 1: Testing the fourth metatarsal by squeezing and spreading the bone with the thumb and fingers (plantar surface).

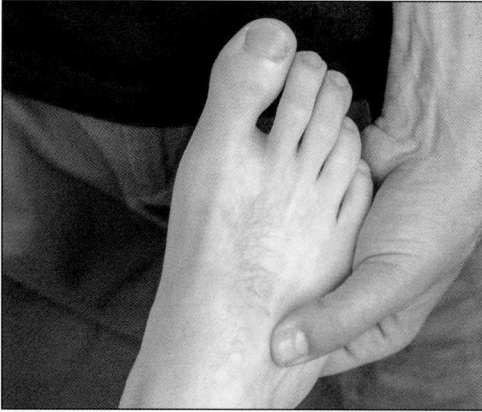

Figure 17.59. Phase 1: Testing the connection between the fourth metatarsal and the cuboid by squeezing and spreading the joint line with the thumb and fingers (plantar surface).

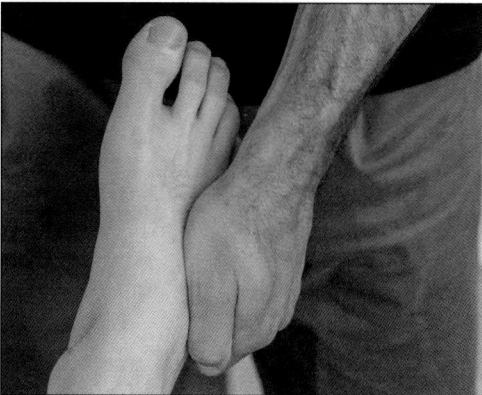

Figure 17.60. Phase 1: Testing the connection between the fourth metatarsal and the bases of the third and fifth metatarsals by squeezing and spreading the joint lines with the thenar eminence and fingers (plantar surface).

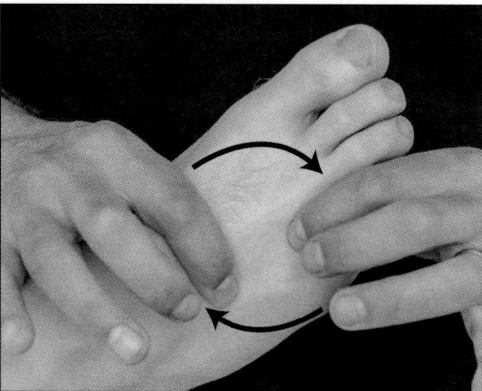

Figure 17.61. Phase 2: Spreading and twisting the fourth metatarsal with the thumbs (plantar surface) and index fingers.

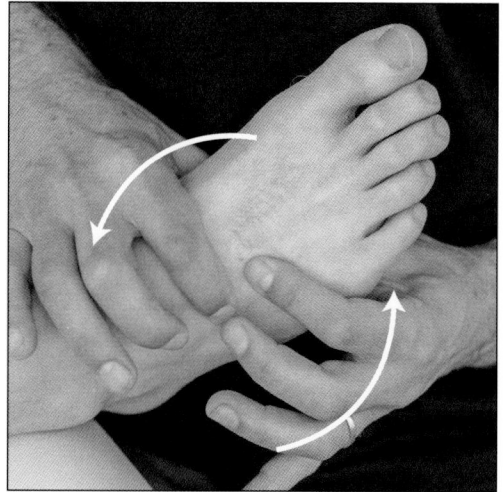

Figure 17.62. Phase 2: Spreading and twisting the connection between the fourth metatarsal and the cuboid with the thumbs (plantar surface) and index fingers.

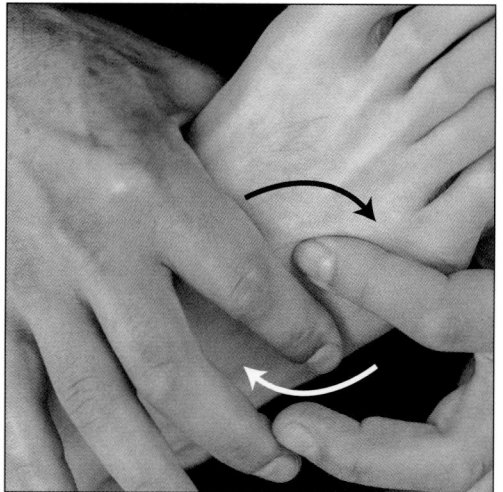

Figure 17.63. Phase 2: Spreading and twisting the connection between the fourth metatarsal and the bases of the third and fifth metatarsals with the thumbs (plantar surface) and index fingers.

Local treatment

An example of a hand position for treatment is shown in figure 17.64. Grasp the bone in a comfortable way and proceed with the six stages of BST treatment (see "Quick Guide to the Six Stages of BST Treatment").

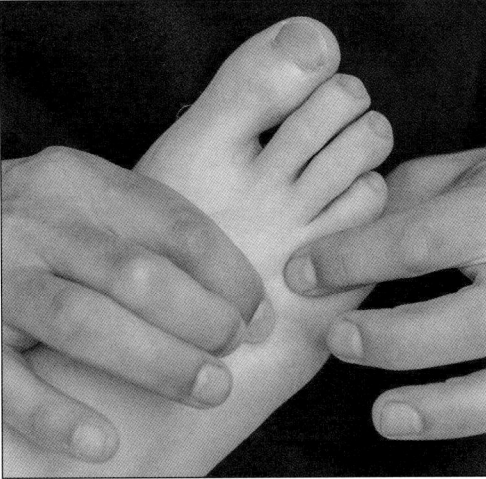

Figure 17.64. Hand position for the local treatment of one section of the shaft of the fourth metatarsal using the thumbs (plantar surface) and index fingers.

Regional treatment

Integrate the local treatment of the fourth metatarsal into the region by using the forefoot gather technique (see "Regional Treatment").

Fifth metatarsal

The fifth metatarsal forms the lateral border of the midfoot. The head of the fifth metatarsal joins the fifth proximal phalanx, and the base of the fifth metatarsal articulates with the cuboid and the base of the fourth metatarsal (figure 17.65). There is a very distinctive tuberosity on the outer side of its base, which can be easily palpated.

Neighbors

Fourth proximal phalanx
Cuboid
Base of fourth metatarsal

Palpation

When you move your fingers proximally from the fifth phalanx over the fifth metatarsophalangeal joint, you will be on

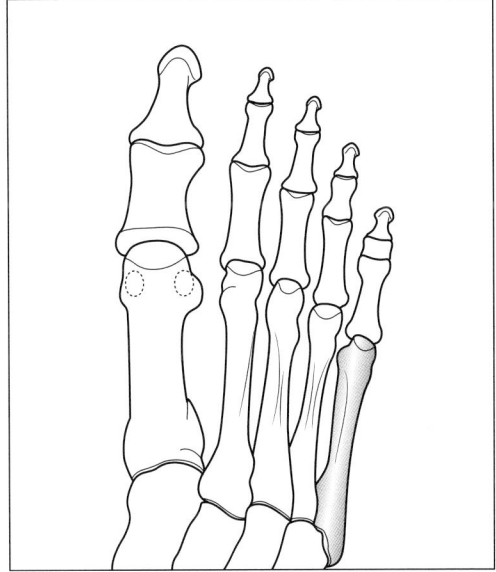

Figure 17.65. Fifth metatarsal.

the head of the fifth metatarsal. Pinch the head of the metatarsal with one hand and wiggle the bone. At the same time, pinch the bone with your other hand, sliding it proximally down the shaft toward the cuboid, monitoring the movement. If you bypass the base of the metatarsal and land on the cuboid or the fourth metatarsal, the wiggling will cease. You can also locate the fifth metatarsal directly by palpating the tuberosity at the base (figure 17.66).

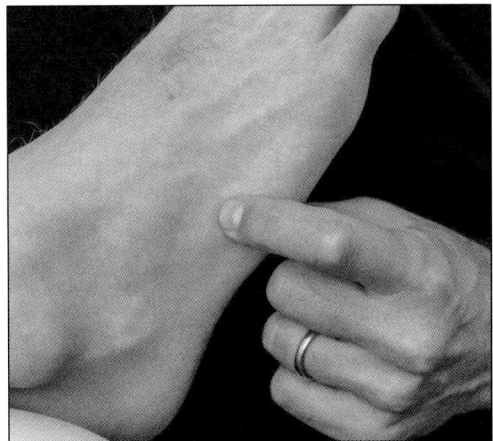

Figure 17.66. Palpating the tuberosity at the base of the fifth metatarsal with the index finger.

Testing

Phase 1: Pinch the fifth metatarsal between your thumb and fingers, squashing and spreading the bone (figure 17.67). Does it feel like wood or concrete?

Now adjust your fingers and test the micromobility between the base of the fifth metatarsal and its neighbors by squeezing the joint lines (figures 17.68 and 17.69).

If both the bone and the connections possess elasticity, move to the next bone to be tested. If the bone feels like concrete or the connective tissue between it and any of its neighbors feels fibrotic, move to phase 2.

Phase 2: Spread and twist the bone(s) in different directions to determine the most rigid pattern within (figure 17.70) or between them (figures 17.71 and 17.72).

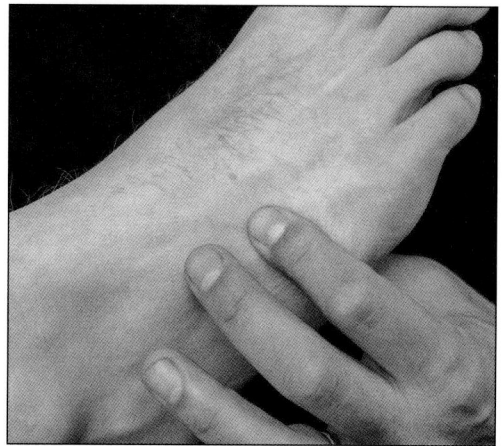

Figure 17.67. Phase 1: Testing the fifth metatarsal by squeezing and spreading the bone with the thumb and fingers (plantar surface).

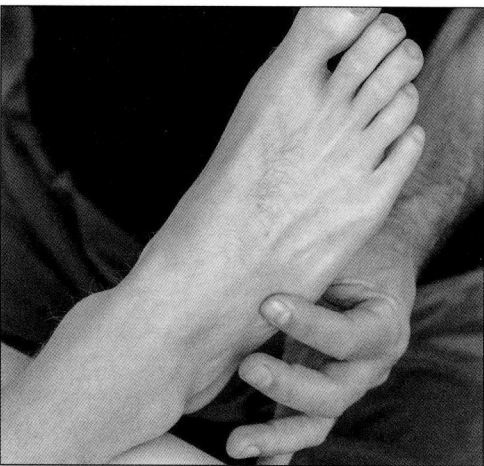

Figure 17.69. Phase 1: Testing the connection between the fifth metatarsal and the base of the fourth metatarsal by squeezing and spreading the joint line with the thumb (plantar surface) and index finger.

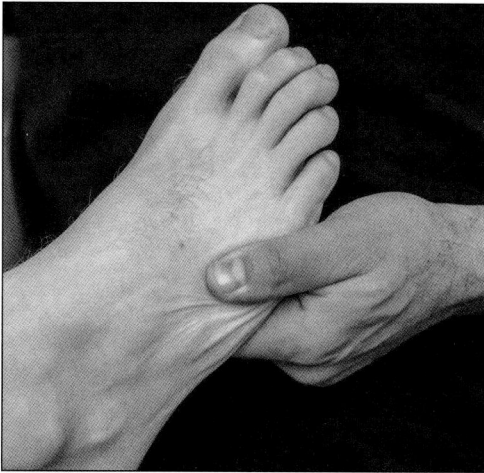

Figure 17.68. Phase 1: Testing the connection between the fifth metatarsal and the cuboid by squeezing and spreading the joint line with the thumb (plantar surface) and index finger.

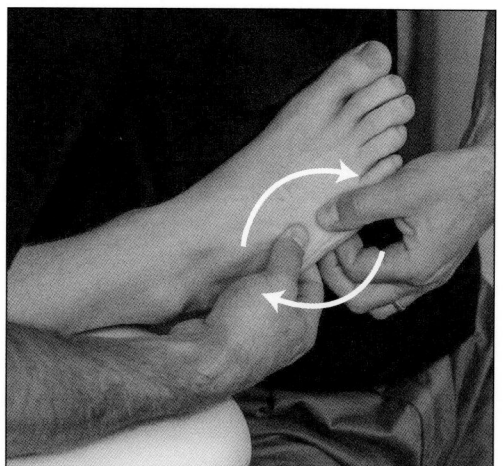

Figure 17.70. Phase 2: Spreading and twisting the fifth metatarsal using the thumbs and fingers (plantar surface).

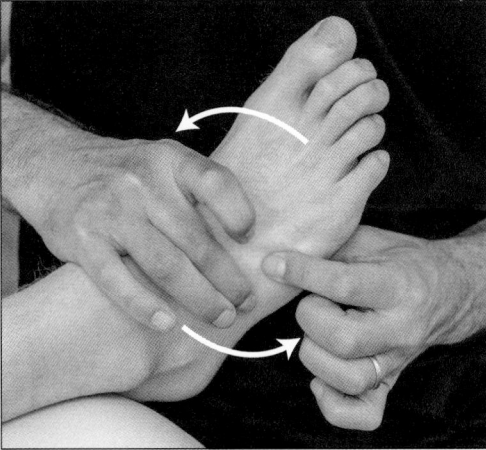

Figure 17.71. Phase 2: Spreading and twisting the connection between the fifth metatarsal and the cuboid using the thumbs (plantar surface) and the index and middle fingers.

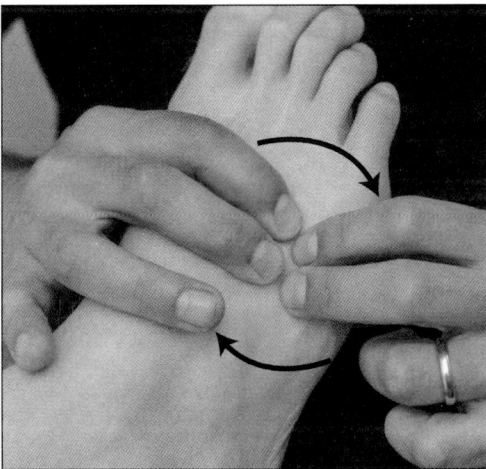

Figure 17.72. Phase 2: Spreading and twisting the connection between the fifth metatarsal and the base of the fourth metatarsal using the thumbs (plantar surface) and the index and middle fingers.

Local treatment

An example of a hand position for treatment is shown in figure 17.73. Grasp the bone in a comfortable way and proceed with the six stages of BST treatment (see "Quick Guide to the Six Stages of BST Treatment").

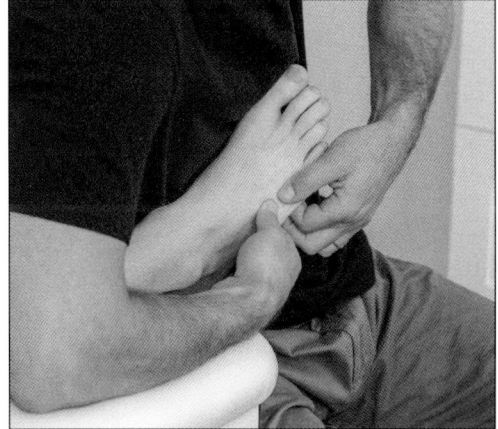

Figure 17.73. Hand position for the local treatment of the fifth metatarsal with the therapist on the medial side of the foot using the thumbs and fingers (plantar surface).

Regional treatment

Integrate the local treatment of the fifth metatarsal into the region by using the forefoot gather technique (see "Regional Treatment").

MIDFOOT

The five bones of the midfoot include the three cuneiforms, the cuboid, and the navicular (figure 17.74). Finding them is more challenging than treating them! But once differentiated from their neighbors, treatment is simple.

Cuneiforms

The three cuneiform bones sit between the navicular, cuboid, and the metatarsals.

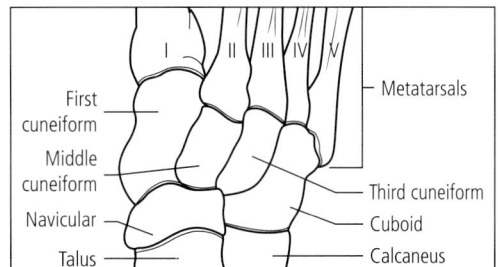

Figure 17.74. Midfoot.

For the testing and treatment protocols for the connections between the cuneiforms and the metatarsals, see "Forefoot."

First cuneiform

The first cuneiform is the largest of the three cuneiforms. It is situated on the medial border of the foot between the base of the first metatarsal and the navicular (figure 17.75).

Neighbors

Bases of first and second metatarsals
Second cuneiform
Navicular

Palpation

Find the first cuneiform by placing the hand on the medial aspect of the foot. With the little finger on the talus and the ring finger on the navicular, the middle finger should rest on the first cuneiform (figure 17.76). Alternatively, all the cuneiforms can be found using the metatarsal wiggle test described above. Pinch the head of the first metatarsal with one hand and wiggle the bone. At the same time, pinch the same metatarsal with

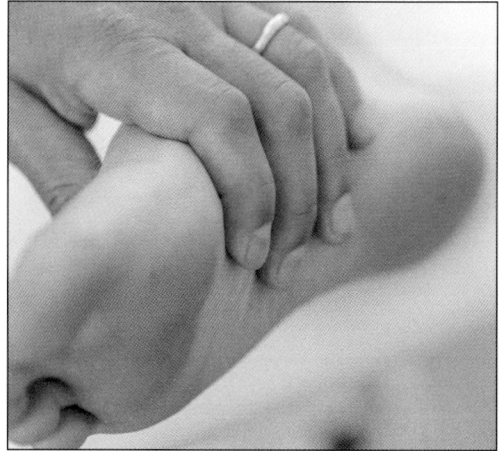

Figure 17.76. Locating the first cuneiform using the generalized medial approach. In this position, the middle finger should rest on the first cuneiform.

the other hand, sliding it down the shaft toward the first cuneiform, monitoring for movement. When the wiggling ceases, you have arrived on the first cuneiform.

Testing

Phase 1: Pinch and spread the first cuneiform, as if pinching a gumdrop from the center (figure 17.77). Does it feel like wood or concrete?

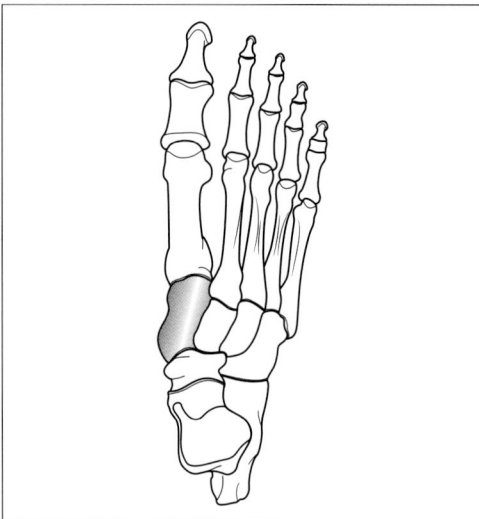

Figure 17.75. First cuneiform.

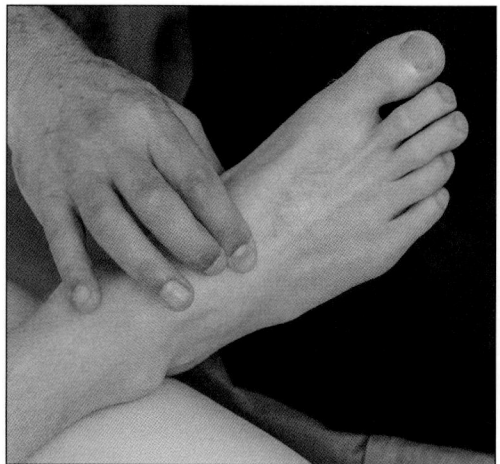

Figure 17.77. Phase 1: Testing the first cuneiform by squeezing and spreading it with the thumb (plantar surface) and index finger.

Now, adjust your fingers and test the micromobility between the first cuneiform and its neighbors by squeezing and spreading the joint lines (figures 17.78 and 17.79).

If both the bone and the connections possess elasticity, move to the next bone to be tested. If the bone feels like concrete or the connective tissue between it and any of its neighbors feels fibrotic, move to phase 2.

Phase 2: Spread and twist the bone(s) in different directions to determine the most rigid torsional pattern within (figure 17.80) or between them (figures 17.81 and 17.82).

Local treatment

An example of a hand position for treatment is shown in figure 17.83. Grasp the bone in a comfortable way and proceed with the

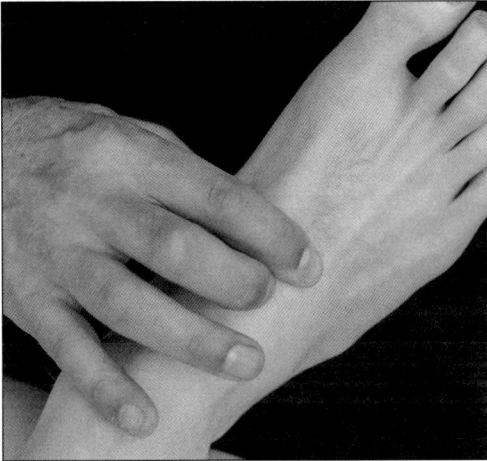

Figure 17.78. Phase 1: Testing the connection between the first and second cuneiforms by squeezing and spreading the joint line with the thumb (plantar surface) and index finger.

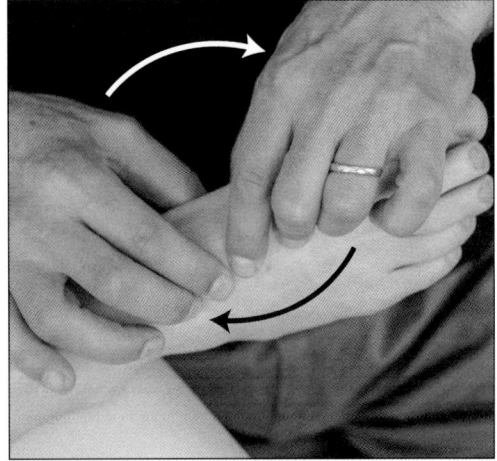

Figure 17.80. Phase 2: Spreading and twisting the first cuneiform using the thumbs (plantar surface) and index fingers.

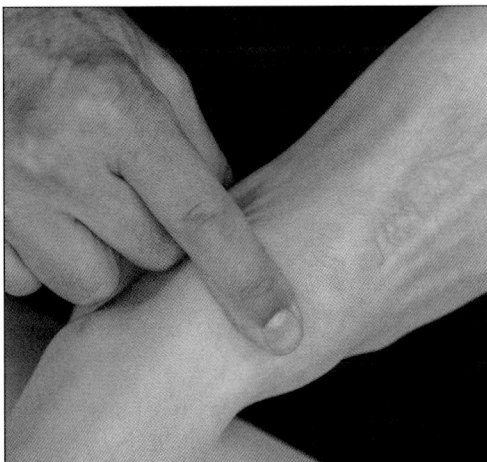

Figure 17.79. Phase 1: Testing the connection between the first cuneiform and the navicular by squeezing and spreading the joint line with the thumb (plantar surface) and index finger.

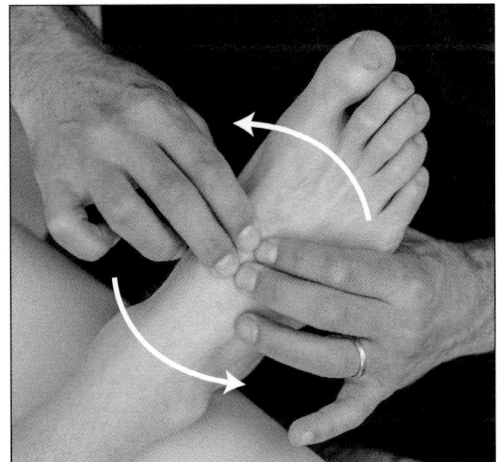

Figure 17.81. Phase 2: Spreading and twisting the connection between the first and second cuneiforms using the thumbs (plantar surface) and index and middle fingers.

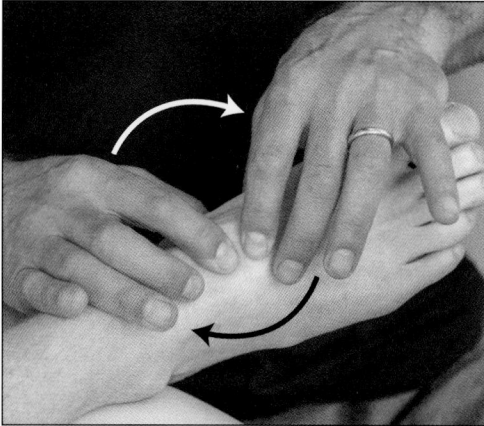

Figure 17.82. Phase 2: Spreading and twisting the connection between the first cuneiform and the navicular using the thumbs (plantar surface) and index fingers.

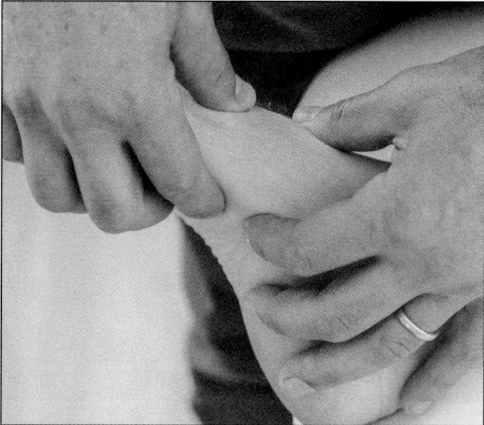

Figure 17.83. Hand position for the local treatment of the first cuneiform with the therapist on the lateral side of the foot using the thumbs and index fingers (plantar surface).

six stages of BST treatment (see "Quick Guide to the Six Stages of BST Treatment").

Regional treatment

Integrate the local treatment of the first cuneiform into the region by using the midfoot gather technique (see "Regional Treatment").

Second cuneiform

The second cuneiform is nestled between the base of the second metatarsal, the navicular, and the first and third cuneiforms (figure 17.84).

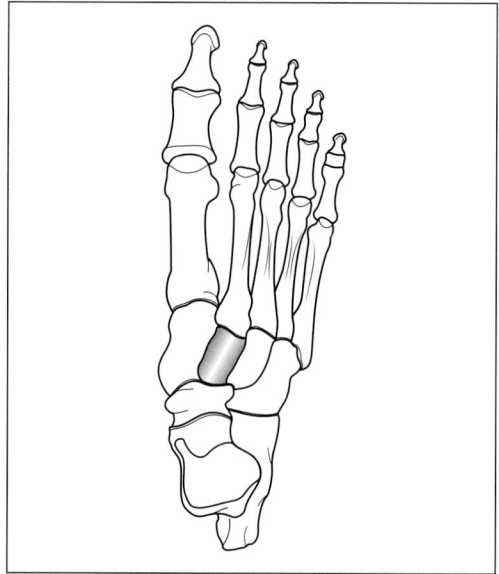

Figure 17.84. Second cuneiform.

It is wedge shaped, with a superior-facing base and an inferior-facing pointed apex.

Neighbors

Base of second metatarsal
First and third cuneiforms
Navicular

Palpation

Pinch the head of the second metatarsal with one hand and wiggle the bone. At the same time, pinch the second metatarsal with your other hand, sliding it proximally down the shaft toward the second cuneiform, monitoring the movement (figure 17.85). If you bypass the base of the metatarsal and land on the second cuneiform, the wiggling will cease.

Testing

Phase 1: Pinch and spread the second cuneiform (figure 17.86). Does it feel like wood or concrete?

Now, adjust your fingers and test the micromobility of the second cuneiform with

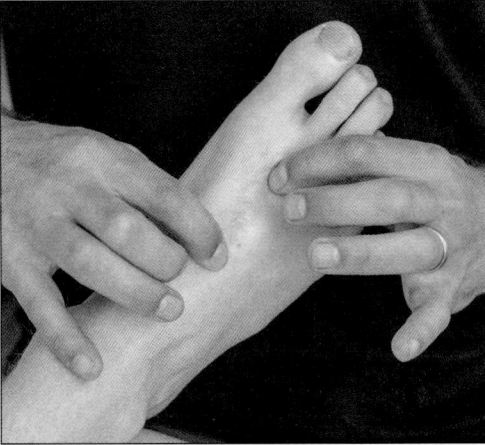

Figure 17.85. Locate the second cuneiform by wiggling the second metatarsal with one hand and sliding down the bone with the other until the movement stops.

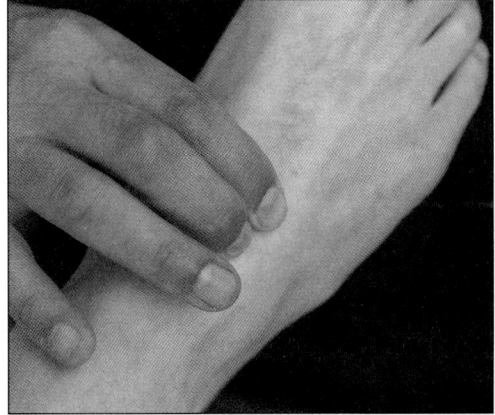

Figure 17.87. Phase 1: Testing the connection between the second cuneiform and the first and third cuneiforms by squeezing and spreading the joint lines using the thumb (plantar surface) and index finger.

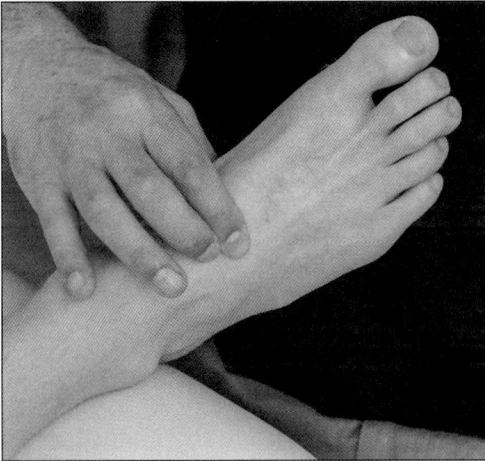

Figure 17.86. Phase 1: Testing the second cuneiform by pinching and spreading the bone with the thumb (plantar surface) and index and middle fingers.

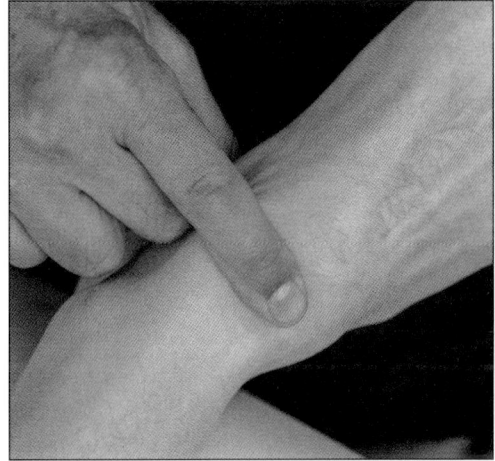

Figure 17.88. Phase 1: Testing the connection between the second cuneiform and the navicular by squeezing and spreading the joint line using the thumb (plantar surface) and index finger.

its neighbors by squeezing and spreading the joint lines (figures 17.87 and 17.88).

If both the bone and the connections possess elasticity, move to the next bone to be tested. If the bone feels like concrete or the connective tissue between it and any of its neighbors feels fibrotic, move to phase 2.

Phase 2: Spread and twist the bone(s) in different directions to determine the most

rigid pattern within (figure 17.89) or between them (figures 17.90 and 17.91). Due to its small size and wedge shape, the spreading and twisting will happen mostly along the base of the bone, since the apex is too narrow and hidden between the other two cuneiforms.

Local treatment

An example of a hand position for treatment is shown in figure 17.92. Grasp the bone in

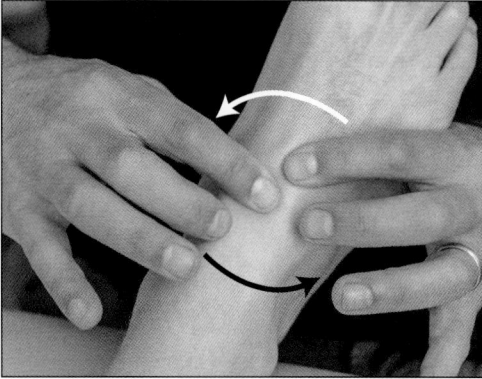

Figure 17.89. Phase 2: Spreading and twisting the second cuneiform with the thumb (stabilizing the apex) and index fingers (along the base of the bone).

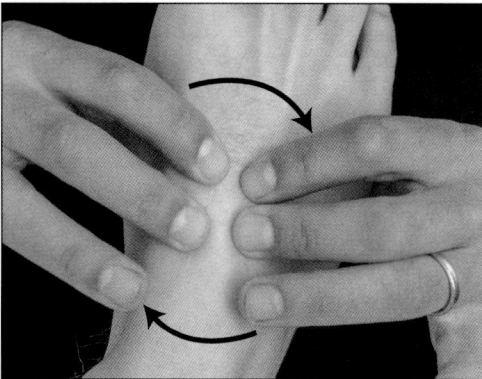

Figure 17.92. Hand position for the local treatment of the second cuneiform using the thumbs (plantar surface) and index fingers.

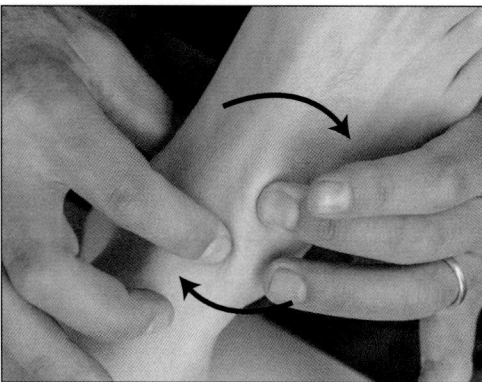

Figure 17.90. Phase 2: Spreading and twisting the connection between the second cuneiform and the first and third cuneiforms using the thumbs (plantar surface) and index fingers.

a comfortable way and proceed with the six stages of BST treatment (see "Quick Guide to the Six Stages of BST Treatment").

Regional treatment

Integrate the local treatment of the second cuneiform into the region by using the midfoot gather technique (see "Regional Treatment").

Third cuneiform

The third cuneiform is smaller than the first but larger than the second. Like the second cuneiform, it is also wedge shaped, with a wider base along the dorsal surface of the midfoot. It's situated between the base of the third metatarsal, the navicular, the second cuneiform, and the cuboid, but also connects to the second and fourth metatarsals (figure 17.93).

Neighbors

Bases of second, third, and fourth metatarsals
Second cuneiform
Navicular
Cuboid

Palpation

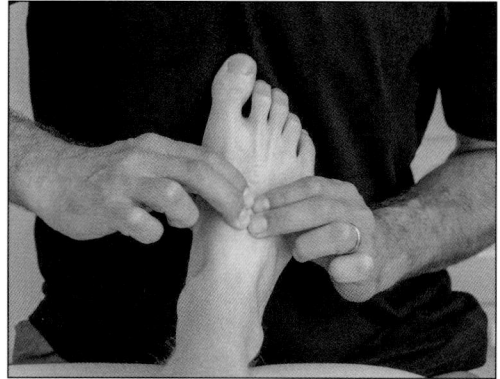

Figure 17.91. Phase 2: Spreading and twisting the connection between the second cuneiform and the navicular with the thumbs (plantar surface) and index fingers.

The cuneiforms can be found using the metatarsal wiggle test described above.

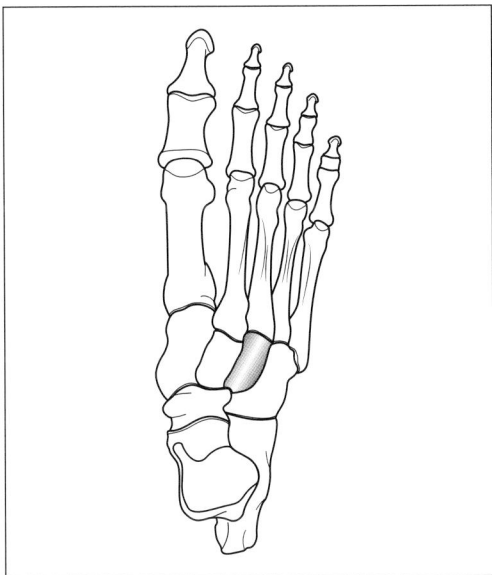

Figure 17.93. Third cuneiform.

Pinch the head of the third metatarsal with one hand and wiggle the bone. At the same time, pinch the third metatarsal with your other hand, sliding it proximally down the shaft toward the third cuneiform, monitoring the movement (figure 17.94). If you bypass the base of the metatarsal and land on the third cuneiform, the wiggling will cease.

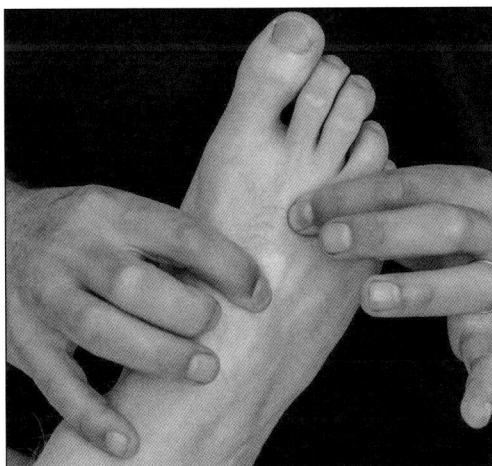

Figure 17.94. Locate the third cuneiform by wiggling the third metatarsal with one hand and sliding down the bone with the other until the movement stops.

Testing

Phase 1: Pinch and spread the third cuneiform (figure 17.95). Does it feel like wood or concrete?

Now, adjust your fingers and test the micromobility of the third cuneiform with its neighbors by squeezing and spreading the joint lines (figures 17.96 to 17.98).

If both the bone and the connections possess elasticity, move to the next bone to be tested.

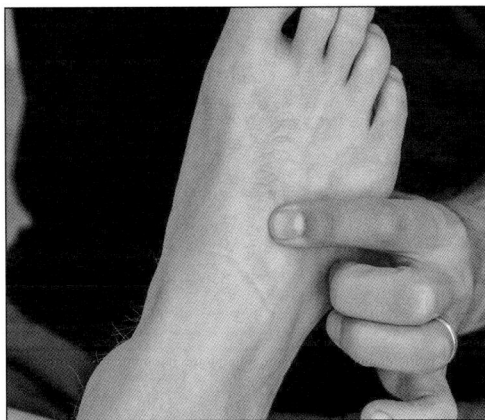

Figure 17.95. Phase 1: Testing the third cuneiform by pinching and spreading the bone with the thumb (plantar surface) and index finger.

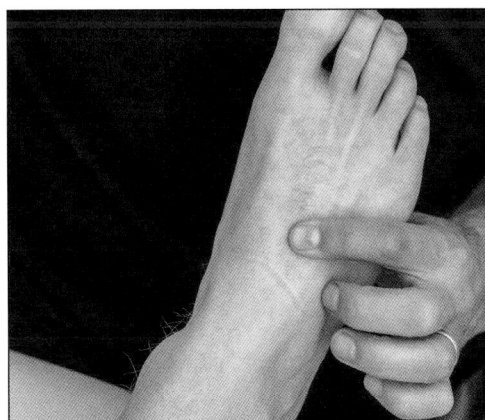

Figure 17.96. Phase 1: Testing the connection between the third cuneiform and the second cuneiform by squeezing and spreading the joint line with the thumb (plantar surface) and index finger.

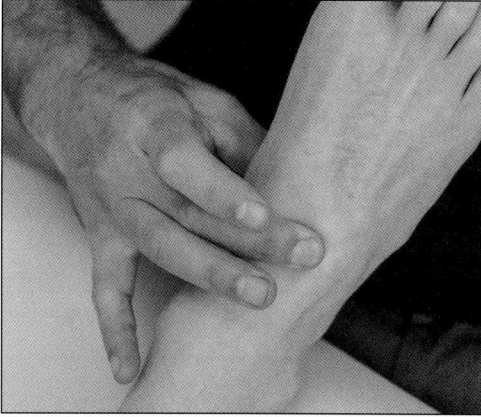

Figure 17.97. Phase 1: Testing the connection between the third cuneiform and the navicular by squeezing and spreading the joint line with the thumb (plantar surface) and middle finger.

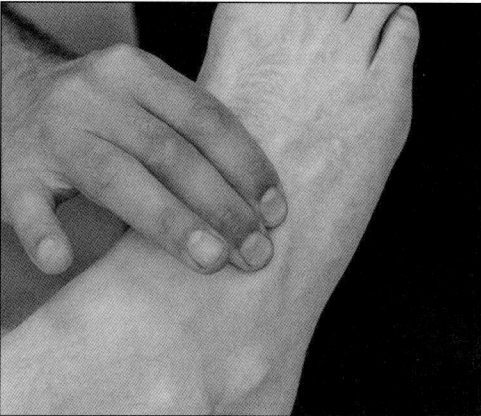

Figure 17.98. Phase 1: Testing the connection between the third cuneiform and the cuboid by squeezing and spreading the joint line with the thumb (plantar surface) and the index and middle fingers.

However, if the bone feels like concrete or the connective tissue between it and any of its neighbors feels fibrotic, move to phase 2.

Phase 2: Spread and twist the bone(s) in different directions to determine the most rigid torsional pattern within (figure 17.99) or between them (figures 17.100 to 17.102) them. Due to its wedge shape, the spreading and twisting will occur mostly along the dorsal base of the bone.

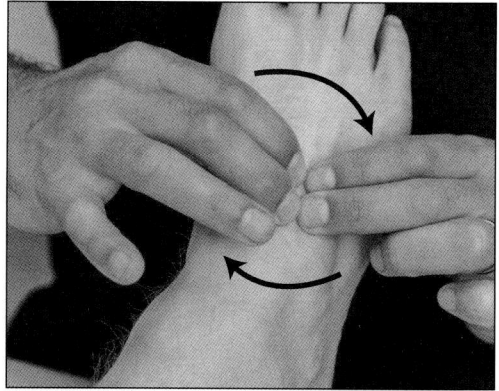

Figure 17.99. Phase 2: Spreading and twisting the third cuneiform with the thumbs (plantar surface) and the index and middle fingers.

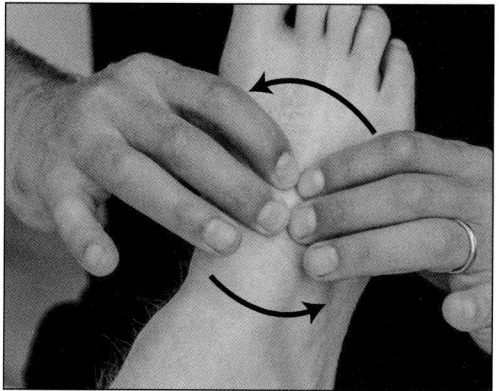

Figure 17.100. Phase 2: Spreading and twisting the connection between the third cuneiform and the second cuneiform with the thumbs (plantar surface) and the index and middle fingers.

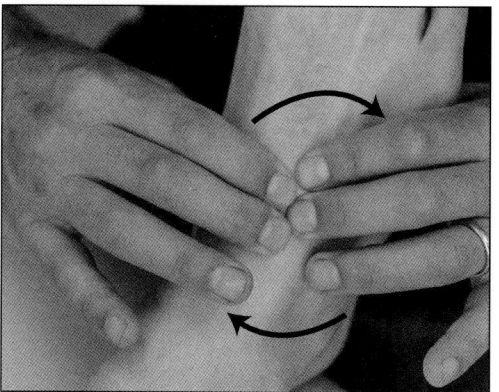

Figure 17.101. Phase 2: Spreading and twisting the connection between the third cuneiform and the navicular with the thumbs (plantar surface) and the index and middle fingers.

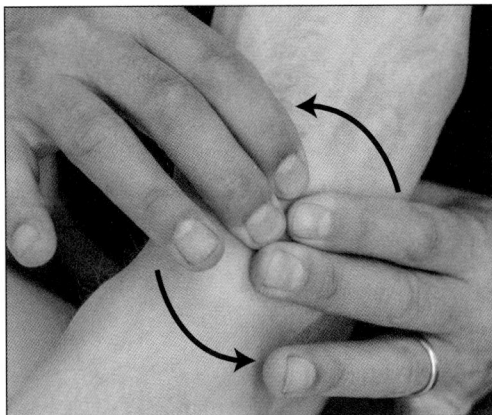

Figure 17.102. Phase 2: Spreading and twisting the connection between the third cuneiform and the cuboid with the thumbs (plantar surface) and the index and middle fingers.

Local treatment

An example of a hand position for treatment is shown in figure 17.103. Grasp the bone in a comfortable way and proceed with the six stages of BST treatment (see "Quick Guide to the Six Stages of BST Treatment").

Regional treatment

Integrate the local treatment of the third cuneiform into the region by using the midfoot gather technique (see "Regional Treatment").

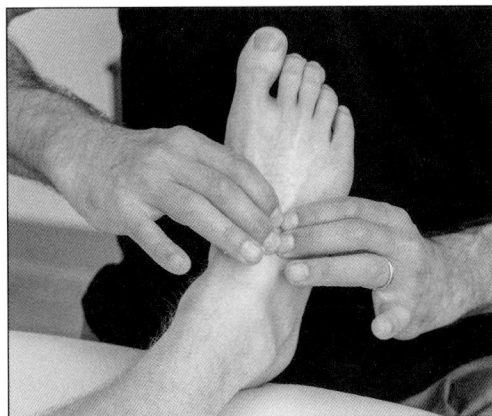

Figure 17.103. Hand position for the local treatment of the third cuneiform using the thumbs (plantar surface) and the index and middle fingers.

Cuboid

The cuboid is on the lateral side of the midfoot (figure 17.104). It's pyramidal shaped with the base pointing superiorly and medially and the apex directed inferiorly and laterally. It has a deep groove in the inferior surface, through which passes the tendon of the peroneus longus muscle. For the testing and treatment protocols for the connections between the cuboid and the metatarsals, see "Forefoot."

Neighbors

Bases of fourth and fifth metatarsals
Third cuneiform
Navicular (occasionally)
Calcaneus

Palpation

Pinch the head of the fourth and/or fifth metatarsal with one hand and wiggle the bone(s). At the same time, pinch the fourth and/or fifth metatarsal with your other hand, sliding it proximally down the shaft(s) toward the cuboid, monitoring the movement.
If you bypass the base of the metatarsals and land on the cuboid, the wiggling will cease.

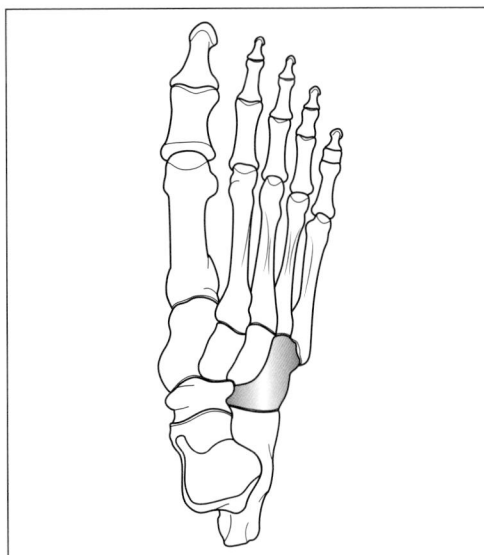

Figure 17.104. Cuboid.

You can also slide a finger down the lateral side of the foot along the fifth metatarsal. Immediately proximal to the tuberosity at its base is the cuboid (figure 17.105).

Testing

Phase 1: Pinch and spread the cuboid (figure 17.106). Does it feel like wood or concrete?

Now, adjust your fingers and test the micromobility of the cuboid with its neighbors by squeezing and spreading the joint lines (figures 17.107 to 17.109). All the neighbors except the calcaneus can be tested without displacing the medial hand. When testing the cuboid with the calcaneus, move your medial hand onto the calcaneus (figure 17.109).

If both the bone and the connections possess elasticity, move to the next bone to be tested. If the bone feels like concrete or the connective tissue between it and any of its neighbors feels fibrotic, move to phase 2.

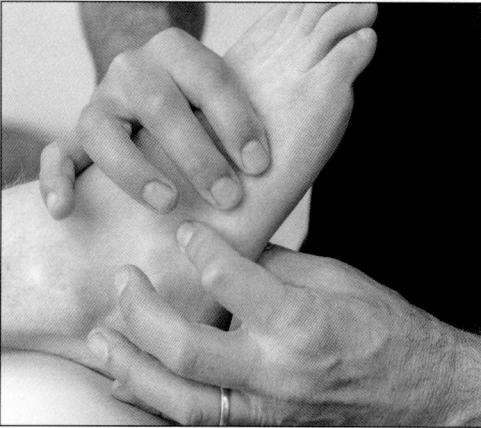

Figure 17.105. Locating the tuberosity on the base of the fifth metatarsal and palpating the cuboid.

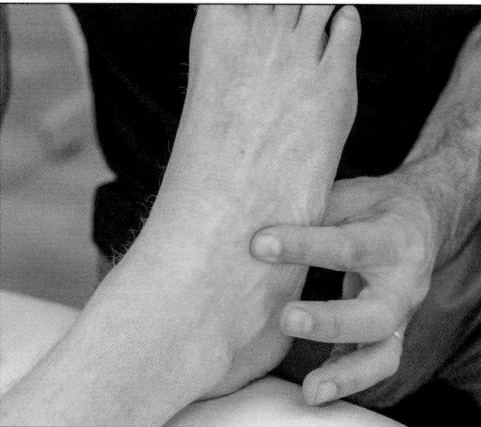

Figure 17.106. Phase 1: Testing the cuboid by pinching and spreading it with the thumb (plantar surface) and index finger.

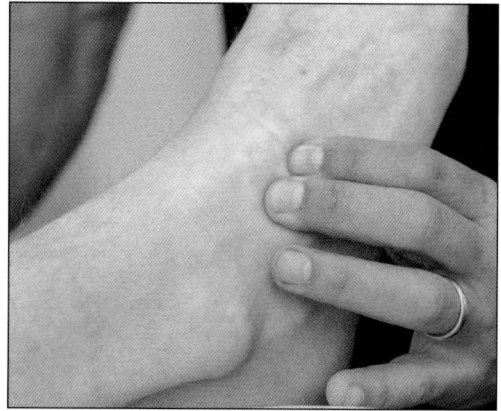

Figure 17.107. Phase 1: Testing the connection between the cuboid and the third cuneiform by squeezing and spreading the joint line with the thumb (plantar surface) and the index and middle fingers.

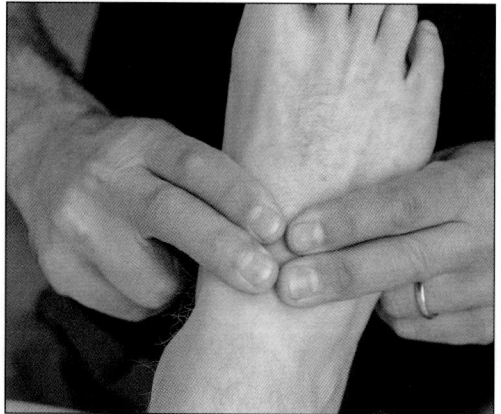

Figure 17.108. Phase 1: Testing the connection between the cuboid and the navicular by squeezing and spreading the joint line with the thumbs (plantar surface) and the index and middle fingers.

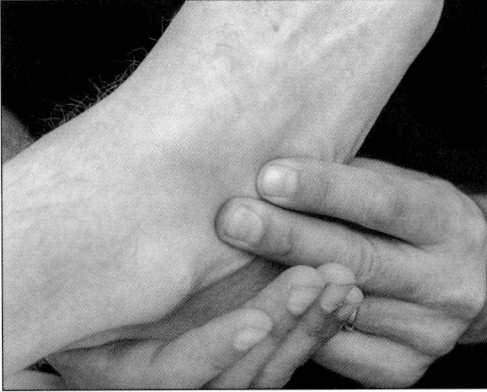

Figure 17.109. Phase 1: Testing the connection between the cuboid and the calcaneus by squeezing and spreading the joint line on the plantar surface (with the thumb) and on the lateral surface (with the index and middle fingers). The calcaneus is supported by cupping it with the other hand.

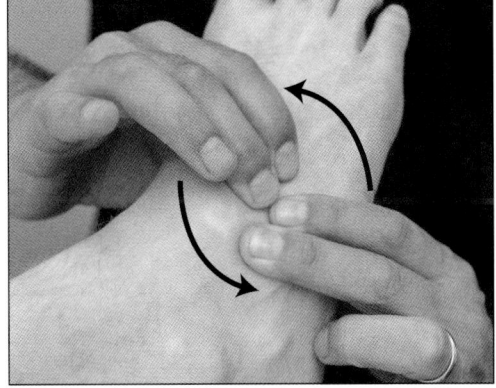

Figure 17.110. Phase 2: Spreading and twisting the cuboid with the thumbs (plantar surface) and the index and middle fingers.

Phase 2: Spread and twist the bone(s) in different directions to determine the most rigid torsional pattern within (figure 17.110) or between them (figures 17.111 to 17.113).

Local treatment

An example of a hand position for treatment is shown in figure 17.114. Grasp the bone in a comfortable way and proceed with the six stages of BST treatment (see "Quick Guide to the Six Stages of BST Treatment").

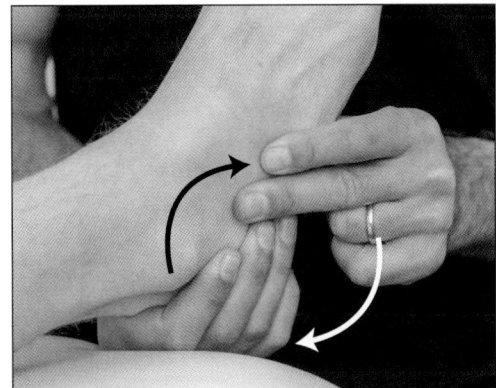

Figure 17.111. Phase 2: Spreading and twisting the connection between the cuboid and the third cuneiform with the thumbs (plantar surface) and the index and middle fingers.

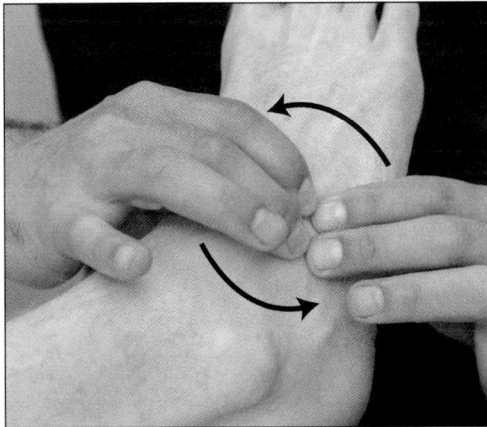

Figure 17.112. Phase 2: Spreading and twisting the connection between the cuboid and the navicular with the thumbs (plantar surface) and the index and middle fingers.

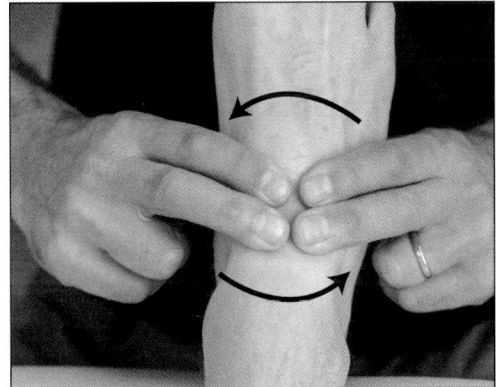

Figure 17.113. Phase 2: Spreading and twisting the connection between the cuboid and the calcaneus with the thumbs (plantar surface) and the index and middle fingers. The calcaneus is secured to the table with the other hand.

131

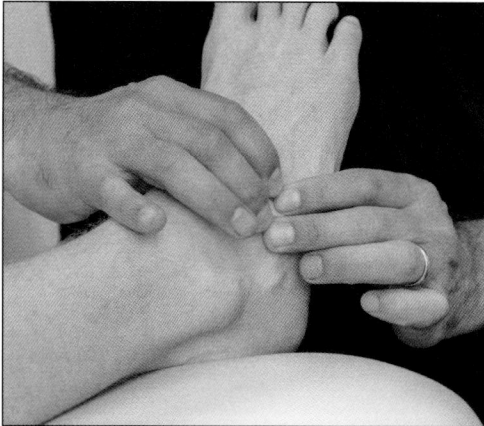

Figure 17.114. Hand position for the local treatment of the cuboid using the thumbs (plantar surface) and the index and middle fingers.

Regional treatment

Integrate the local treatment of the cuboid into the region by using the midfoot gather technique (see "Regional Treatment").

Navicular

Shaped almost like a boat—concave on the plantar surface and convex on the dorsal surface—the navicular forms part of the medial midfoot (figure 17.115).

Neighbors

First, second, and third cuneiforms
Cuboid (occasionally)
Talus

Palpation

One can generally find the navicular by placing the hand on the medial aspect of the foot. If your little finger is on the talus, your ring finger should be on the navicular (figure 17.116). Another neat way to find the navicular is to ask the subject to plantar flex and adduct the foot. Follow the tendon of the tibialis posterior muscle from behind the medial malleolus to where it inserts on the navicular (figure 17.117).

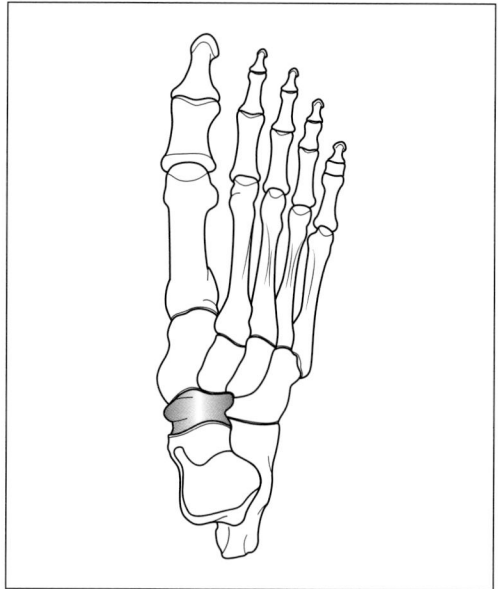

Figure 17.115. Navicular.

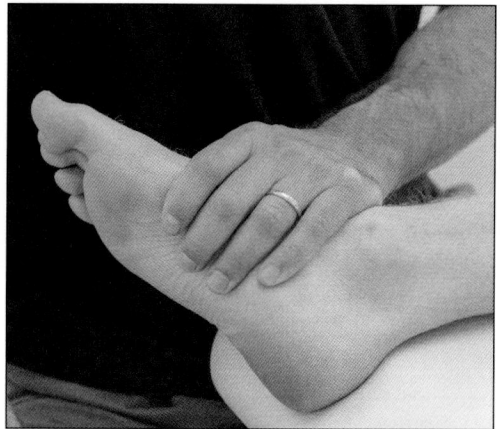

Figure 17.116. By placing the hand on the medial aspect of the foot, the little finger rests on the talus, and the ring finger rests on the navicular.

Testing

Phase 1: Pinch and spread the navicular (figure 17.118). Does it feel like wood or concrete?

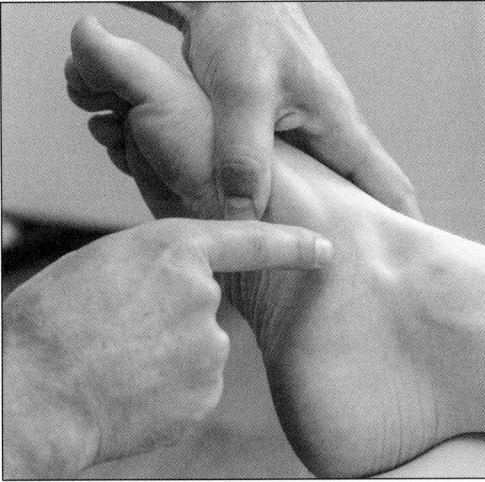

Figure 17.117. Finding the navicular by following the tendon of the tibialis posterior muscle to where it inserts on the bone.

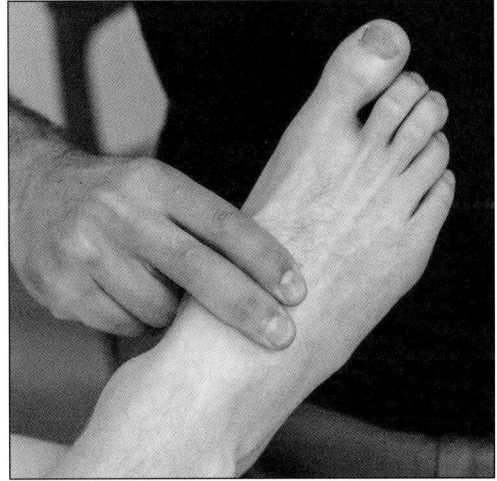

Figure 17.118. Phase 1: Testing the navicular by pinching and spreading the bone with the thumb and index finger.

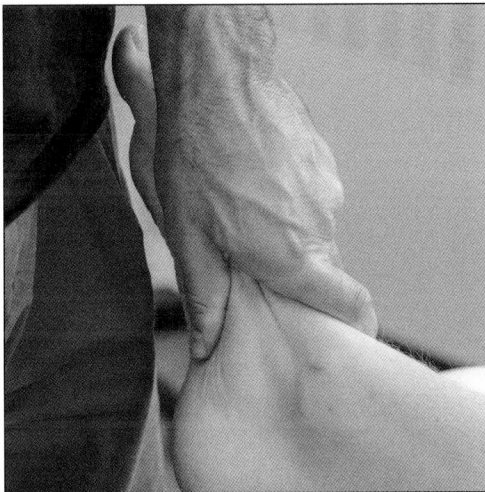

Figure 17.119. Phase 1: Testing the connection between the navicular and the first, second, and third cuneiforms by squeezing and spreading the joint lines with the thumb (plantar surface) and the index and middle fingers.

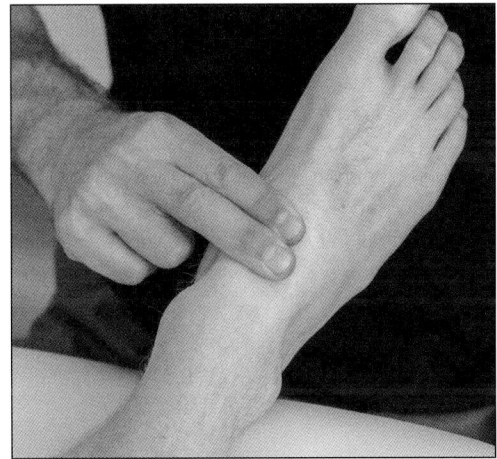

Figure 17.120. Phase 1: Testing the connection between the navicular and the talus by squeezing and spreading the joint line with the thumb (plantar surface) and the index and middle fingers.

Now, adjust your fingers and test the micromobility between the navicular and its neighbors by squeezing and spreading the joint lines (figures 17.119 and 17.120).

If both the bone and the connections possess elasticity, move to the next bone to be tested. If the bone feels like concrete or the connective tissue between it and any of its neighbors feels fibrotic, move to phase 2.

Phase 2: Spread and twist the bone(s) in different directions to determine the most rigid pattern within (figure 17.121) or between them (figures 17.122 and 17.123).

Local treatment

An example of a hand position for treatment is shown in figure 17.124. Grasp the bone in

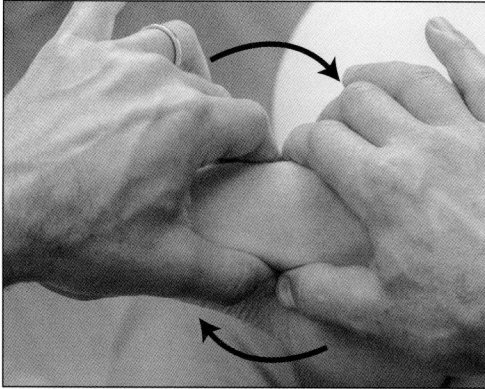

Figure 17.121. Phase 2: Spreading and twisting the navicular.

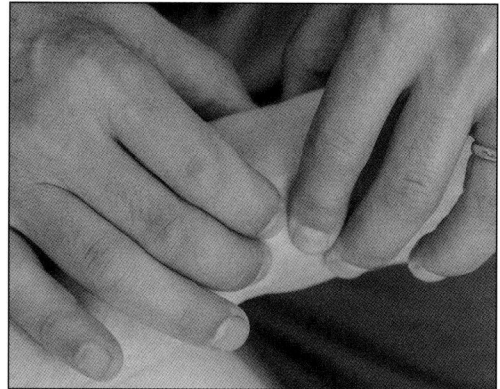

Figure 17.122. Phase 2: Spreading and twisting the connection between the navicular and the first, second, and third cuneiforms with the thumbs (plantar surface) and the index and middle fingers.

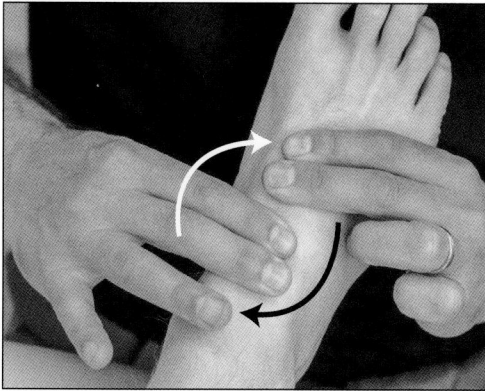

Figure 17.123. Phase 2: Spreading and twisting the connection between the navicular and the talus with the thumbs (plantar surface) and the index and middle fingers.

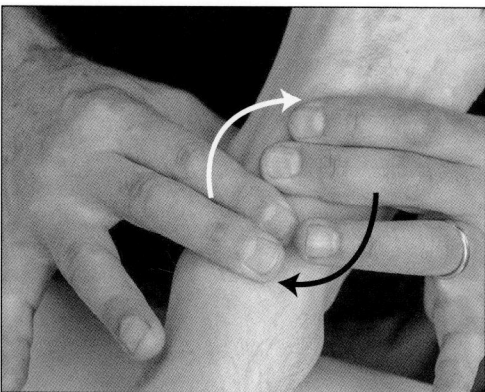

Figure 17.124. Hand position for the local treatment of the navicular with the foot turned onto the lateral side and with the therapist using the thumbs (plantar surface) and mostly the index fingers.

a comfortable way and proceed with the six stages of BST treatment (see "Quick Guide to the Six Stages of BST Treatment").

Regional treatment

Integrate the local treatment of the navicular into the region by using the midfoot gather technique (see "Regional Treatment").

HINDFOOT

The talus and the calcaneus make up the hindfoot (figure 17.125). These are larger bones than those of the forefoot and midfoot, so we can thoroughly test them from different directions and angles. The shape and size of these two bones allow us to compress

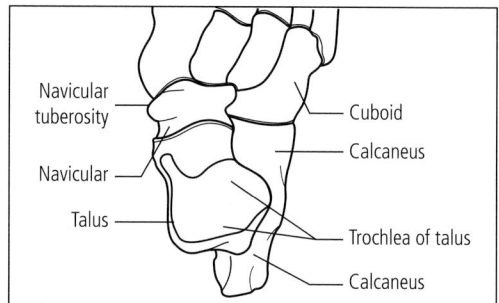

Figure 17.125. Hindfoot.

and spread them without altering our hand positions too much, but I have also included treatment variations for specific parts of each bone, and these variations may require alternate hand or finger positions.

Talus

The talus is the bony link between the leg and the foot. It has a head, neck, and body (figure 17.126). The head of the talus articulates with the navicular, and the body supports the tibia and articulates with both the medial and lateral malleoli.

Neighbors

Navicular
Tibia
Fibula
Calcaneus

Palpation

The talus can be palpated both segmentally and globally.

Head: Locate the navicular by following the tendon of the tibialis posterior muscle as described above for the navicular. If you slide your finger just behind the navicular tuberosity, you will feel the flat, smooth surface of the medial head of the talus (figure 17.127).

Neck: To palpate the medial neck, imagine a line drawn from the navicular tuberosity to the medial malleolus. The neck of the talus is located at the approximate midway point of the line. Also, you can use the tendons of the tibialis anterior and tibialis posterior muscles to guide you. Have the patient dorsiflex and supinate the foot. The medial portion of the neck is located in between the insertion points of the two tendons on the first cuneiform and metatarsal and navicular, respectively (figure 17.128).

To palpate the lateral neck, place a finger on the anterior border of the lateral malleolus, then move the finger distally and medially (figure 17.129).

Body: The body of the talus has two lateral processes that are relatively easy to find: the posterolateral and posteromedial processes. The posterolateral process is located directly

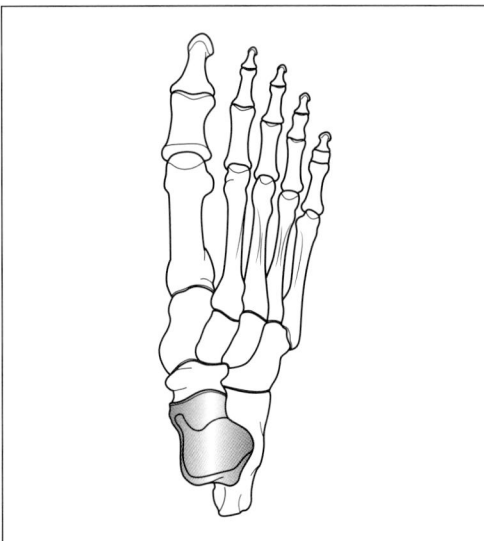

Figure 17.126. Talus.

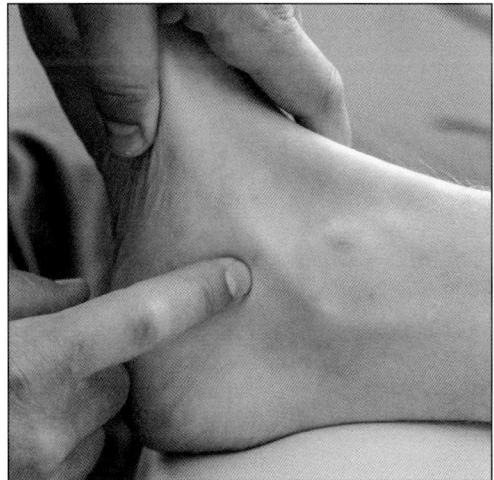

Figure 17.127. Palpating the medial aspect of the head of the talus (located just behind the navicular tuberosity) with the index finger.

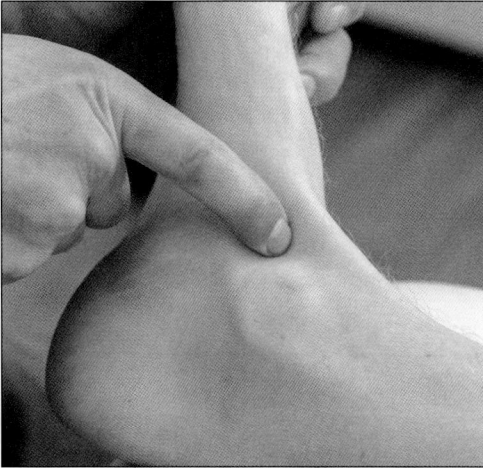

Figure 17.128. Palpating the medial neck of the talus (located between the insertion points of the tendons of tibialis anterior and tibialis posterior muscles on the first cuneiform and metatarsal and navicular) with the index finger.

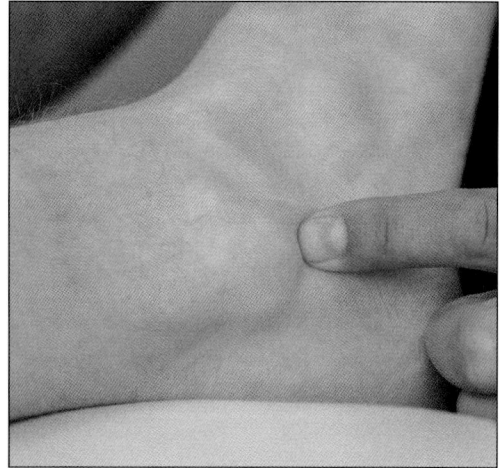

Figure 17.130. Palpating the posterolateral process of the talus (located directly below the lateral malleolus and immediately above the articulation between the talus and calcaneus) with the index finger.

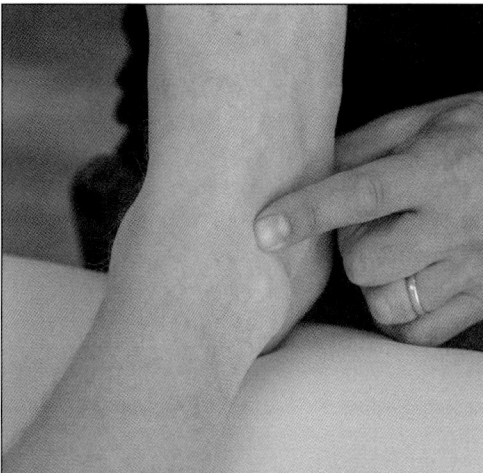

Figure 17.129. Palpating the lateral neck of the talus (distally and medially to the lateral malleolus) with the index finger.

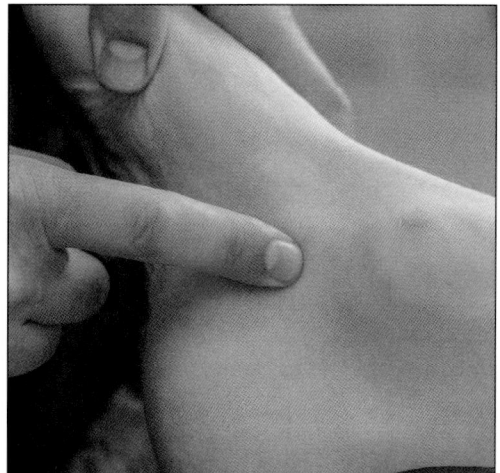

Figure 17.131. Palpating the posteromedial process of the talus (located directly below the medial malleolus and directly above the talocalcaneal line) with the index finger.

below the lateral malleolus and immediately above the articulation between the talus and calcaneus (figure 17.130).

The posteromedial process is located directly below the medial malleolus and directly above the talocalcaneal line. To palpate it, start at the Achilles tendon at the level of the medial malleolus and move distally onto the bone (figure 17.131).

Global: Sit facing the foot. Slide your lateral hand down the shaft of the tibia until you reach the neck of the talus. Grasp the neck and head with your index or middle finger, with the thumb wrapped around the midfoot. With the thumb and index finger of your medial hand, grasp both the posterolateral and posteromedial processes, with the other fingers resting on the calcaneus (figure 17.132).

136

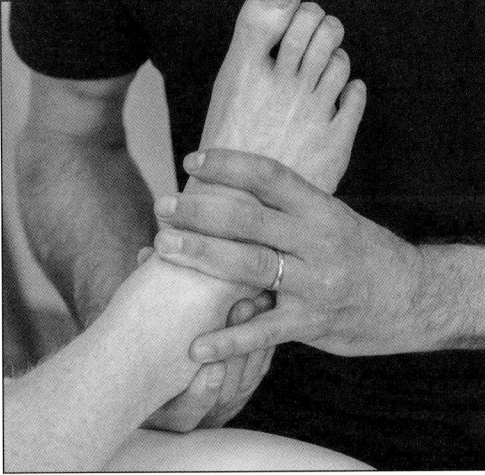

Figure 17.132. Global palpation of talus. The thumb of the lateral hand is on the plantar surface and hidden from view.

Testing

Global: Begin by testing the talus globally (and directly with the spreading and twisting phase) to find (*a*) if the bone is compacted and (*b*) the specific torsional pattern of compaction. Sit facing the foot, holding talus as described above. Spread the bone:

- in an anteroposterior direction (one hand moving toward the toes and one hand moving toward the heel, then reverse and repeat), twisting in both directions (figure 17.133).
- in a mediolateral direction (one hand moving medially and one hand moving laterally, then reverse and repeat), twisting in both directions (figure 17.134).
- in a superoinferior direction (one hand moving proximally and one hand moving distally, then reverse and repeat), twisting in both directions (figure 17.135).

This combination of tests should provide a clear idea of the pattern of compaction.

Now, test the connections between the talus and its neighbors by applying a spreading

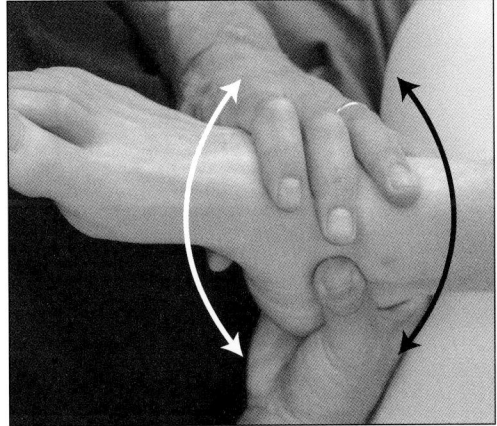

Figure 17.133. Anteroposterior spreading and twisting of the talus.

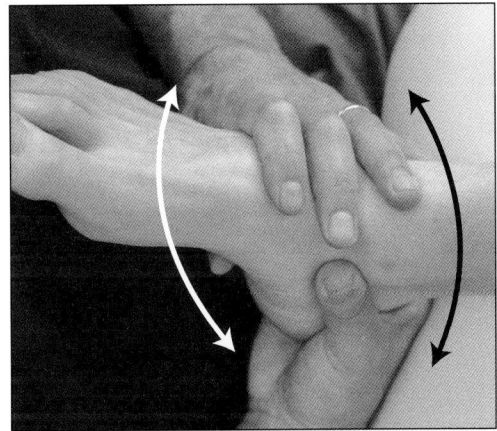

Figure 17.134. Mediolateral spreading and twisting of the talus.

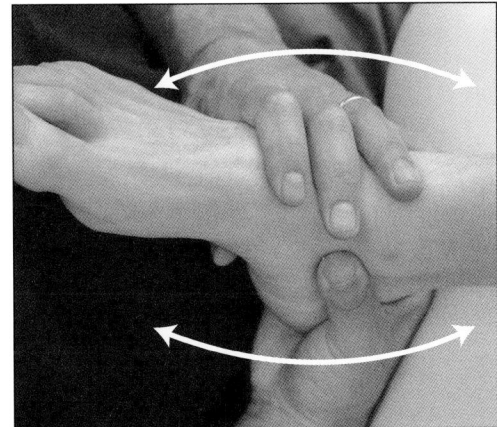

Figure 17.135. Superoinferior spreading and twisting of the talus.

137

and twisting force between the talus and the tibia (figure 17.136), navicular (figure 17.137), and calcaneus (figure 17.138). To test the connection with the fibula, grasp the medial side of the talus with your medial hand and place your lateral hand on the lateral malleolus (figure 17.139).

Does the talus or any of the connections with its neighbors feel like wood or concrete in any direction? Is there one segment that feels more compacted than another? If the whole bone feels more like wood, move to the next bone to be tested. If the whole talus, any segments of the talus, or any of the connections with its neighbors feels more like concrete or is fibrotic, either move directly to treatment or specifically retest the head, neck, and body for more localized compacted tissue.

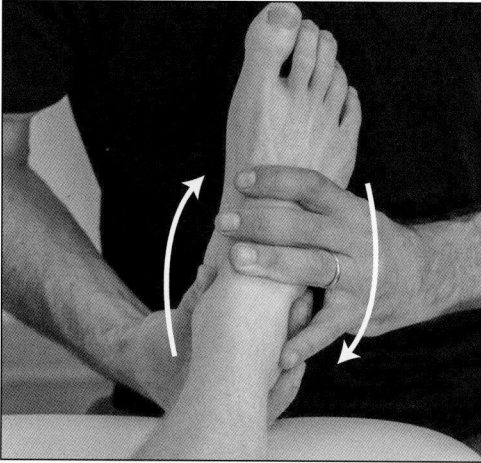

Figure 17.136. Spreading and twisting the connection between the talus and the tibia. The thumb of the lateral hand is on the plantar surface and hidden from view.

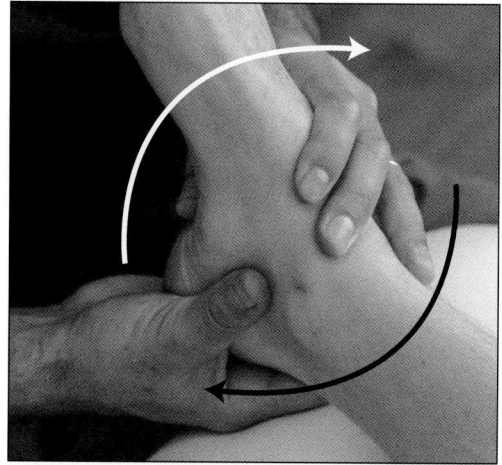

Figure 17.138. Spreading and twisting the connection between the talus and the calcaneus.

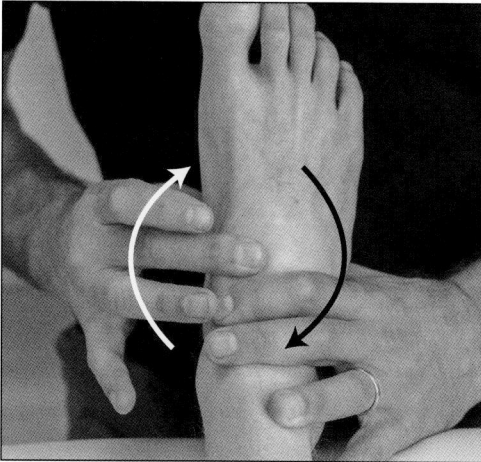

Figure 17.137. Spreading and twisting the connection between the talus and the navicular with the thumbs (plantar surface) and the index and middle fingers.

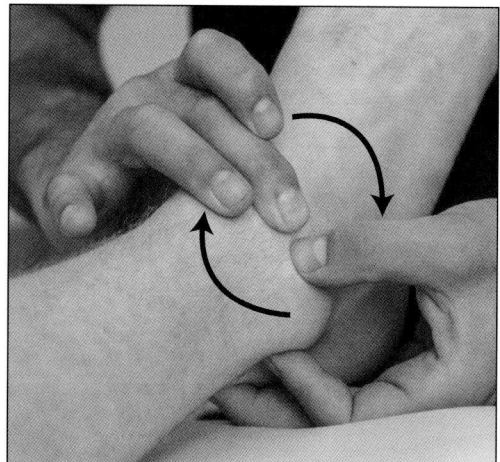

Figure 17.139. Spreading and twisting the connection between the talus and the fibula.

Local treatment

Grasp the bone in a comfortable way and proceed with the six stages of BST treatment (see "Quick Guide to the Six Stages of BST Treatment"). Local treatment can be applied from either the global hold (figure 17.140) or more specifically to any segments of the bone. If one or more of the segments of the talus are compacted, and if the global approach is insufficiently specific, change positions to apply the six stages of treatment with corresponding hand positions to the head and neck (figure 17.141), medial body (figure 17.142), lateral body (figure 17.143), or posterior body (figure 17.144).

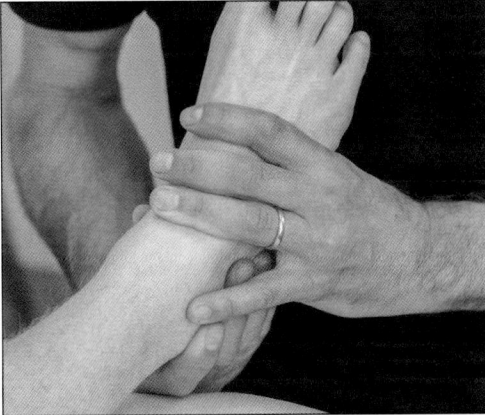

Figure 17.142. Hand positions for the specific treatment of the medial body of the talus using the thumbs, index fingers, and the thenar space.

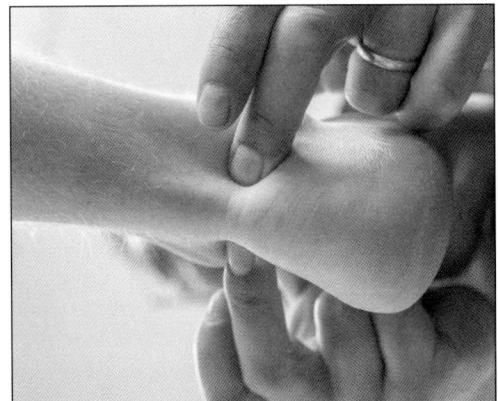

Figure 17.143. Hand positions for the specific treatment of the lateral body of the talus using the thumbs, index fingers, and the thenar space.

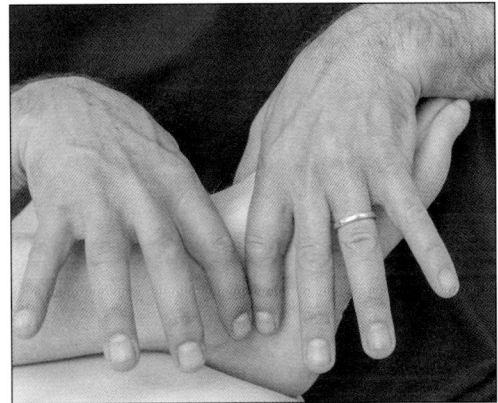

Figure 17.140. Local treatment of the talus using the global hold.

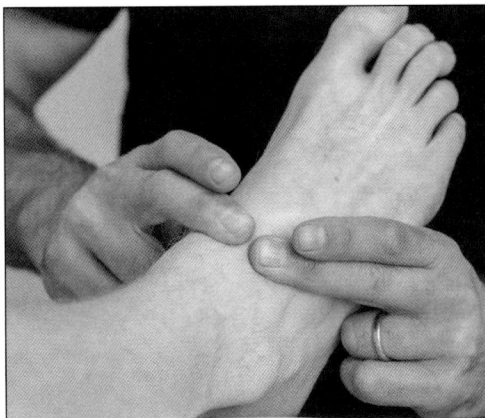

Figure 17.141. Hand positions for the specific treatment of the head and neck of the talus using the middle fingers.

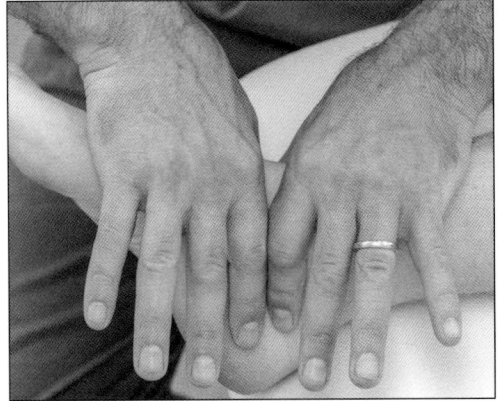

Figure 17.144. Hand positions for the specific treatment of the posterior body of the talus using the middle fingers. Here, the foot is extended off the end of the table for a better view.

Regional treatment

Integrate the local treatment of the talus into the region by using the hindfoot gather technique (see "Regional Treatment").

Calcaneus

The calcaneus is the irregular-shaped heel bone at the back of the foot that accommodates the insertion of the Achilles tendon upon the posterior surface (figure 17.145). On its medial surface, it has a small posteromedial tuberosity called the sustentaculum tali, which resembles a small cliff overhanging the concave bone valley below it. At the floor of the valley sits a posteromedial knob, the calcaneal tuberosity. Less prominent but still palpable, the lateral calcaneal tuberosity is situated on the other side of the posterior calcaneus.

Neighbors

Navicular
Cuboid

Palpation

Global: Sit at the foot. Cup the posterior part of the calcaneus with the medial hand and pinch the anterior part with the lateral thumb and fingers. To find the anterior segment, locate the cuboid on the lateral side of the foot, then slide your thumb posteriorly and just across the calcaneocuboid joint (figure 17.146).

Lateral surface: Locate the calcaneocuboid joint line and follow the bone along the lateral surface toward the end of the heel (figure 17.147).

Sustentaculum tali: The sustentaculum tali sits on the medial side of the calcaneus approximately one finger's width below the medial malleolus (figure 17.148).

Medial surface and posteromedial calcaneal tuberosity: Below the sustentaculum tali is the concave medial surface, which is bordered by the posteromedial calcaneal tuberosity (figure 17.149).

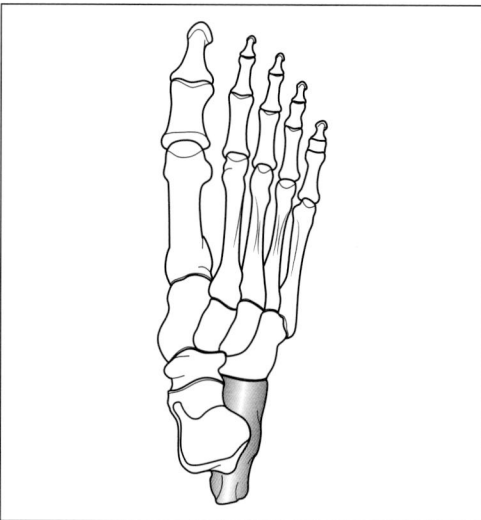

Figure 17.145. Calcaneus.

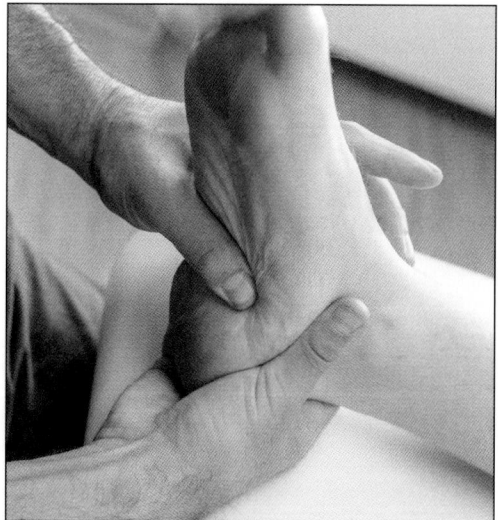

Figure 17.146. Global palpation of the calcaneus.

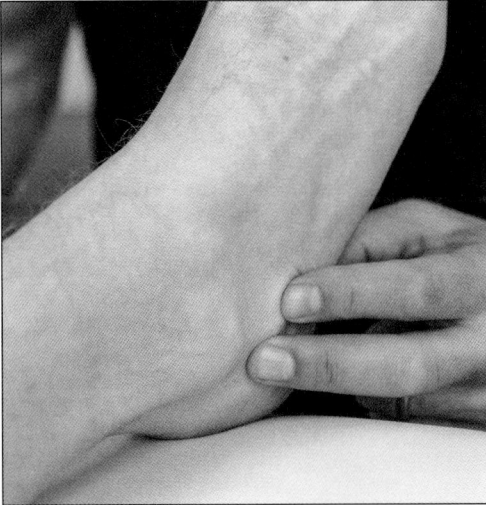

Figure 17.147. Palpating the lateral surface of the calcaneus with the index and middle fingers.

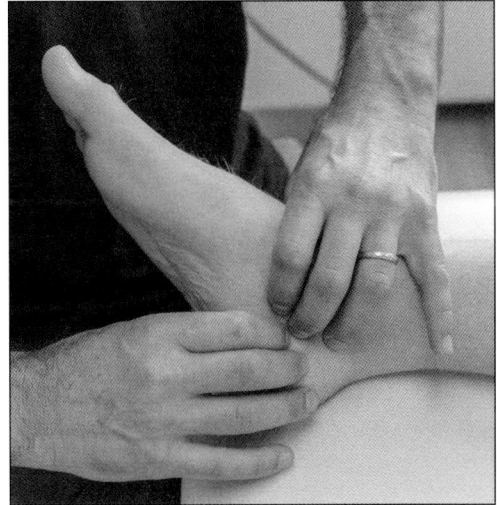

Figure 17.149. Palpating the concave medial surface and posteromedial tuberosity of the calcaneus with the index and middle fingers.

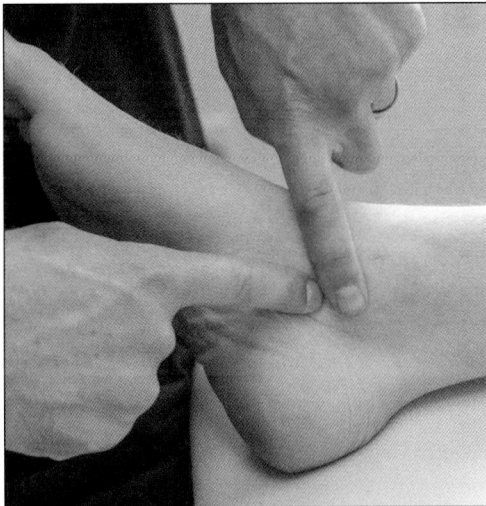

Figure 17.148. Palpating the sustentaculum tali with the right index finger. The left index is shown measuring the space between the medial malleolus and sustentaculum tali.

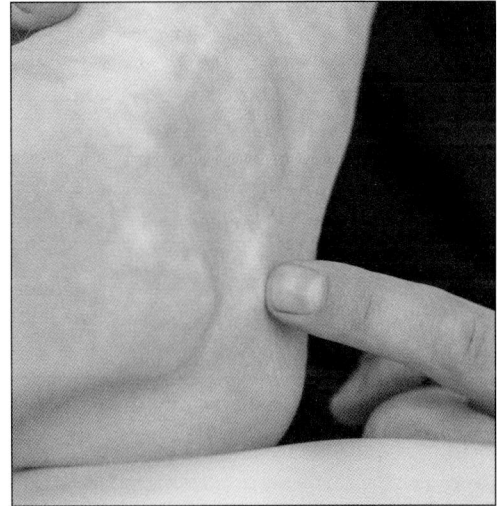

Figure 17.150. Palpating the posterolateral calcaneal tuberosity with the index finger.

Posterolateral calcaneal tuberosity: The posterolateral calcaneal tuberosity sits on the lateral side of the posterior calcaneus (figure 17.150).

Testing

Global: As with the talus described above, begin by testing the calcaneus globally (and directly with the spreading and twisting phase) to find (*a*) if the bone is compacted

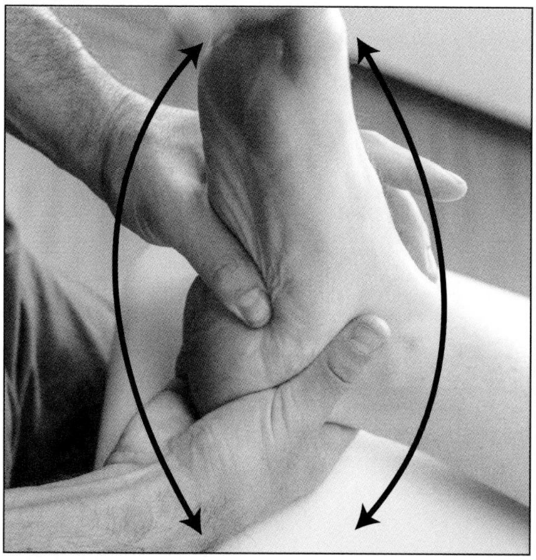

Figure 17.151. Anteroposterior spreading and twisting of the calcaneus.

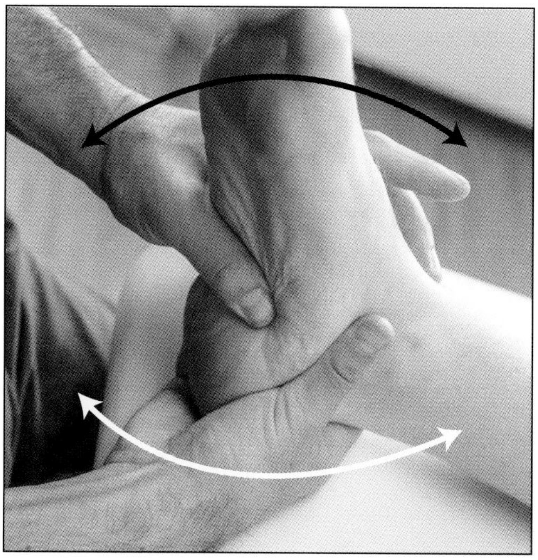

Figure 17.153. Superoinferior spreading and twisting of the calcaneus.

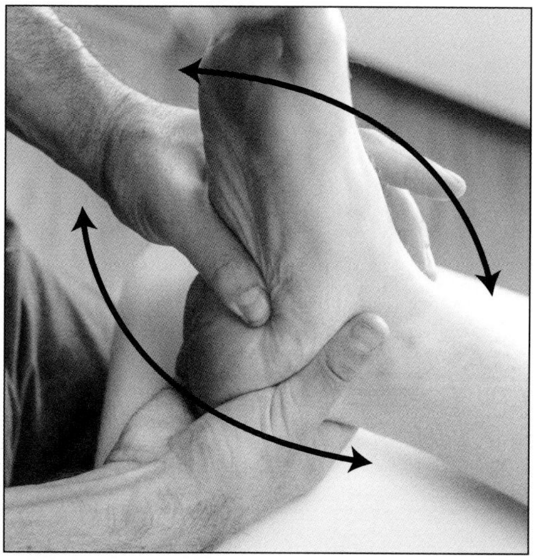

Figure 17.152. Mediolateral spreading and twisting of the calcaneus.

- in a mediolateral direction (one hand moving medially and one hand moving laterally, then reverse and repeat), twisting in both directions (figure 17.152).
- in a superoinferior direction (one hand moving proximally and one hand moving distally, then reverse and repeat), twisting in both directions (figure 17.153).

Now, test the connections between the calcaneus and its neighbors by applying a spreading and twisting force between the calcaneus and the talus (figure 17.154) and between the calcaneus and cuboid (figure 17.155).

Does the calcaneus or any of the connections with its neighbors feel like wood or concrete in any direction? Is there one part of the bone that feels more compacted than another? If the whole bone feels more like wood, move to the next bone to be tested. If the whole calcaneus, any segments of the calcaneus, or any of the connections with its neighbors feels more like concrete or is fibrotic, either move directly to treatment or retest specific segments.

and (*b*) the specific pattern of compaction. Sit facing the foot, holding calcaneus in the global grip described above. Spread the calcaneus:

- in an anteroposterior direction (one hand moving toward the toes and one hand moving toward the heel, then reverse and repeat), twisting in both directions (figure 17.151).

142

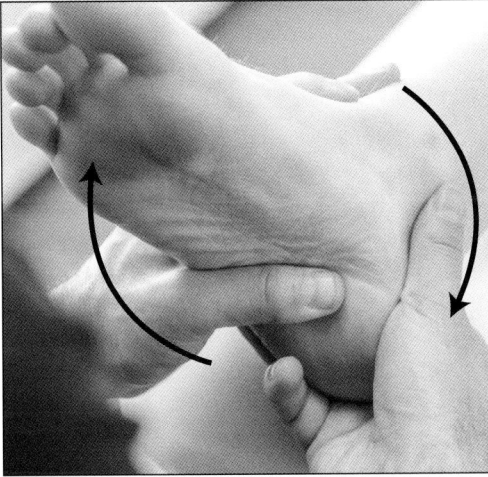

Figure 17.154. Spreading and twisting the connection between the calcaneus and the talus. The top, lateral hand "suctions" the talus away from the calcaneus, which is stabilized by the medial, bottom hand.

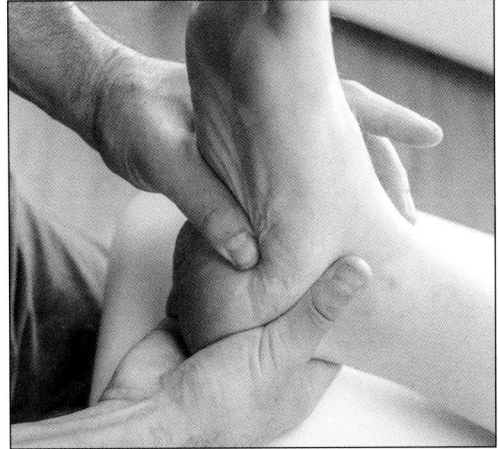

Figure 17.155. Spreading and twisting the connection between the calcaneus and the cuboid. The lateral hand pinches the cuboid with the thumb and index finger while the medial hand stabilizes the calcaneus.

Local treatment

Grasp the bone in a comfortable way and proceed with the six stages of BST treatment (see "Quick Guide to the Six Stages of BST Treatment"). Local treatment of the calcaneus can be applied from either

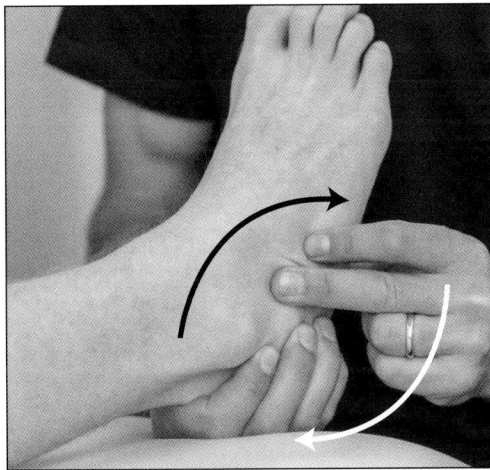

Figure 17.156. Local treatment of the calcaneus using the global hold.

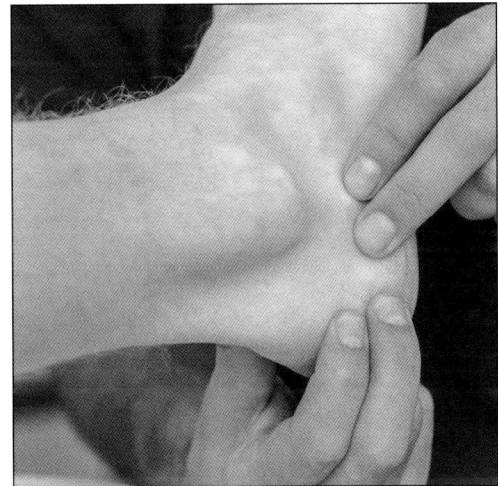

Figure 17.157. Hand positions for the specific treatment of the lateral surface of the calcaneus using the thumb (medial surface) and index and middle fingers.

the global hold (figure 17.156) or more specifically to any of the segments. If one or more of the segments of the calcaneus are compacted, or if the global approach is insufficient, change hand positions to apply the six stages of treatment specifically to the lateral surface of the calcaneus (figure 17.157), medial surface and posteromedial calcaneal tuberosity (figure 17.158), sustentaculum tali

143

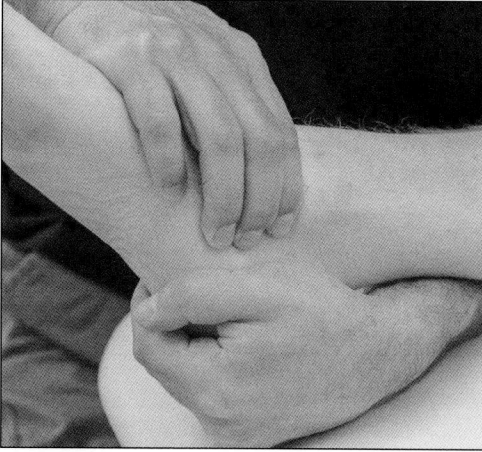

Figure 17.158. Hand positions for the specific treatment of the medial surface and posteromedial calcaneal tuberosity using the hand and thenar eminence of one hand and the index, middle, and ring fingers of the other.

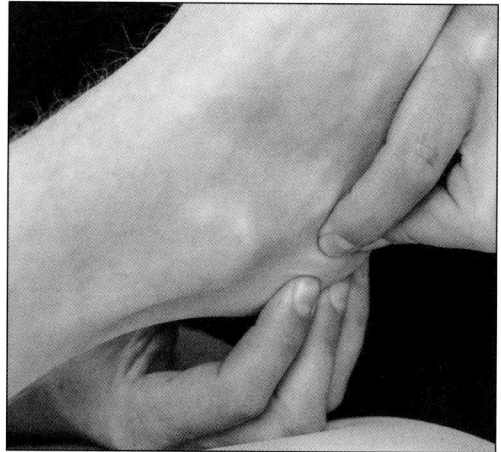

Figure 17.160. Hand positions for the specific treatment of the posterolateral calcaneal tuberosity using the thumbs (stabilizing the bone on the medial surface) and the index and middle fingers.

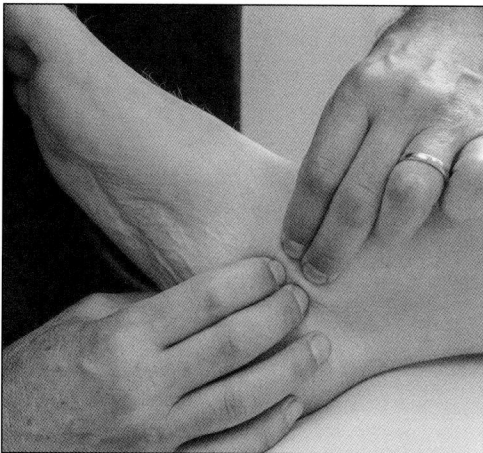

Figure 17.159. Hand positions for the specific treatment of the sustentaculum tali using the index and middle fingers of both hands.

(figure 17.159), or posterolateral calcaneal tuberosity (figure 17.160).

Regional treatment

Integrate the local treatment of the calcaneus into the region by using the hindfoot gather technique (see "Regional Treatment").

LOWER EXTREMITY

Excluding the bones of the feet, each lower extremity contains four bones: the fibula, tibia, patella, and femur (figure 17.161).

Tibia

After the femur, the tibia is the second largest bone in the body. It has three segments: a distal end, which includes the medial malleolus and articulates with the talus and the lateral malleolus, a subcutaneous shaft, and a proximal end, which joins the femur and head of the fibula (figure 17.162).

Neighbors

Talus
Fibula
Femur

Palpation

Global: Locate the extremities of the tibia by placing one hand just below the joint

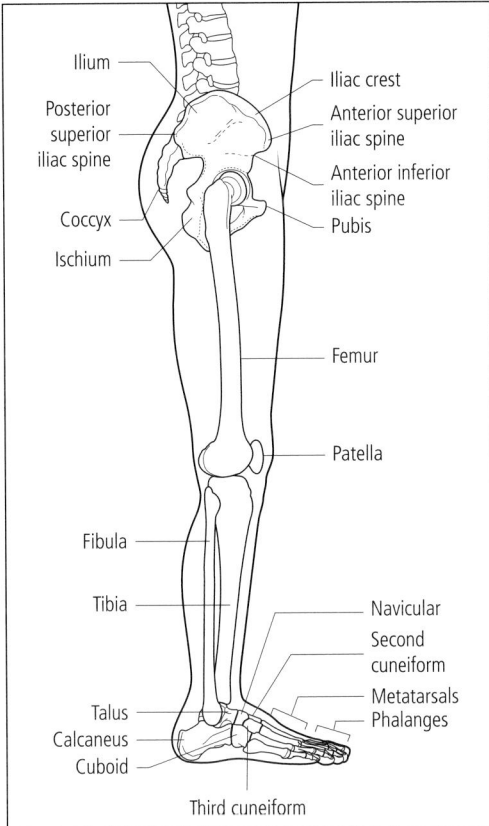

Figure 17.161. Lower extremity.

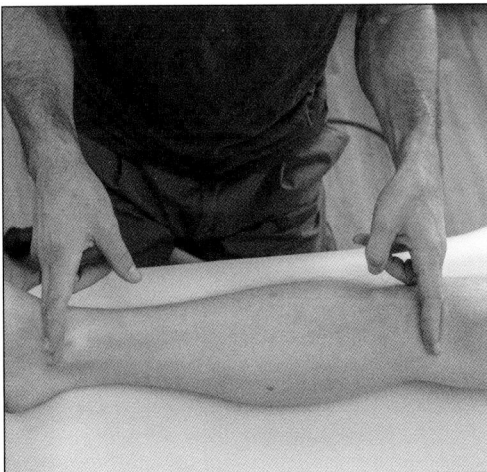

Figure 17.162. Tibia.

line with the femur and the other hand just above the joint line with the talus (figure 17.163).

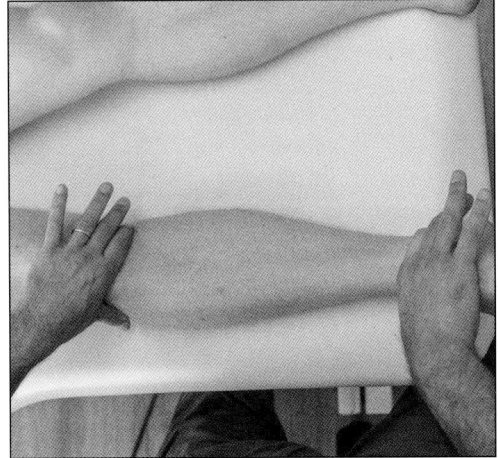

Figure 17.163. Global palpation of the tibia.

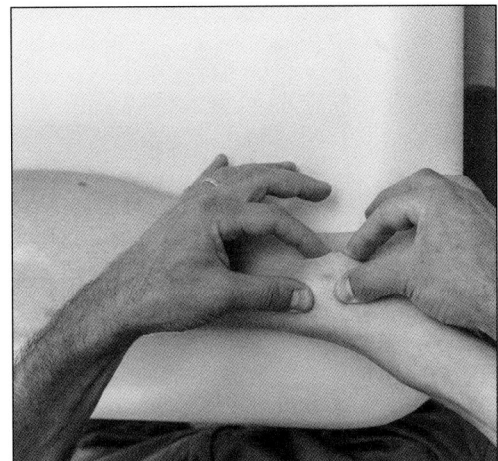

Figure 17.164. Palpating the medial malleolus of the tibia.

Medial malleolus: Follow the bone down its protuberance on the medial side of the foot (figure 17.164).

Distal end: From the medial malleolus, follow the medial border of the tibia all around the distal end of the bone until the articulation with the fibula. If you hold the distal end of the tibia with one hand and plantar flex and dorsiflex the foot with the other hand, the demarcation between the talus and the tibia will become even clearer (figure 17.165). You can also surround the ankle with both hands and ask the subject to wiggle their foot.

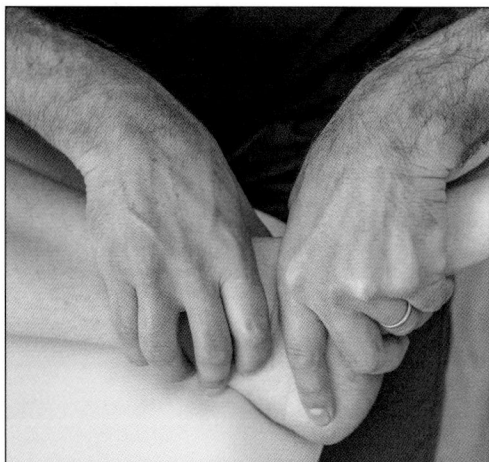

Figure 17.165. Palpating the distal end of the tibia with the proximal hand.

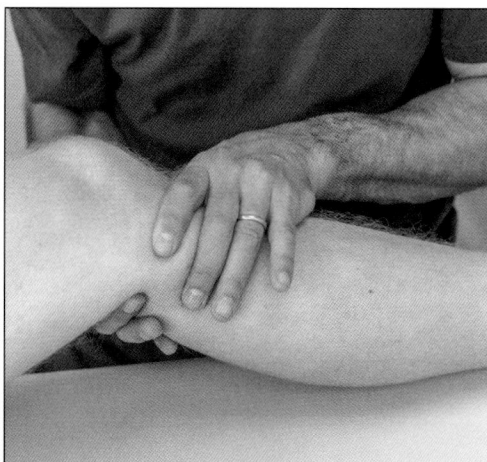

Figure 17.167. Palpating the proximal end of the tibia.

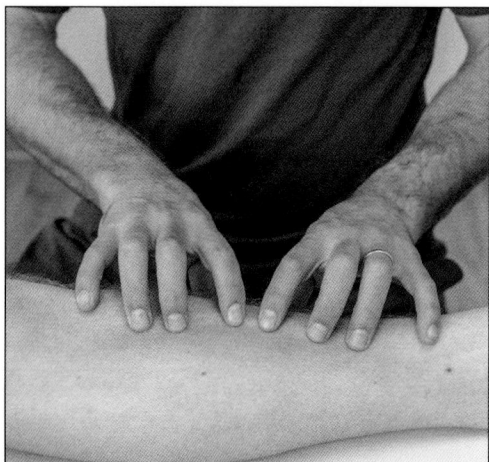

Figure 17.166. Palpating the shaft of the tibia.

Shaft: Follow the shaft of the bone back up toward the knee (figure 17.166).

Proximal end: Once at the knee, palpate around the joint line between the tibia and femur, then move back down onto the wider proximal end, or tibial plateau (figure 17.167). To find the joint line, palpate the line with one hand and with the other hand flex and extend the knee until the demarcation becomes clear.

Testing

As with other larger bones, global testing usually precedes more specific testing and can be done in phases. For the connections between the tibia and its neighbors, (and since the bones are relatively large), instead of performing a preliminary joint test, jump right into the spreading and twisting phase—this will give you the necessary information in one step.

Phase 1: Perform a global transverse scan. Starting at the medial malleolus, apply firm pressure transversely and in series, moving up the tibia toward the proximal end, evaluating the texture of the bone (figure 17.168). The scan is a quick way to test the bone's ability to flex. Take note of any specific compacted areas, including within the medial malleolus, distal end, shaft, and proximal end.

Phase 2: Perform a global longitudinal test. Place one hand just distal to the joint line of the knee. Place the other hand just proximal to the joint line with the talus. Apply a longitudinal tensile force into the bone,

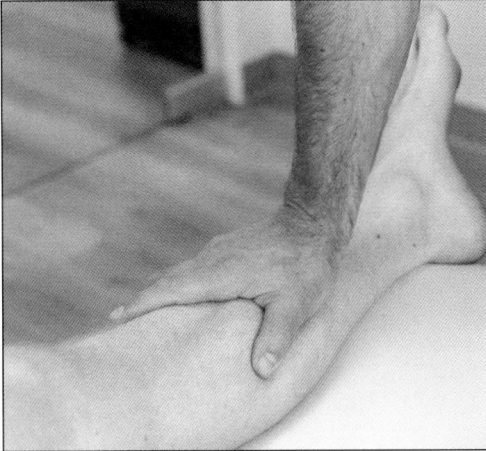

Figure 17.168. Phase 1: Global transverse scan of the tibia. Apply firm pressure into the shaft of the bone, moving up from distal to proximal.

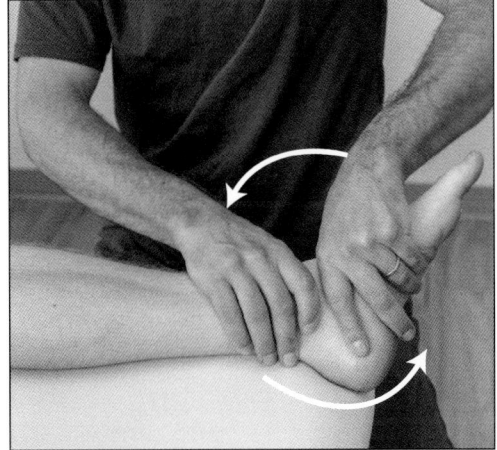

Figure 17.170. Phase 2: Spreading and twisting the connection between the tibia and the talus using the thenar spaces of each hand.

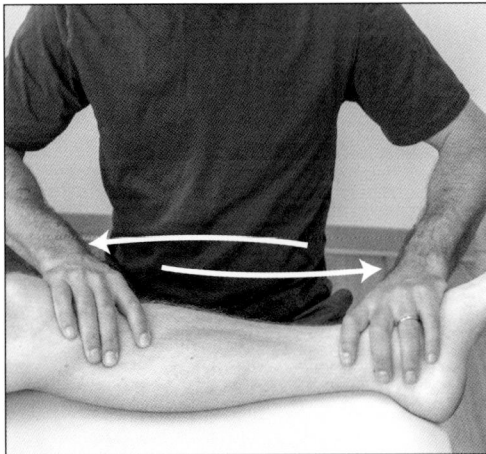

Figure 17.169. Phase 2: Global longitudinal test of the tibia. Spread and twist the bone in different directions. In this photo, the spreading action of the distal hand is being applied mainly with the index and middle fingers, with the other two fingers resting passively on the foot.

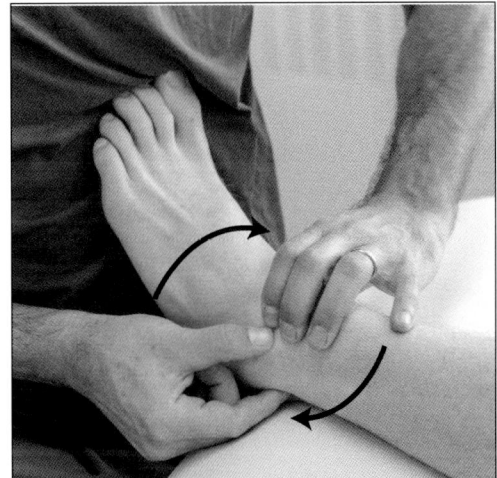

Figure 17.171. Phase 2: Spreading and twisting the connection between the tibia and the lateral malleolus.

lateral malleolus (figure 17.171), and between the tibia and the femur (figure 17.172).

twisting it in both directions (figure 17.169). Take note of any compacted areas, including within the distal end, medial malleolus, shaft, and proximal end.

Now, spread and twist the connections between the tibia and the talus (figure 17.170), between the tibia and the

If the bone and its connections possess elasticity, move to the next bone to be tested. If the entire tibia, any segments, or any of the connections with its neighbors feels more like concrete than like wood or is fibrotic, move directly to treatment, or retest specific segments, if necessary.

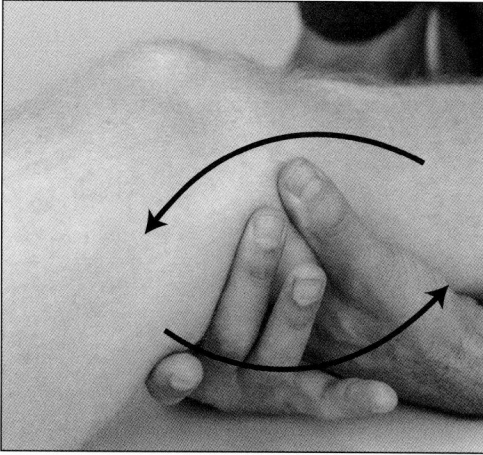

Figure 17.172. Phase 2: Spreading and twisting the connection between the tibia and the femur.

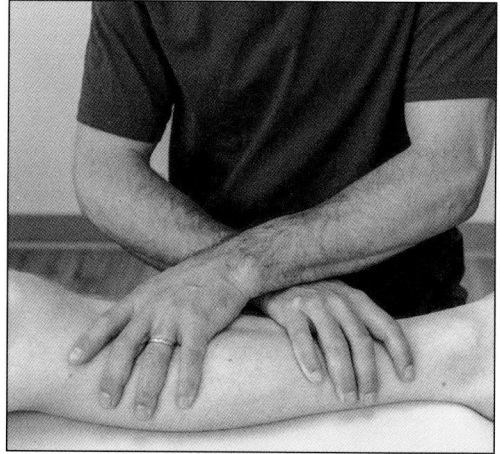

Figure 17.174. Hand position for the spreading and integration stages of local treatment of the tibia.

Local treatment

Grasp the bone in a comfortable way and proceed with the six stages of BST treatment (see "Quick Guide to the Six Stages of BST Treatment"). As with most of the larger bones, local treatment can be applied from either the global hold or from more specific holds to any of the segments or connections.

Global: Grasp the tibia in the global hold described above (figure 17.173). This position

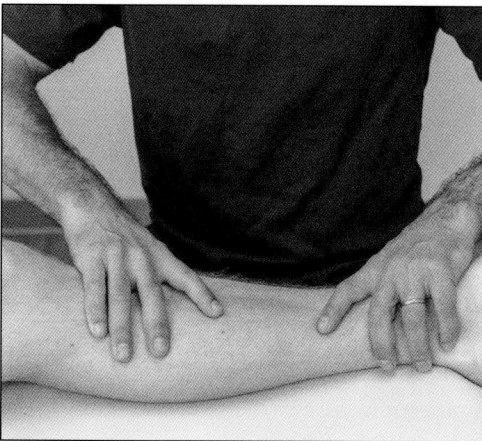

Figure 17.173. Global hand position for the cocooning, compression, dialogue, and augmentation stages of local treatment of the tibia.

is great for the cocooning, compression, dialogue, and augmentation stages of treatment.

For the spreading and integration stages, you may wish to cross your hands to more efficiently apply a spreading force to the bone (figure 17.174).

Specific segments: If one or more of the segments of the tibia are compacted, and if the global approach is insufficient, change positions to apply the six stages of treatment specifically to the medial malleolus (figure 17.175), distal end (figure 17.176), specific parts of the shaft (figure 17.177), or tibia plateau (figure 17.178).

Regional treatment

Integrate the local treatment of the tibia into the region by using the lower extremity gather technique (see "Regional Treatment").

Fibula

The fibula is the other bone of the lower leg, and is more slender than the tibia. It has three

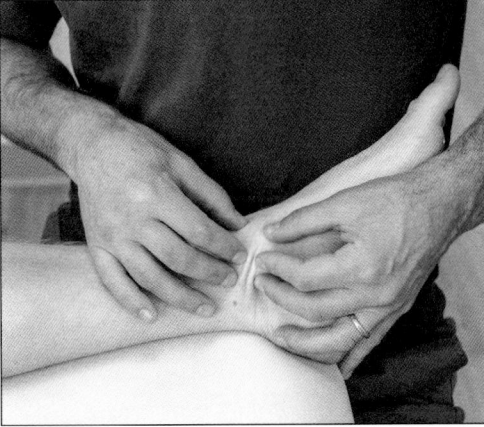

Figure 17.175. Hand position for the specific treatment of the medial malleolus.

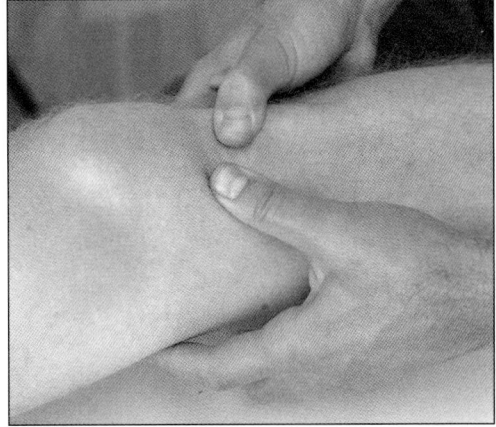

Figure 17.176. Hand position for the specific treatment of the distal end of the tibia.

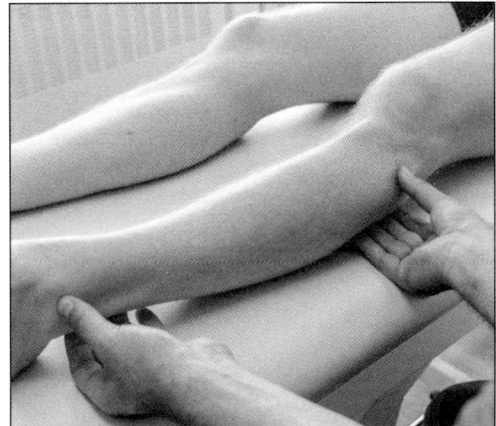

Figure 17.177. Hand position for the treatment of a specific part of the shaft of the tibia.

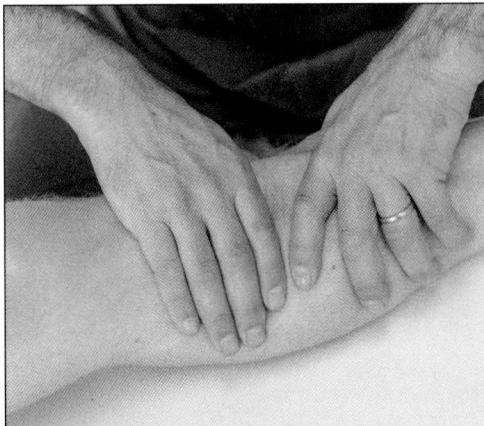

Figure 17.178. Hand position for the treatment of the tibial plateau, using the thumbs to treat a specific section of the plateau.

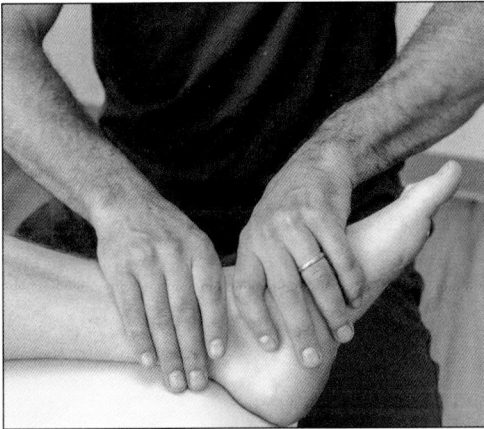

Figure 17.179. Fibula.

segments: the proximal end, the shaft, and the lateral malleolus (figure 17.179).

Neighbors

Talus
Tibia

Palpation

Global: Locate the extremities of the fibula by placing one hand on the distal end at the lateral malleolus on the external side of the ankle and the other hand on the proximal end just below the knee joint (figure 17.180).

149

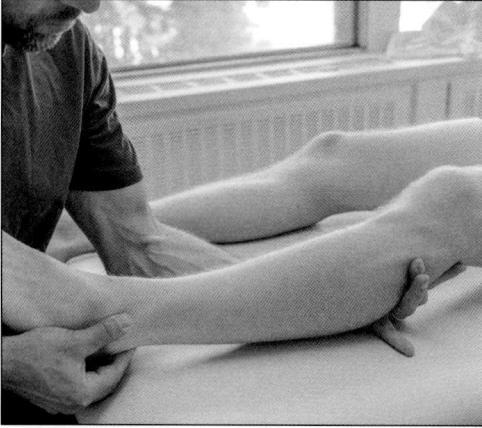

Figure 17.180. Global palpation of the fibula.

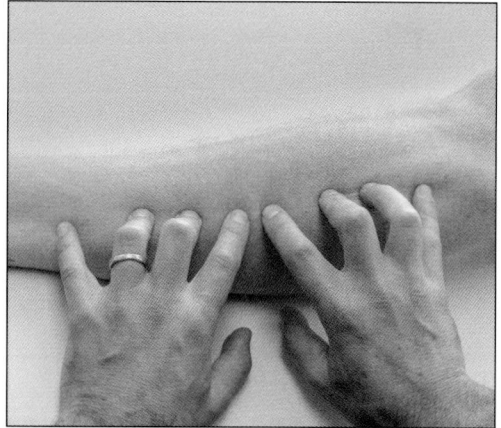

Figure 17.182. Palpating the shaft of the fibula.

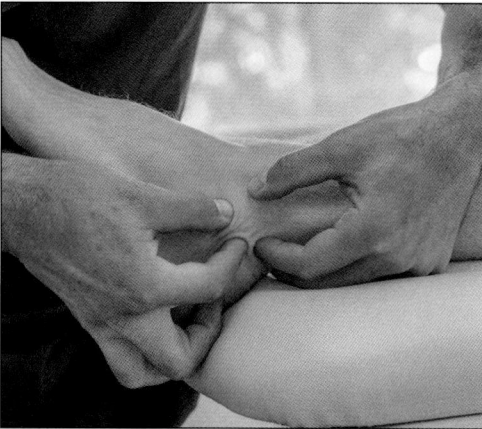

Figure 17.181. Palpating the lateral malleolus of the fibula with the thumbs and index fingers.

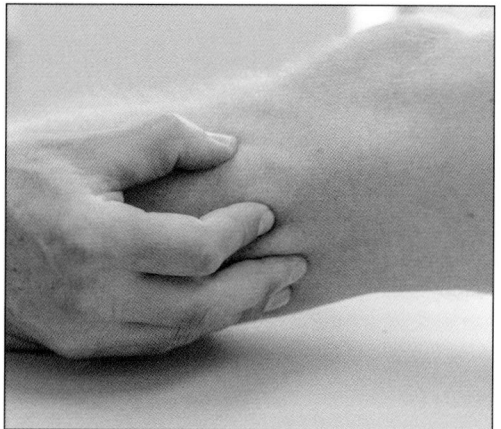

Figure 17.183. Palpating the proximal end of the fibula with the thumb and index finger.

Lateral malleolus: Follow the bone down its protuberance on the lateral side of the ankle (figure 17.181).

Shaft: Follow the shaft of the bone back up toward the knee (figure 17.182).

Proximal end: Palpate the bony protuberance on the lateral side of the lower leg just below the knee joint line (figure 17.183).

Testing

As with other large bones, global testing usually precedes more specific testing, and can be done in phases, if necessary. For the connections between the fibula and its neighbors, and since the bones are relatively large, instead of performing a preliminary joint test, jump right into the spreading and twisting phase—this will give you the necessary information in one step.

Phase 1: Have the subject lie on the opposite side to be tested. Perform a global transverse scan. Starting at the lateral malleolus, apply firm pressure transversely into the fibula and in series, moving up the bone toward the proximal end, evaluating the texture of the bone (figure 17.184). The scan is a quick way to test the bone's ability to flex. Take note of any specific compacted areas, including within the lateral malleolus, shaft, and proximal end.

Phase 2: Have the subject return to supine. Perform a global longitudinal test. With one hand, grasp the proximal end of the fibula, and with the other hand, hold the lateral malleolus. Apply a longitudinal tensile force into the bone, twisting it in both directions (figure 17.185). Again, take note of any

compacted areas, including within the lateral malleolus, shaft, and proximal end.

Spread and twist the connections between the lateral malleolus and the talus (figure 17.186), between the lateral malleolus and the distal tibia (figure 17.187), between the shaft of the fibula and the shaft of the tibia (figure 17.188), and between the proximal

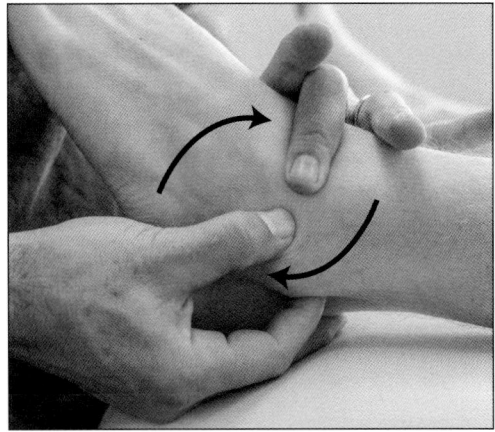

Figure 17.186. Spreading and twisting the connection between the lateral malleolus and the talus, pinching the lateral malleolus with the thumb and index finger of the lateral hand and stabilizing the talus with the middle finger of the medial hand.

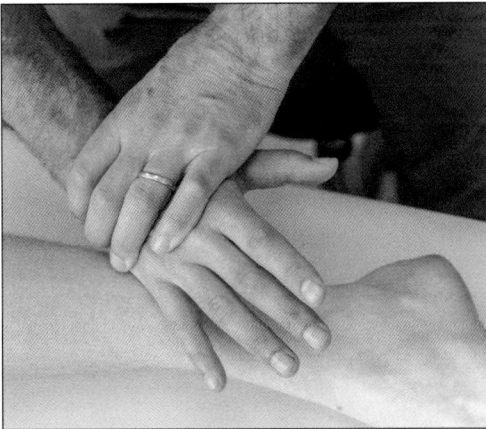

Figure 17.184. Phase 1: Global transverse scan of the fibula. Apply firm pressure into the shaft toward the table, moving in series from distal to proximal.

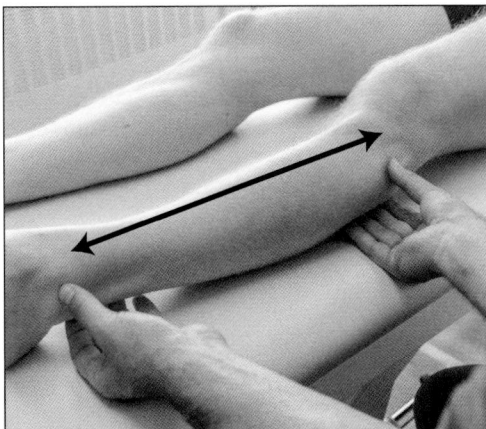

Figure 17.185. Phase 2: Global longitudinal test of the fibula using the thumbs and index fingers.

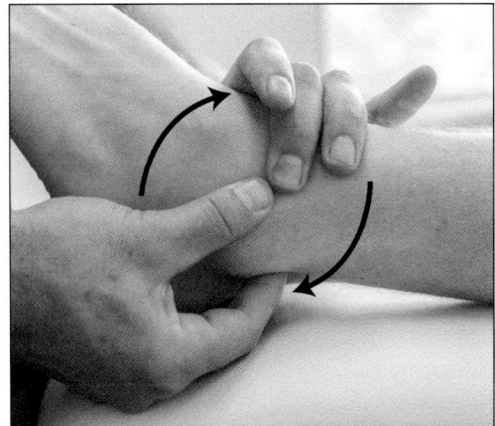

Figure 17.187. Spreading and twisting the connection between the lateral malleolus and the distal tibia, pinching the lateral malleolus with the thumb and index finger of the lateral hand and stabilizing the tibia with the middle finger of the medial hand.

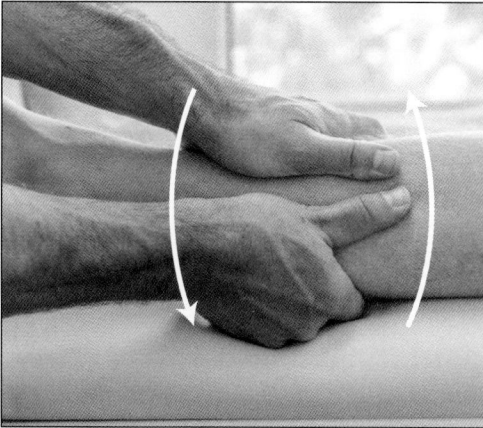

Figure 17.188. Spreading and twisting the connection between the shaft of the fibula and the shaft of the tibia using the thenar eminences of each hand to spread the bones apart. This can be repeated in series along the shaft of the bones.

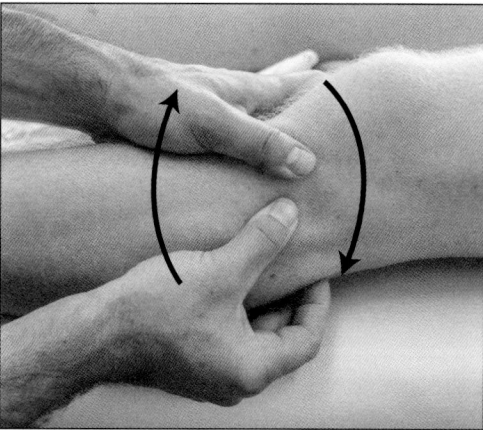

Figure 17.189. Spreading and twisting the connection between the proximal fibula and the proximal tibia using primarily the thumbs.

end of the fibula and the proximal end of the tibia (figure 17.189).

If the whole bone and its connections possess sufficient elasticity, move to the next bone(s) to be tested. If the entire fibula, any segments, or any of the connections with the fibula and its neighbors feels more like concrete than like wood or is fibrotic, move directly to treatment, or retest specific segments, if necessary.

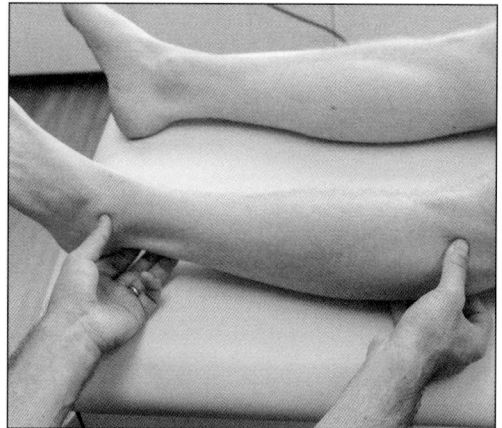

Figure 17.190. Global hand position for the cocooning, compression, dialogue, and augmentation stages of local treatment of the fibula.

Local treatment

Grasp the bone in a comfortable way and proceed with the six stages of BST treatment (see "Quick Guide to the Six Stages of BST Treatment"). As with most of the larger bones, local treatment can be applied from either the global hold or from more specific holds to any of the segments or connections.

Global: Grasp the fibula in the global hold (figure 17.190).

For the next two stages, you may wish to cross your hands to more efficiently apply a spreading force to the bone (figure 17.191).

Specific segments: If one or more of the segments of the fibula is compacted, and if the global approach is insufficient, change positions to apply the six stages of treatment to the lateral malleolus (figure 17.192), specific parts of the shaft (figure 17.193), or proximal end (figure 17.194).

Regional treatment

Integrate the local treatment of the fibula into the region by using the lower extremity gather technique (see "Regional Treatment").

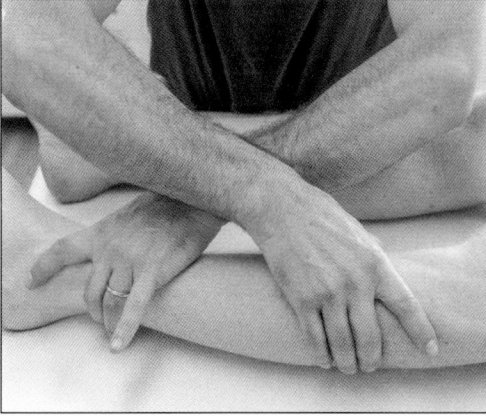

Figure 17.191. Crossed-hand position for the spreading and integration stages of local treatment of the fibula.

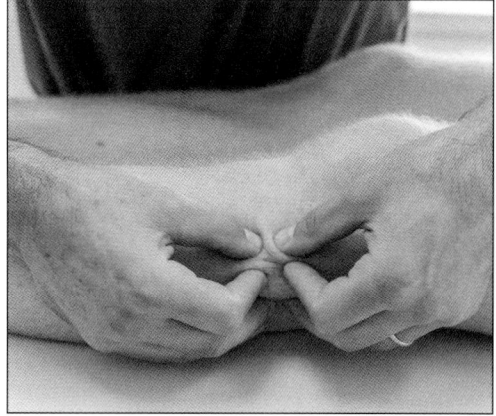

Figure 17.192. Hand position for the specific treatment of the lateral malleolus using the thumbs and middle fingers.

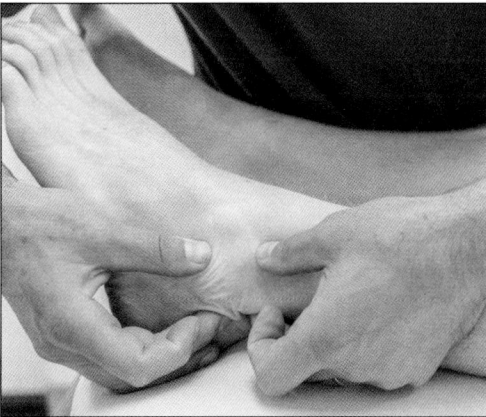

Figure 17.193. Hand position for the treatment of a specific part of the shaft of the fibula using the thumbs and index fingers.

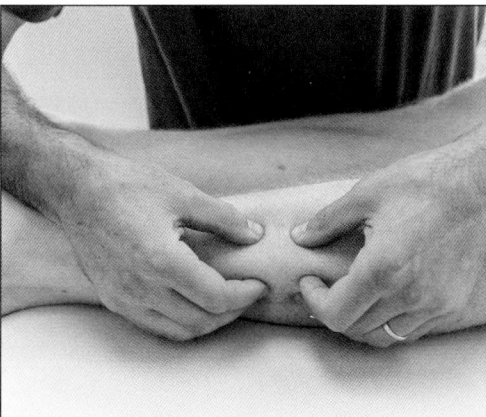

Figure 17.194. Hand position for the specific treatment of the proximal end of the fibula using the thumbs and index fingers.

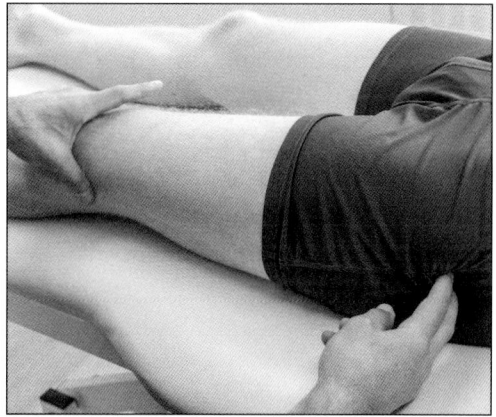

Figure 17.195. Femur.

Femur

The femur is the longest and strongest bone in the body. It has four segments: the distal end, the shaft, the greater trochanter, and the head and neck (figure 17.195).

Neighbors

Tibia
Patella
Iliac

Palpation

Besides the greater trochanter, and unlike the tibia and fibula, which are subcutaneous,

153

all segments of the femur are well surrounded by muscle tissue. For this reason, really take your time descending through the muscle until you reach the bone.

Global: Locate the extremities of the femur by placing one hand on the distal end where it meets the tibia. With the other hand, follow the femur up toward the pelvis to the greater trochanter, the bony prominence on the lateral side of the pelvis (figure 17.196).

Distal end: Follow the bone back down to the medial and lateral protuberances just above the knee joint line. Flex and extend the knee of the subject to palpate the distal end more clearly (figure 17.197).

Shaft: Follow the shaft of the bone up toward the hip. Practice descending through the quadriceps muscles to the bony level. Go slowly—too much force here can be uncomfortable for the subject (figure 17.198).

Greater trochanter: Palpate the bony protuberance on the lateral side of the upper leg (figure 17.199).

Testing

As with other larger bones, global testing usually precedes more specific testing.

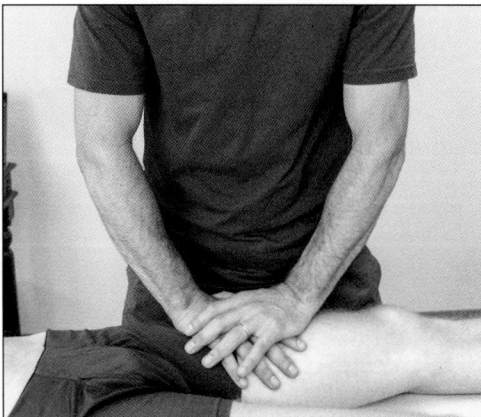

Figure 17.197. Palpating the distal end of the femur with the thumb and middle finger.

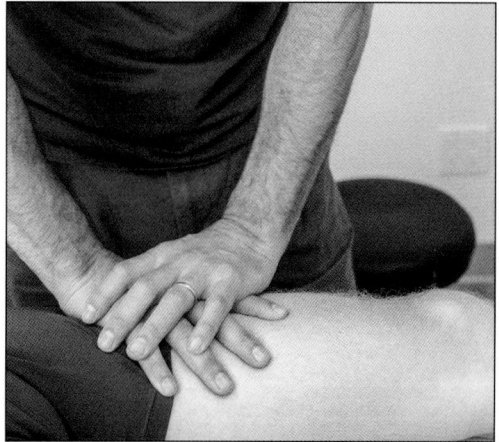

Figure 17.198. Palpating the shaft of the femur.

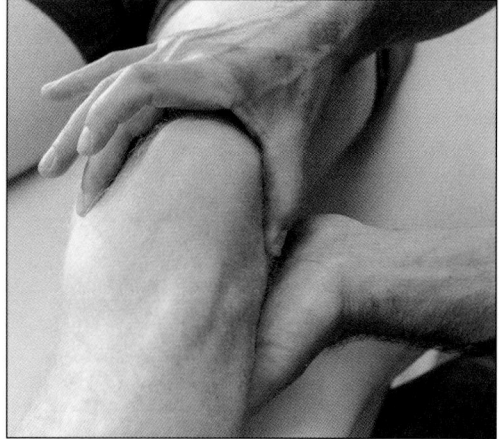

Figure 17.196. Global palpation of the femur.

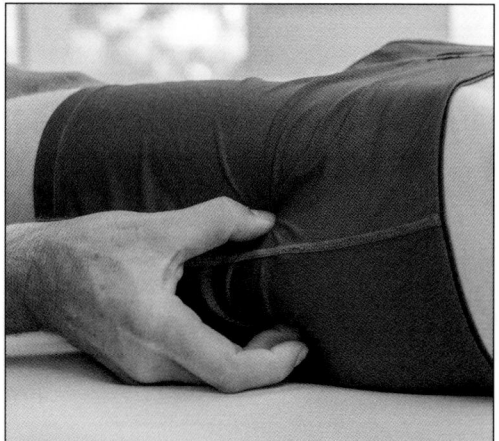

Figure 17.199. Palpating the greater trochanter of the femur with the thumb and middle finger.

For the connections between the femur and its neighbors, and since the bones are relatively large, I suggest directly performing the spreading and twisting phase, since this will give you the necessary information in one step.

Phase 1: Perform a global transverse scan. Starting at the distal end of the femur just proximal to the patella, apply firm pressure transversely into the bone and in series, moving up toward the proximal end. Descend slowly until you reach the bone, evaluating the texture of the shaft (figure 17.200). The scan is a quick way to test the bone's ability to flex. Take note of any specific compacted areas, including within the distal end, the shaft, and the greater trochanter.

Phase 2: Perform a global longitudinal test. With one hand, grasp the distal end of the femur, and with the other hand, hold the greater trochanter. This hand position is identical to the global palpation test described above. Apply a longitudinal tensile force into the bone, twisting it in both directions (figure 17.201). Take note of any compacted areas.

Now, spread and twist the connections between the distal end of the femur and the tibia (figure 17.202), between the distal end of the femur and the patella (figure 17.203), and between the head of the femur and the acetabulum of the iliac. One way to test the connection between the head of the femur and the acetabulum is to place the leg of the subject over your shoulder, grasp the upper thigh with both arms, and apply a tensile force parallel to the angle of the femoral neck (figure 17.204).

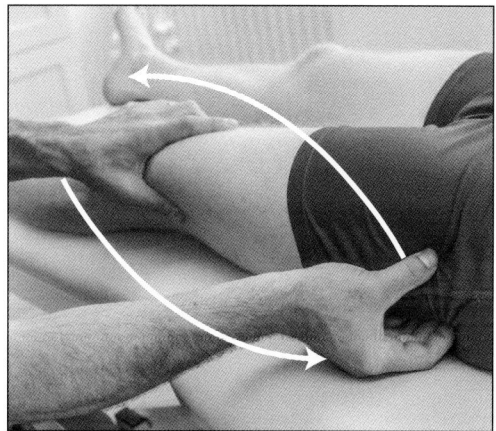

Figure 17.201. Phase 2: Global longitudinal test of the femur. Spread and twist the bone in different directions.

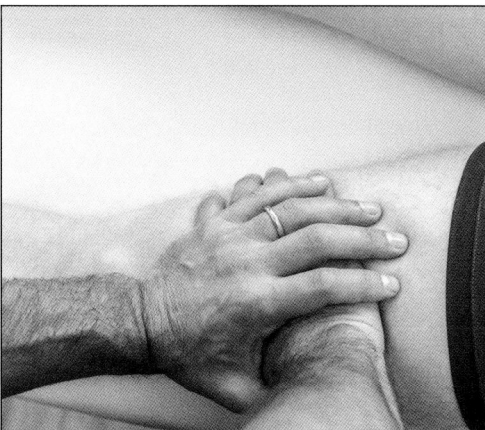

Figure 17.200. Phase 1: Global transverse scan of the femur. Descend slowly until you reach the bone, evaluating the texture of the shaft.

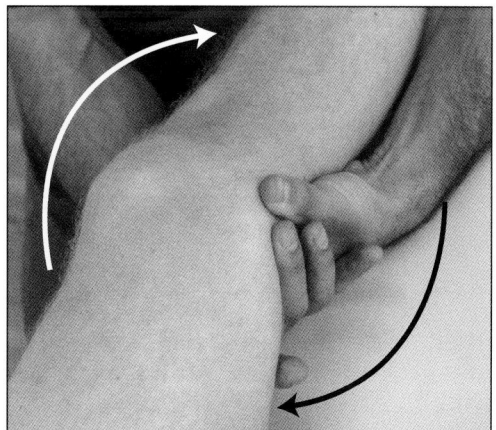

Figure 17.202. Spreading and twisting the connection between the distal end of the femur and the tibia with both hands on the posterior side of the leg.

155

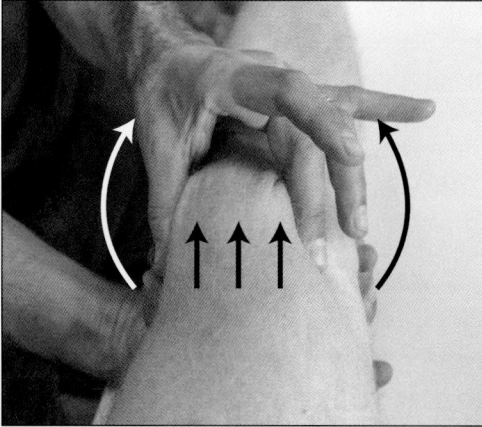

Figure 17.203. Spreading and twisting the connection between the patella and the distal end of the femur. Stabilize the femur with the bottom hand and lift the patella away from the bone with the thumb and index finger.

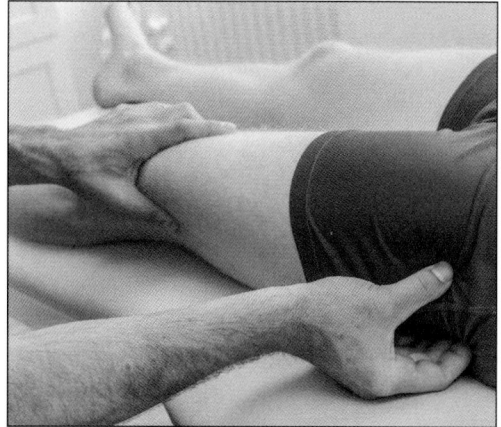

Figure 17.205. Global hand position for the cocooning, compression, dialogue, and augmentation stages of local treatment of the femur.

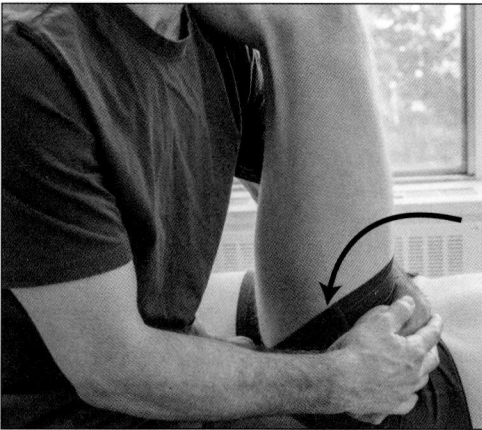

Figure 17.204. Spreading and twisting the connection between the femoral head and the acetabulum.

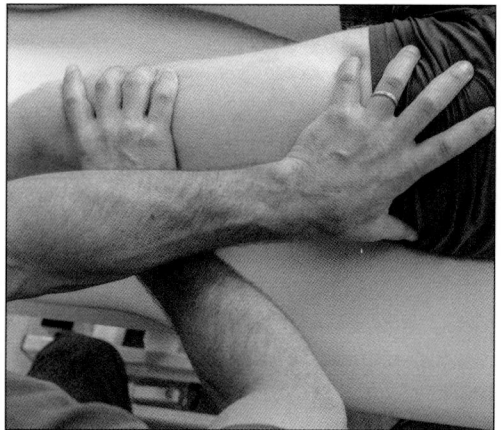

Figure 17.206. Crossed-hand position for the spreading and integration stages of local treatment of the femur.

If the whole bone and its connections possess sufficient elasticity, move to the next bone to be tested. If the entire femur, any segments, or any of the connections between the femur and its neighbors feels more like concrete than like wood or is fibrotic, move directly to treatment, or retest specific segments, if necessary.

Local treatment

Grasp the bone in a comfortable way and proceed with the six stages of BST treatment (see "Quick Guide to the Six Stages of BST Treatment"). As with most of the larger bones, local treatment can be applied from either the global hold or from more specific holds to any of the segments or connections.

Global: For the first four stages, grasp the femur (figure 17.205).

For the spreading and integration stages, you may wish to cross your hands to more efficiently apply a spreading force to the bone (figure 17.206).

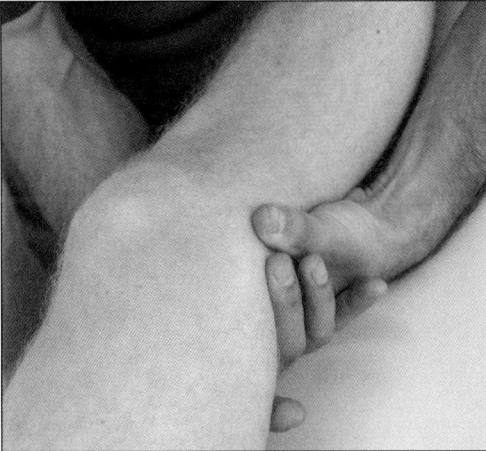

Figure 17.207. Hand position for the specific treatment of the distal end of the femur.

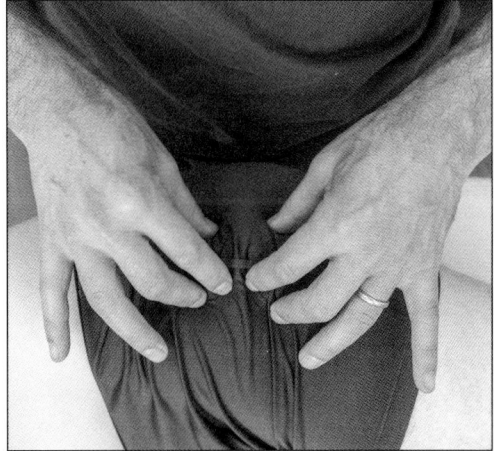

Figure 17.209. Hand position for the specific treatment of the greater trochanter.

Specific segments: If one or more of the segments of the femur is compacted, and if the global approach is insufficient, change hand positions to apply the six stages of treatment specifically to the distal end (figure 17.207), specific parts of the shaft (figure 17.208), or greater trochanter (figure 17.209).

Regional treatment

Integrate the local treatment of the femur into the region by using the lower extremity gather technique (see "Regional Treatment").

For the femoral head and neck and its articulation with the acetabulum, the pelvic gather will also work.

Patella

The patella is embedded within the quadriceps and patellar tendons, making it the largest sesamoid bone in the body. It is triangular in shape and sits between the two distal condyles of the femur (figure 17.210).

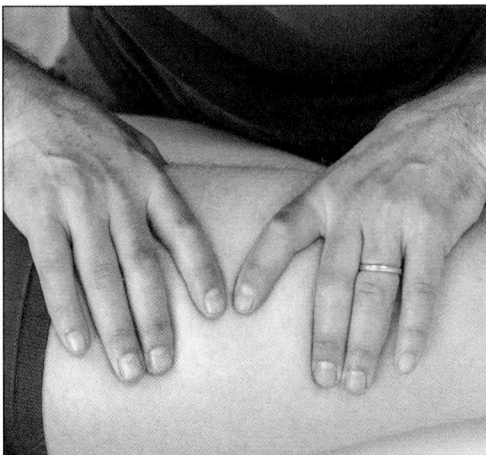

Figure 17.208. Hand position for the treatment of a specific part of the shaft of the femur.

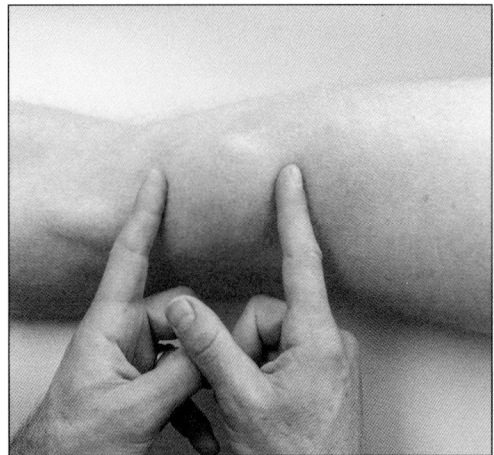

Figure 17.210. Patella.

157

Neighbor

Femur

Testing

Make sure that the leg of the subject is fully extended on the table to give the patella and quadriceps tendons slack. Grasp the patella with both sets of fingers and spread and twist the bone in different directions to determine if it is compacted and in which specific direction (figure 17.211).

Now, gently apply a lifting force to evaluate the connection with the femur (figure 17.212).

If the whole bone and its connections possess sufficient elasticity, move to the next bone to be tested. If the patella or its connections feel more like concrete than like wood or are fibrotic, move to treatment.

Local treatment

An example of a hand position for local treatment of the patella is shown in figure 17.213. Grasp the bone in a comfortable way and proceed with the six stages of BST treatment (see "Quick Guide to the Six Stages of BST Treatment").

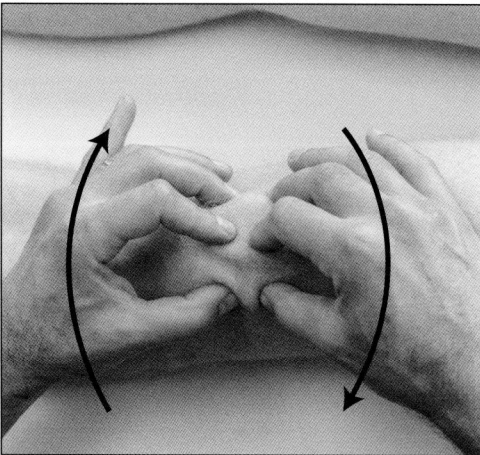

Figure 17.212. Spreading and twisting the connection between the patella and the femur by lifting the patella toward the ceiling with the thumb and index finger and stabilizing the femur with the other hand.

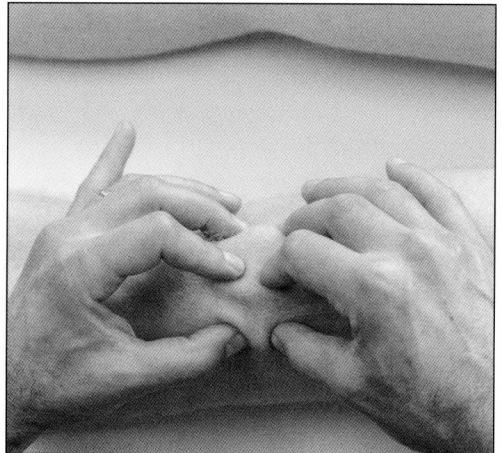

Figure 17.213. Hand position for treatment of the patella using the thumbs and index fingers.

Regional treatment

Integrate the local treatment of the femur into the region by using the lower extremity gather technique (see "Regional Treatment").

PELVIS

The pelvis comprises four bones: the two innominate bones, the sacrum, and the coccyx (figure 17.214).

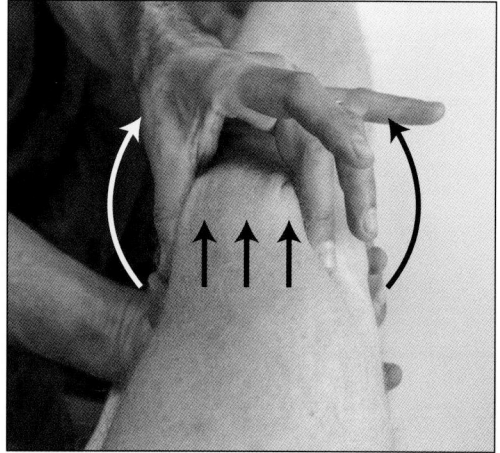

Figure 17.211. Spreading and twisting the patella.

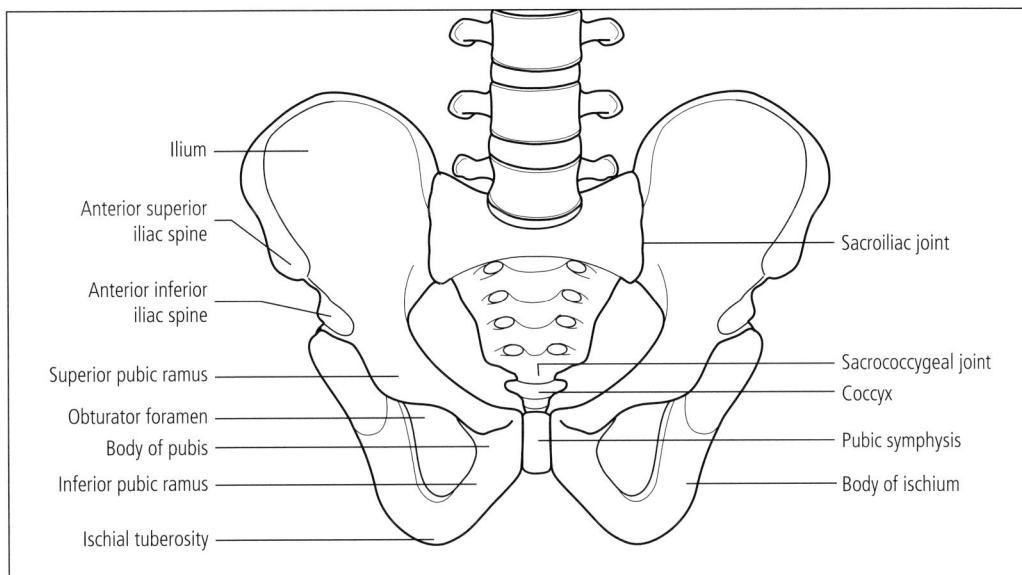

Figure 17.214. Pelvis.

Labels (left side, top to bottom): Ilium; Anterior superior iliac spine; Anterior inferior iliac spine; Superior pubic ramus; Obturator foramen; Body of pubis; Inferior pubic ramus; Ischial tuberosity

Labels (right side, top to bottom): Sacroiliac joint; Sacrococcygeal joint; Coccyx; Pubic symphysis; Body of ischium

Innominates

The innominate bone has three sections: the ilium, ischium, and pubis. The ilium is the large, dish-shaped blade above and behind the acetabulum, the round fossa that receives the head of the femur (figure 17.215). The ischium (figure 17.226) expands downward from the acetabulum into the

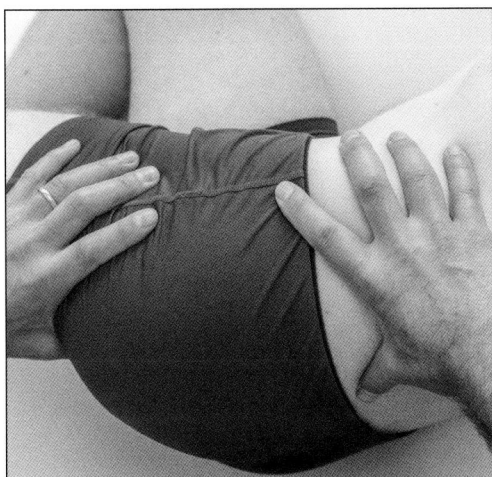

Figure 17.215. Ilium.

ischial tuberosity, then curves back up toward the pubis (figure 17.235). The superior pubic ramus extends inward from the acetabulum, running horizontally, where it joins the opposite pubis at the pubic symphysis.

The ilium is delineated by the iliac crest above, the upper border of the acetabulum below, and by its posterior and anterior edges. The crest is bookended on each side by the anterior and posterior superior iliac spines. Below each spine is a notch, and below the notches are the anterior and posterior inferior iliac spines, respectively. The ischium has two parts; a body and a ramus. The body includes the ischial tuberosity, otherwise known as the "sit bone." Below, we'll discuss the palpation, testing, and local treatment of each segment separately. There are many ways to approach the innominates. This is one suggestion for an ilium-ischium-pubis sequence that I find works quite well.

159

Neighbors

Sacrum
Opposite innominate
Femur

Ilium

All three steps (palpation, testing, and treatment) can be done with the subject in a side-lying position.

Palpation

With the patient lying on the side opposite the one to be treated, locate the crest and then follow it in each direction toward the anterior and posterior superior spines and down toward the upper rim of the acetabulum (figure 17.216).

Testing

Phase 1: With hands crossed on the upper section of the ilium, apply a tensile force to the section of bone between the anterior and posterior superior iliac spines (figure 17.217). With hands still crossed, move the palm of one hand into the concavity of the ilium and the other hand

to the ischial tuberosity (figure 17.218). Even though the ischial tuberosity is not technically part of the ilium, it gives us a solid handle for the testing and treatment of the posteroinferior section. Apply a tensile force between your hands, testing the bone. Have the subject turn over and repeat on the other side. Does the bone feel normal? If yes, move to the next section to be tested. If the bone is compacted, move to phase 2.

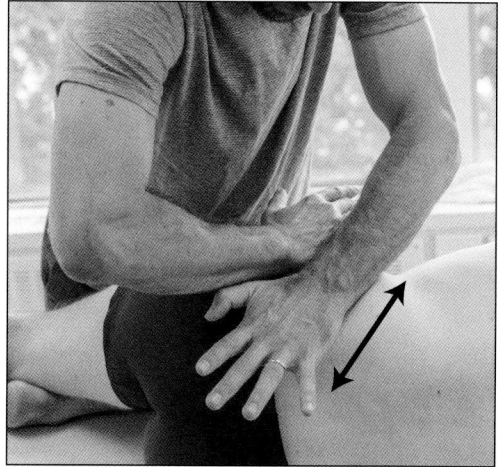

Figure 17.217. Phase 1: Testing the upper section of the ilium.

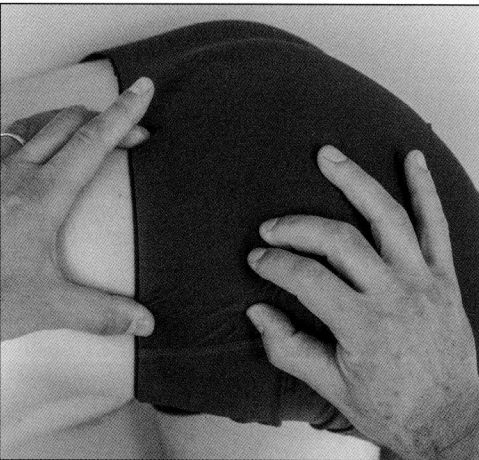

Figure 17.216. Palpating the ilium.

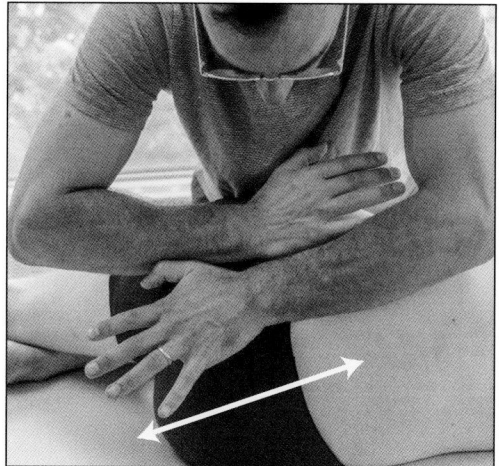

Figure 17.218. Phase 1: Testing the posteroinferior section of the ilium.

Phase 2: Spread and twist the compacted upper (figure 17.219) or posteroinferior (figure 17.220) segment of the ilium to determine the most rigid torsional pattern of compaction.

Local treatment

Grasp the upper (figures 17.221 and 17.223) or posteroinferior (figures 17.222 and 17.224) sections of the ilium and proceed with the six stages of BST treatment (see "Quick Guide to the Six Stages of BST Treatment").

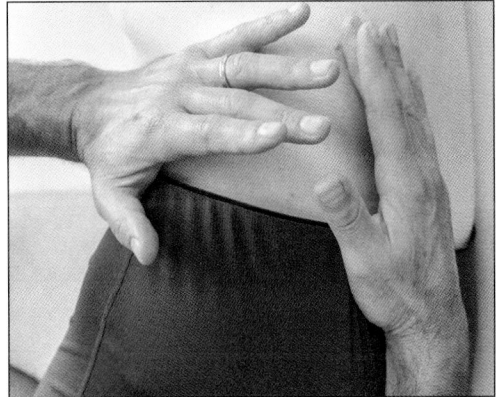

Figure 17.221. Hand position for the cocooning, compression, dialogue, and augmentation stages of local treatment of the upper section of the ilium.

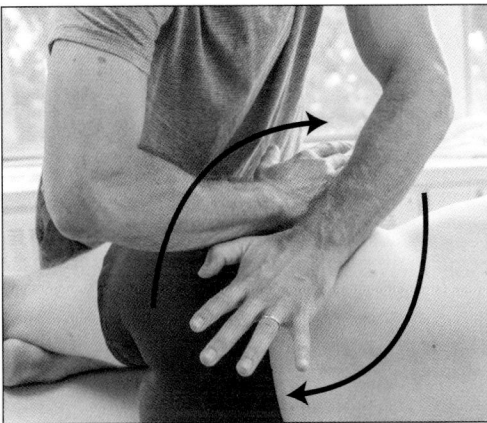

Figure 17.219. Phase 2: Spreading and twisting the upper section of the ilium.

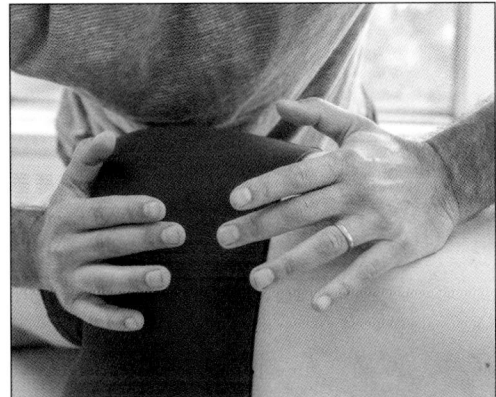

Figure 17.222. Hand position for the cocooning, compression, dialogue, and augmentation stages of local treatment of the posteroinferior section of the ilium.

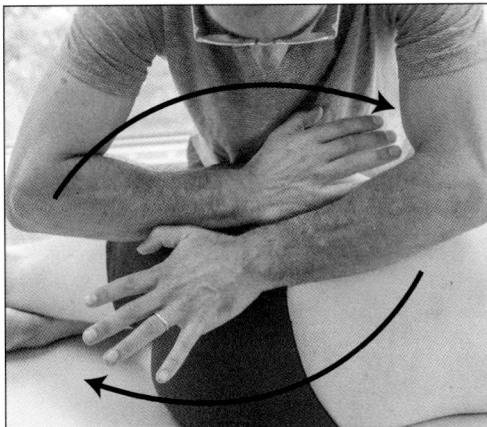

Figure 17.220. Phase 2: Spreading and twisting the posteroinferior section of the ilium.

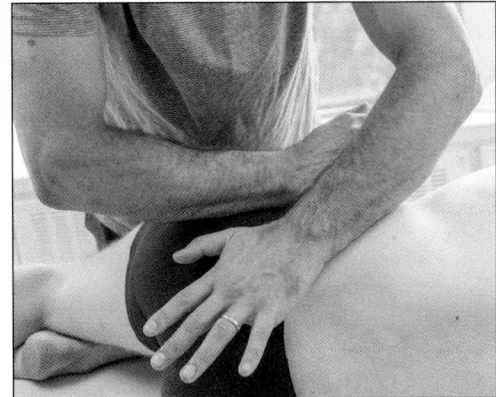

Figure 17.223. Hand position for the spreading and integration stages of local treatment of the upper section of the ilium.

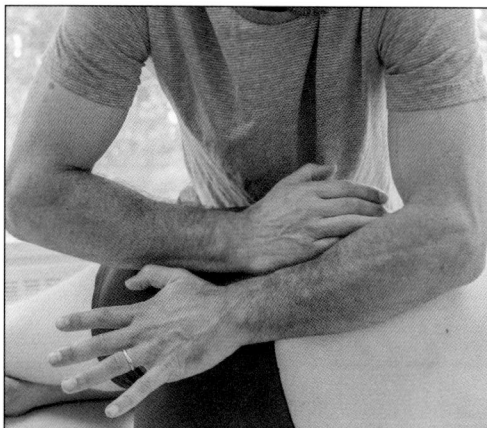

Figure 17.224. Hand position for the spreading and integration stages of local treatment of the posteroinferior section of the ilium.

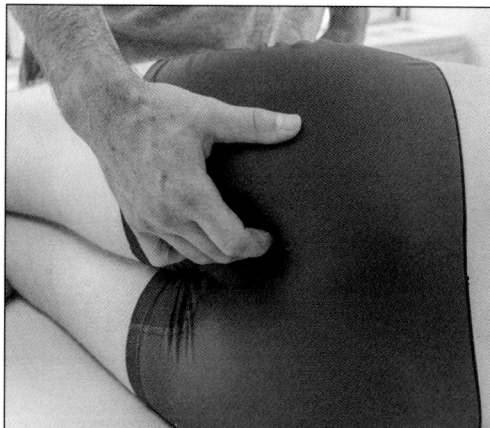

Figure 17.225. Ischium.

For the spreading and integration stages, return to the crossed-hand positions (figures 17.223 and 17.224).

Regional treatment

Integrate the local treatment of the ilium into the region by using the pelvic gather technique (see "Regional Treatment").

Ischium

As with the ilium, palpation, testing, and treatment of the ischium can be done with the patient in a side-lying position (figure 17.225).

Palpation

Follow the ilium down behind the greater trochanter of the femur toward the lateral side of the ischium (figure 17.226). From there, palpate the body of the ischium and ischial tuberosity by curling the fingers around the bone (figure 17.227).

Testing

With the subject on the same side as above, test the lateral side of the *same* ischium. Then, without having the subject change sides

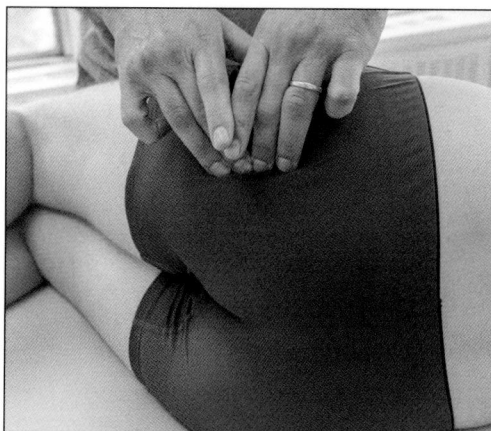

Figure 17.226. Palpating the ischium by following the bone down from behind the greater trochanter.

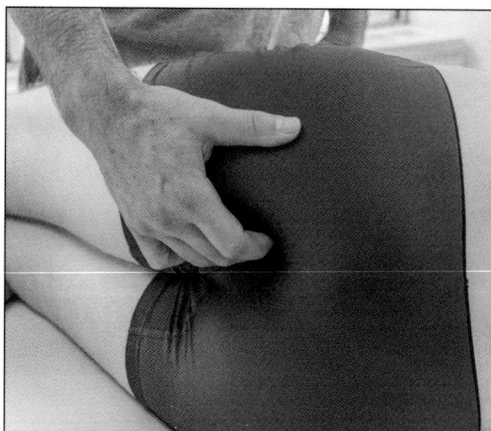

Figure 17.227. Palpating the ischial tuberosity by hooking the fingers underneath the bone.

and by staggering their legs accordingly, test the ischial tuberosity on the *opposite* side.

Phase 1: Move one hand to a global position along the ilium, with the other on the lateral part of the ischial tuberosity (figure 17.228). Apply a tensile force between your hands. Now, have the subject stagger their legs to expose the medial aspect of the opposite ischial tuberosity. With both hands, apply a tensile force to the bone (figure 17.229). Have the subject turn onto the other side and repeat both steps. Do the bones feel normal? If yes, move to the next section to be tested. If either of the bones is compacted, move to phase 2.

Phase 2: Spread and twist the compacted segment to determine the most rigid torsional pattern of compaction (figures 17.230 and 17.231).

Local treatment

Grasp the ischium (figure 17.232) or opposite ischial tuberosity (figure 17.233) and proceed with the six stages of BST treatment (see "Quick Guide to the Six Stages of BST Treatment"). For the spreading and integration stages of treatment of the ischium, and to apply a more efficient spreading force, return to the crossed-hand position used for

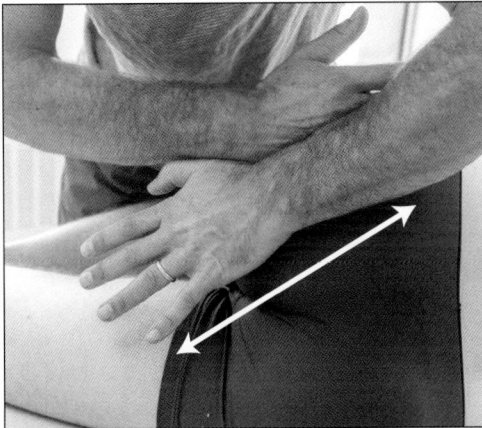

Figure 17.228. Phase 1: Testing the ischium.

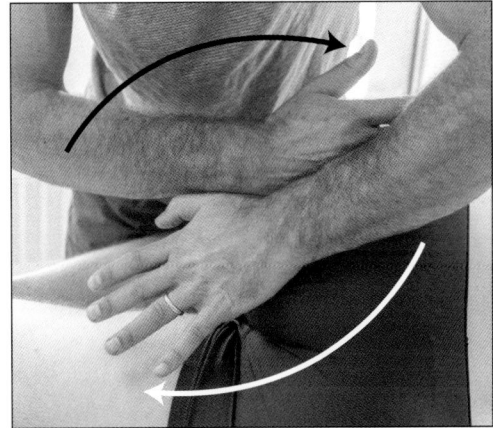

Figure 17.230. Phase 2: Spreading and twisting the ischium.

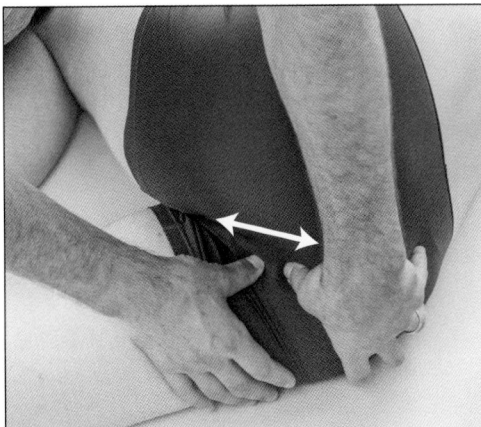

Figure 17.229. Phase 1: Testing the opposite ischial tuberosity with the thumbs.

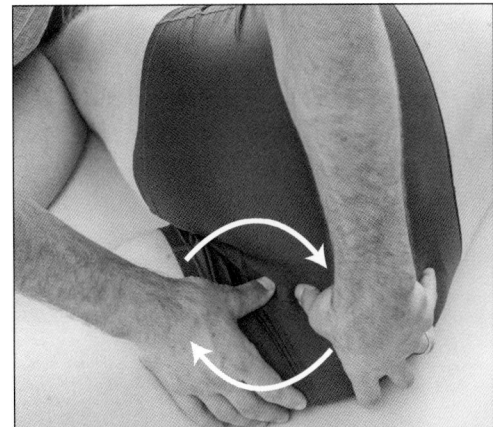

Figure 17.231. Phase 2: Spreading and twisting the opposite ischial tuberosity with the thumbs.

testing (figure 17.234). For the tuberosity, adjust the hands if necessary.

Regional treatment

Integrate the local treatment of the ischium into the region by using the pelvic gather technique (see "Regional Treatment").

Pubis

For the testing and treatment of the pubis, have the subject turn to supine (figure 17.235).

Palpation

Slide the heel of the hand down the abdomen to the pubic symphysis (figure 17.236) and then onto the superior pubic ramus on each side (figure 17.237).

Testing

Phase 1: With the subject supine, test each pubic ramus (figure 17.238) and the symphysis (figure 17.239) by spreading the bone(s). Then, cross the hands, place one hand on the iliac crest and the other on the

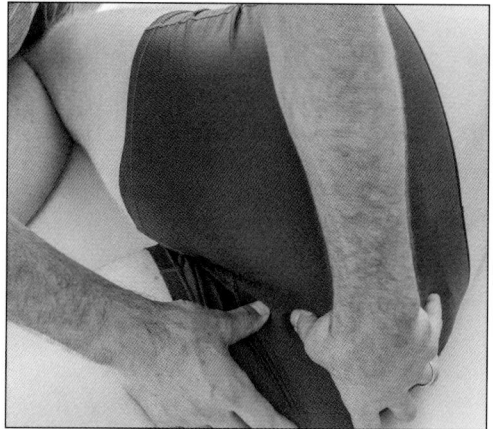

Figure 17.232. Hand position for the cocooning, compression, dialogue, and augmentation stages of local treatment of the ischium using the palms of each hand.

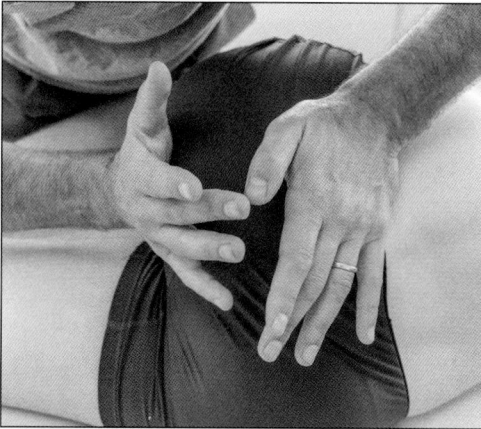

Figure 17.234. Hand position for the local treatment of the ischial tuberosity with the thumbs.

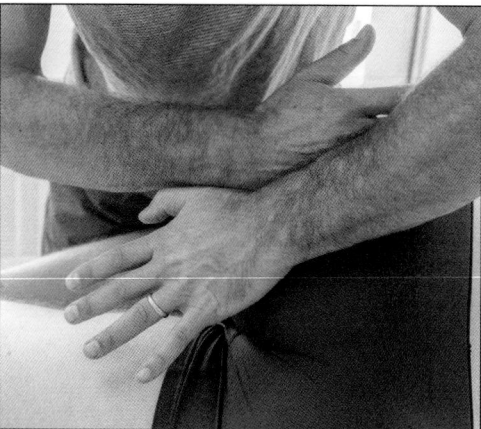

Figure 17.233. Hand position for the spreading and integration stages of local treatment of the ischium.

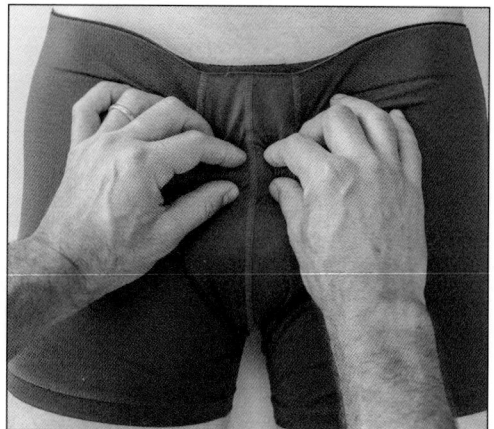

Figure 17.235. Pubis.

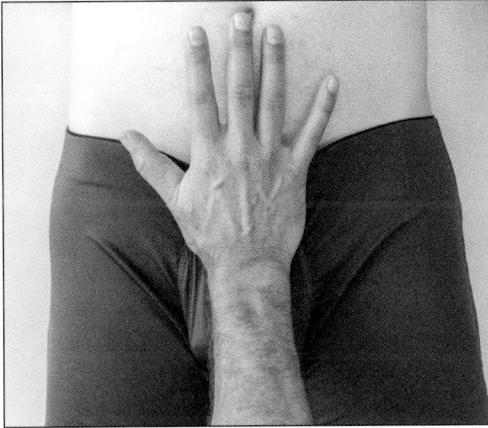

Figure 17.236. Palpating the pubic symphysis by sliding the heel of the hands down the abdomen onto the bone.

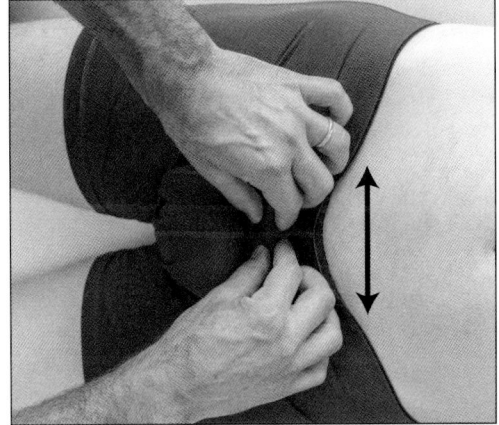

Figure 17.239. Phase 1: Testing the pubic symphysis by applying a tensile force between the two bones.

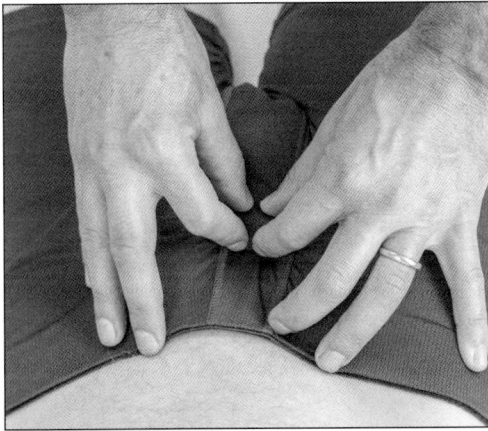

Figure 17.237. Palpating the right superior pubic ramus with the thumbs and index fingers.

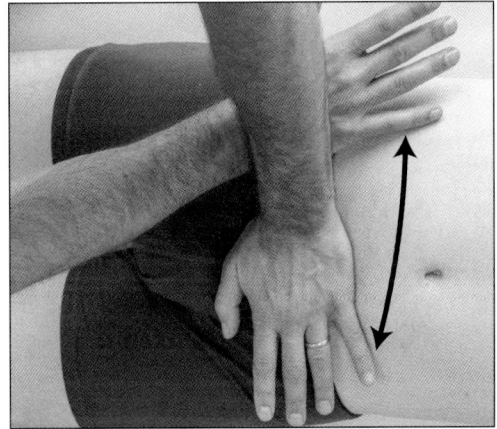

Figure 17.240. Phase 1: Testing the right pubis with the ilium by applying a tensile force with the palms of the hands.

same pubic ramus (figure 17.240). Apply a tensile force between the hands to test the iliopubic segment, including the superior pubic ramus where it ascends to meet the ilium. Repeat on both sides.

Do the bones feel normal? If yes, move to the next segment to be tested. If either of the bones is compacted, move to phase 2.

Phase 2: Spread and twist the compacted segment to determine the most rigid torsional pattern of compaction (figures 17.241–17.243).

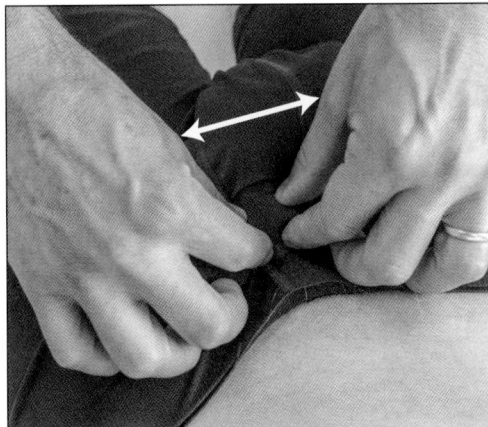

Figure 17.238. Phase 1: Testing the left pubic ramus with the thumbs and index fingers.

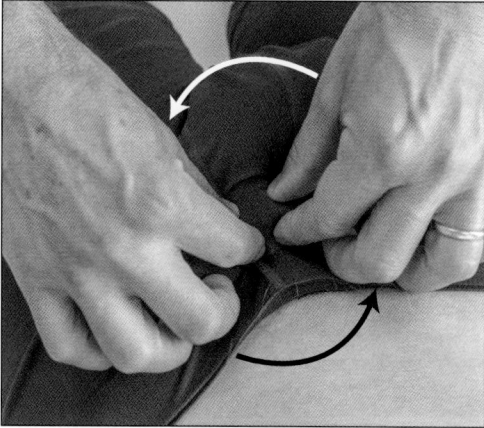

Figure 17.241. Phase 2: Spreading and twisting the left pubic ramus with the thumbs and index fingers.

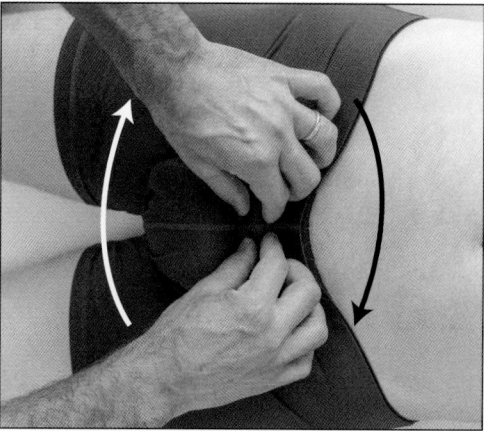

Figure 17.242. Phase 2: Spreading and twisting the symphysis with the thumbs and index fingers.

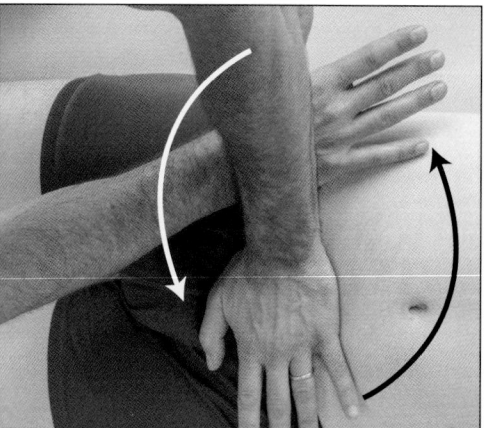

Figure 17.243. Phase 2: Spreading and twisting the right pubis and ilium.

Local treatment

Grasp the pubic ramus (figure 17.244), pubic symphysis (figure 17.245), or the iliopubic segment (figure 17.246), and proceed with the six stages of BST treatment (see "Quick Guide to the Six Stages of BST Treatment"). For the spreading and integration stages of treatment for the iliopubic segment, and to apply a more efficient spreading force, recross the hands as was done during testing (figure 17.246). For the pubic rami and symphysis, adjust the hands if necessary.

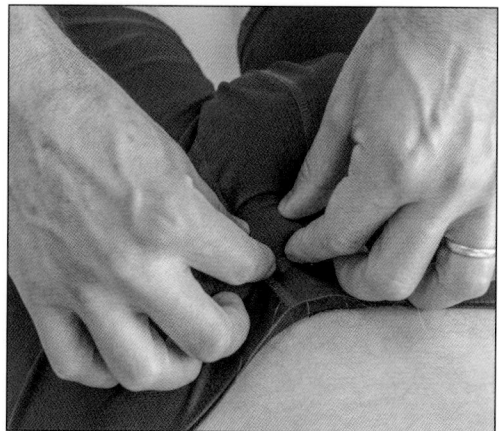

Figure 17.244. Hand position for the local treatment of the pubic ramus.

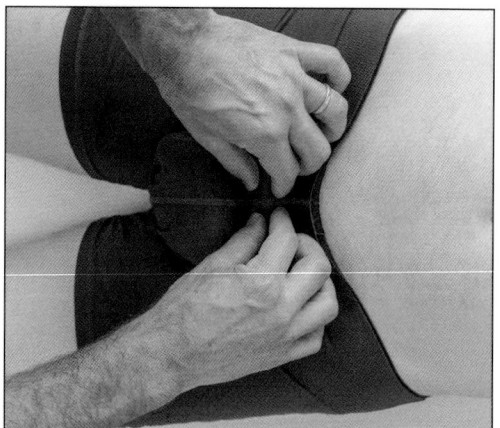

Figure 17.245. Hand position for the local treatment of the pubic symphysis.

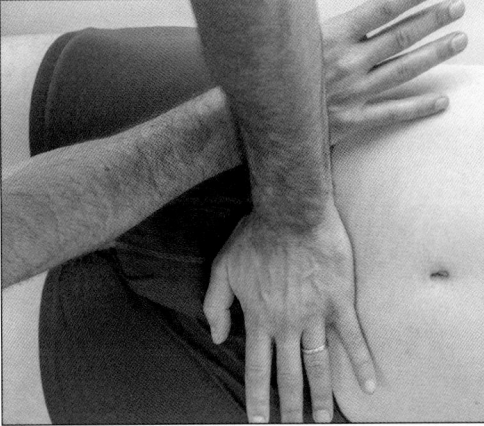

Figure 17.246. Hand and position for the local treatment of the iliopubic segment. This photo depicts the crossed-hand position, which can be used for all six stages or just the spreading and integration stages.

Regional treatment

Integrate the local treatment of the pubis into the region by using the pelvic gather technique (see "Regional Treatment").

Sacrum and coccyx

The sacrum is a triangular bone that sits at the base of the spine and between the fifth lumbar vertebra (L5), the two ilia, and the coccyx. Along with the coccyx, the sacrum forms the inferior posterior border of the pelvic bowl (figure 17.247). It has a prominent medial crest running from its proximal base to its distal apex, where it articulates with the coccyx. The sacrum sits obliquely in relation to L5, forming the oblique promontory angle at the sacrolumbar joint. The degree of the obliquity can vary considerably from one person to the next. The posterior surface of the sacrum is convex and bumpy, displaying three or four prominent tubercles forming the ridge of the medial crest. Lateral to the spinous tubercles are the sacral laminae, and lateral to the laminae are another set of bumpy articular processes. The uppermost pair of articular processes articulate with the inferior articular process of L5, and the distal couple of articular processes form the sacral cornua, which join the corresponding cornua of the coccyx. Lateral still to the articular processes are the four sacral foramina, small holes that accommodate the exit of the sacral nerves.

The coccyx is a sort of scaled-down version of the sacrum. If the sacrum were an upside-down Christmas tree, the coccyx would be the triangle-shaped tree-topper ornament. Like the sacrum, the coccyx has a lumpy convex posterior surface with vestiges of tubercles and articular processes. The coccygeal cornua join the corresponding

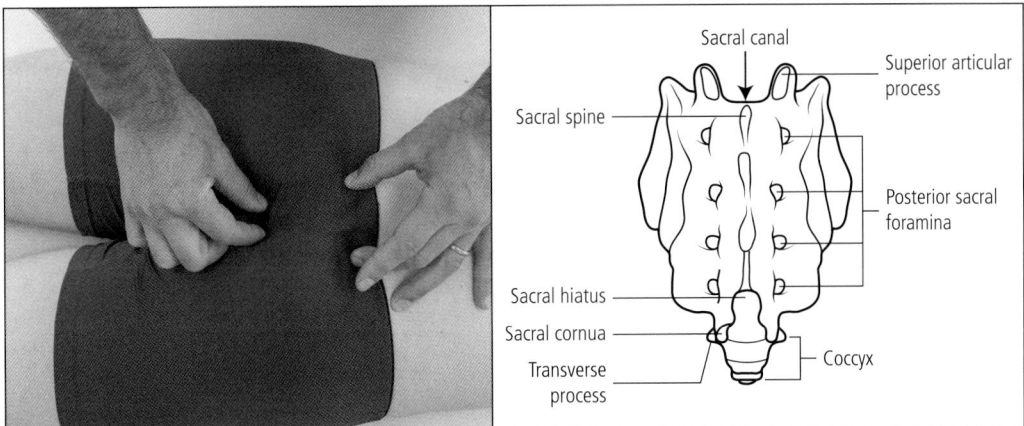

Figure 17.247. Sacrum and coccyx.

sacral cornua, mentioned earlier. The lateral borders of the coccyx give attachment to various ligaments and their expansions, which connect the coccyx to the sacrum and indirectly to each ilium.

Neighbors

Sacrum:
Coccyx
Both ilia
Fifth lumbar vertebra

Coccyx:
Sacrum

Palpation

With the subject prone, find the spinous process of L5, then descend to the next bony prominence, which is the base of the sacrum (figure 17.248). Alternately, from a superolateral approach, follow the iliac crest toward the posterior superior iliac spines, medial to which sits the base of the sacrum (figure 17.249). Follow the medial crest down toward the coccyx, where the sacral hiatus, the space between and just above the two sacral cornua, marks the sacrococcygeal joint (figure 17.250). To find the distal tip of the

coccyx, sometimes it's necessary to gently dig a little into the soft tissue at its distal extremity (figure 17.251).

Testing

Phase 1: With the subject prone and with your hands superimposed, perform a series of compressions or microspreading movements to test the quality of the sacrum and coccyx (figure 17.252), as well as their

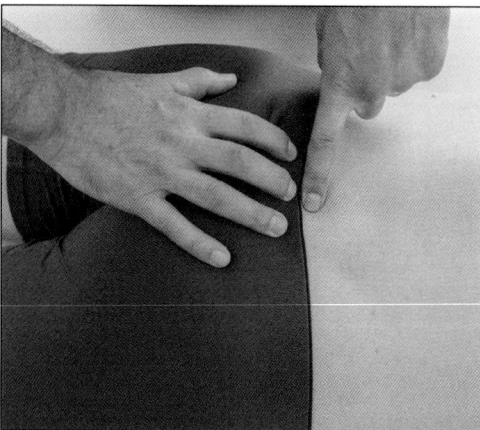

Figure 17.249. Palpating the sacrum from the right posterior superior iliac crest. The hypothenar eminence of the proximal hand is palpating the right superior crest, while the fingers of the distal hand slide medially onto the sacrum.

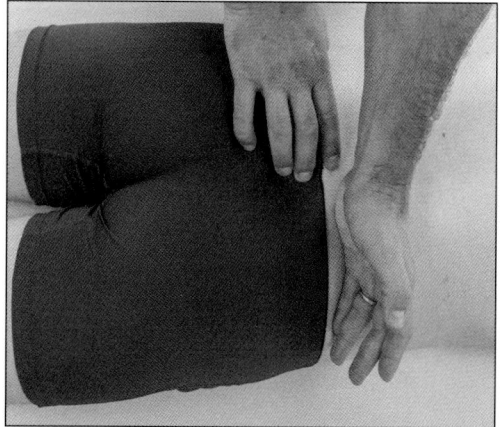

Figure 17.248. Palpating L5 and the sacrum. The proximal index is palpating the spinous process of L5, and the fingers of the distal hand slide distally onto the next bony eminence.

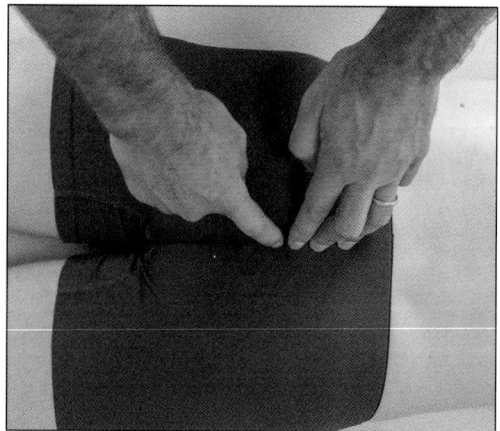

Figure 17.250. Palpating the sacrococcygeal joint from the sacral hiatus and cornua. Follow the medial crest down toward the coccyx, where the sacral hiatus marks the sacrococcygeal joint.

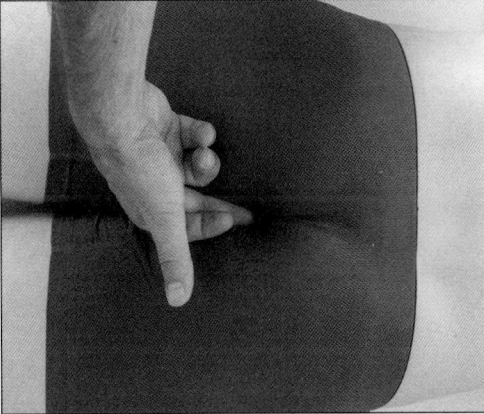

Figure 17.251. Palpating the tip of the coccyx with the tip of the middle finger. Sometimes it's necessary to gently dig into the soft tissue distal to the tip of the coccyx to palpate the very tip of the bone.

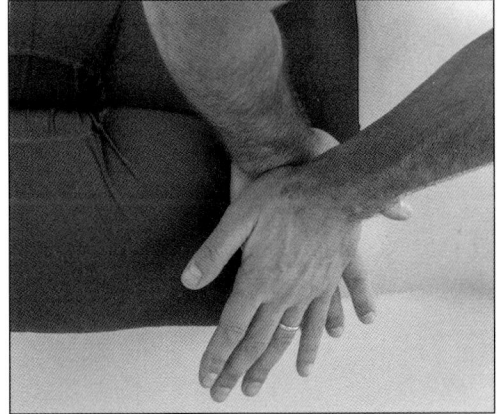

Figure 17.253. Phase 1: Testing the right sacroiliac joint. Perform a series of compressions or microspreading movements along each sacroiliac joint to test the quality of the joint.

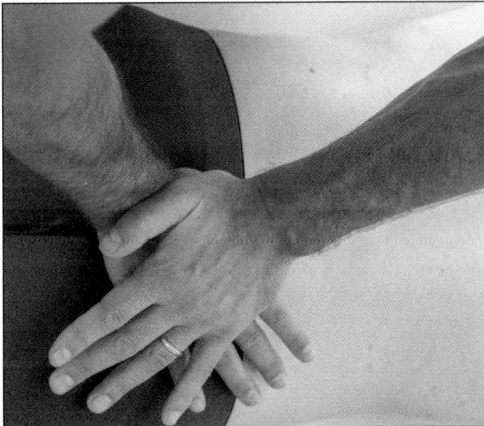

Figure 17.252. Phase 1: Testing the sacrum and coccyx. Perform a series of compressions or microspreading movements to test the quality of the bone.

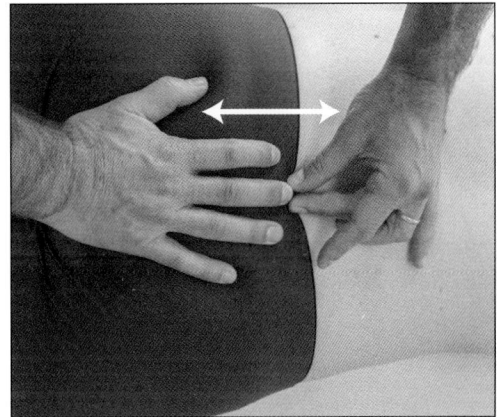

Figure 17.254. Phase 1: Testing the connection between L5 and the sacrum by spreading the bones.

connections with both ilia (figure 17.253). For the connection between the sacrum and L5, pinch the spinous process of L5 with one hand and grasp the sacrum with the other and spread the bones apart (figure 17.254). Once at the coccyx, test the sacrococcygeal joint as well as the coccyx itself (figure 17.255). While the sacrum is quite robust, the coccyx is more fragile, so make sure the coccygeal compressions are not too forceful.

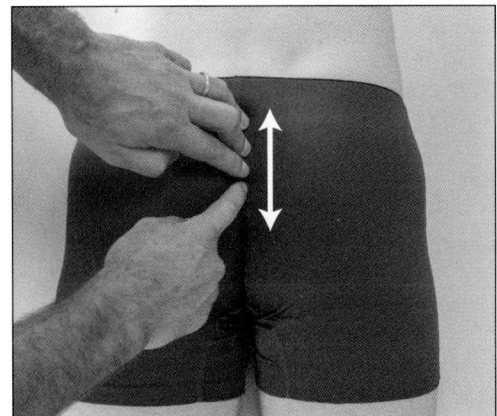

Figure 17.255. Phase 1: Testing the sacrococcygeal joint between the sacrum and the coccyx by spreading the bones.

If both the bones and their connections possess elasticity, move to the next bone to be tested. If the bones or any specific areas feel more like concrete than like wood, or if the connections feel fibrotic, move to phase 2 of testing.

Phase 2: If compacted, spread and twist the sacrum and/or coccyx (figures 17.256 and 17.257) and/or its connections: sacrum with coccyx (figure 17.258), sacrum with both ilia (figure 17.259), and sacrum with L5 (figure 17.260).

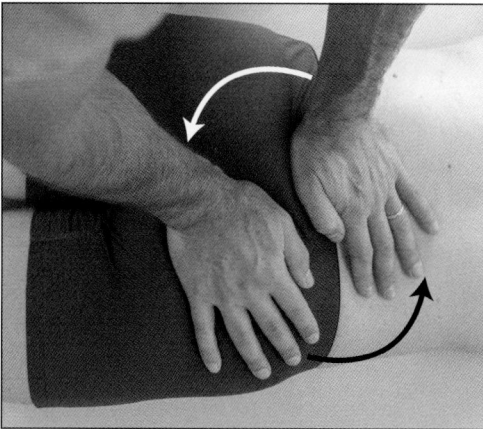

Figure 17.256. Phase 2: Spreading and twisting the sacrum in an oblique pattern with the palms of each hand. Hand placement will vary here depending on the quality of the bone.

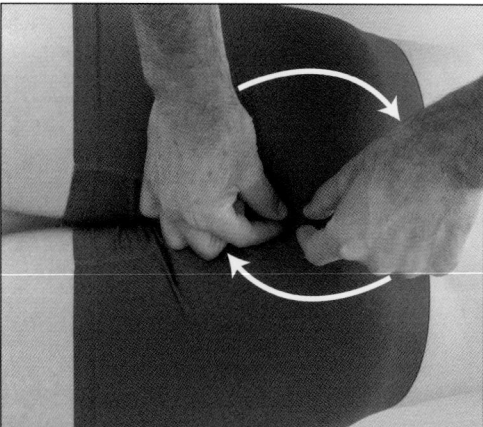

Figure 17.257. Phase 2: Spreading and twisting the coccyx with the thumb and index fingers.

Local treatment

A similar treatment approach can be applied to both the sacrum and coccyx, so they are grouped together here. Grasp the sacrum (figure 17.261) or coccyx (figure 17.262) and proceed with the six stages of BST treatment (see "Quick Guide to the Six Stages of BST Treatment").

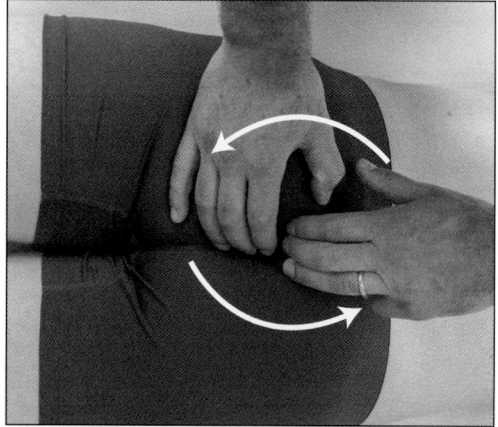

Figure 17.258. Phase 2: Spreading and twisting the connection between the sacrum and the coccyx.

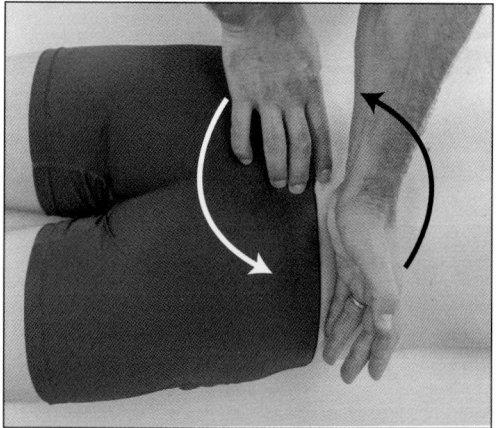

Figure 17.259. Phase 2: Spreading and twisting the connections between the sacrum and right ilium. This photo depicts the proximal hand on the superior iliac crest, but make sure to test the connections along the entire length of each sacroiliac joint.

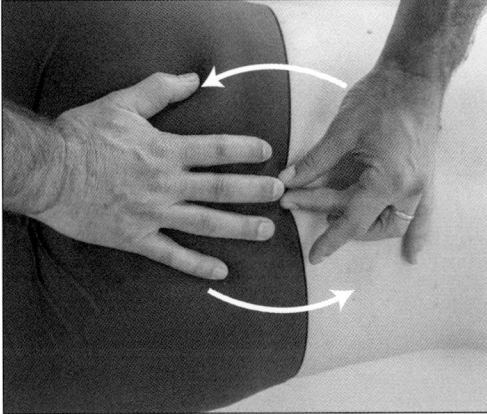

Figure 17.260. Phase 2: Spreading and twisting the connection between the sacrum and L5.

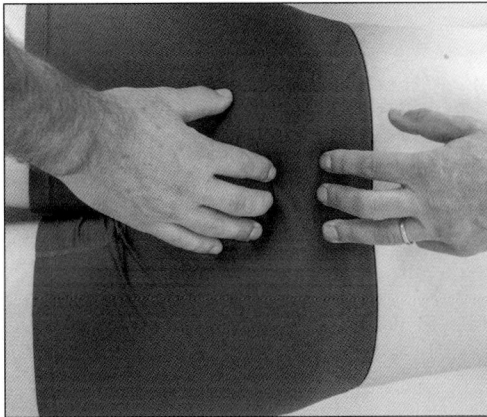

Figure 17.261. Hand position for the local treatment of the sacrum using the fingers. This can also be done using the palms or the thenar or hypothenar eminences.

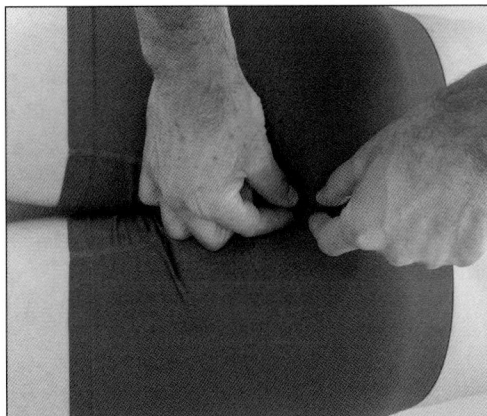

Figure 17.262. Hand position for the local treatment of the coccyx using the thumbs and index fingers.

Regional treatment

Integrate the local treatment of the sacrum/coccyx into the region by using the pelvic gather technique (see "Regional Treatment").

LUMBAR SPINE

The five lumbar vertebrae are the largest components of the vertebral column (figure 17.263). Each lumbar vertebra has numerous segments: the body, pedicles, laminae, and transverse and spinous processes. Only the posterior segments (all segments except the body) can be *directly* treated with BST. The evaluation of the lumbar vertebrae (as well as that of the thoracic vertebrae, to be discussed next) happens in series and is nearly identical from one vertebra to the next. Likewise, the local treatment of each vertebra is very similar. With this in mind, we'll discuss the particulars of L5, and then group the other four together.

Fifth lumbar vertebra

The body of L5 (figure 17.264) is massive and broad, and compared with other lumbar vertebrae, the spinous process is smaller,

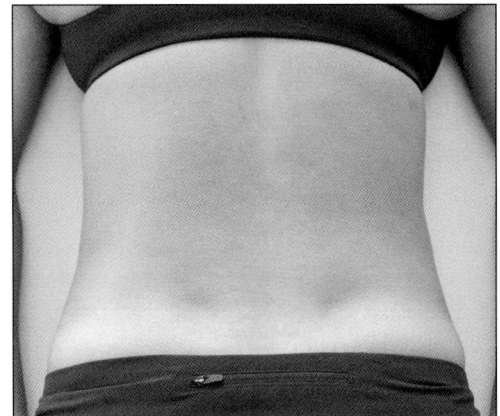

Figure 17.263. Lumbar spine.

171

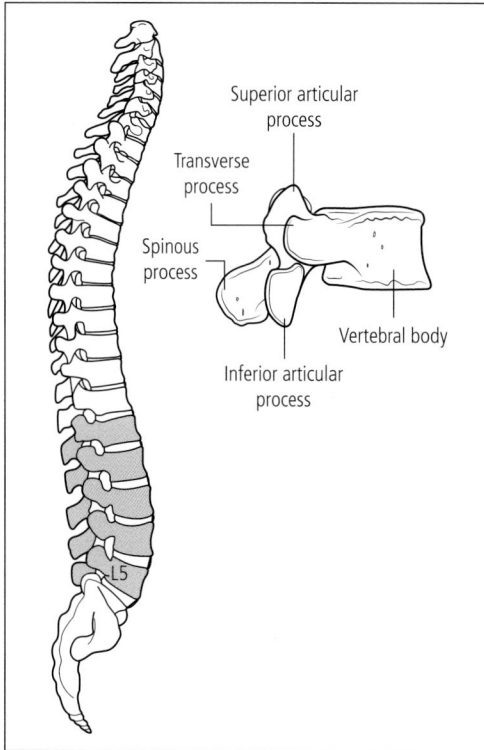

Figure 17.264. Lumbar vertebrae and (inset) L5 (lateral view).

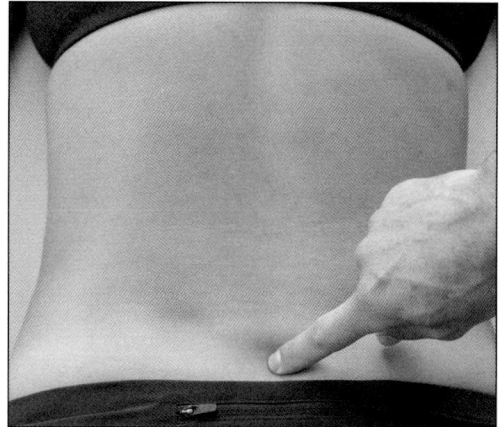

Figure 17.265. Palpating the spinous process of L5.

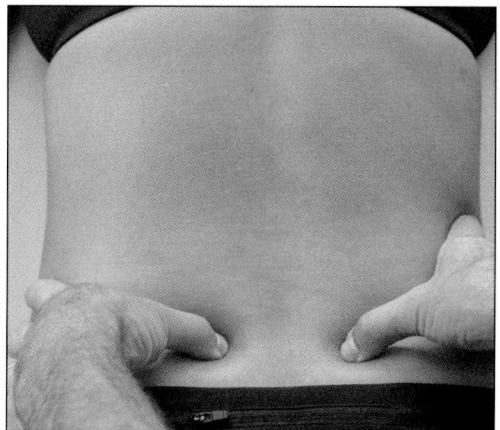

Figure 17.266. Palpating the transverse process of L5 with the thumbs.

and the transverse processes are thicker. The superior articular processes articulate with the inferior articular processes of the fourth lumbar vertebra (L4) above it.

Neighbors

Sacrum
L4

Palpation

To locate the spinous process of L5, follow the sacral base proximally into a small central depression. The bony prominence immediately proximal to the depression is the spinous process of L5 (figure 17.265).

The lumbar transverse processes sit roughly at the same level as the spinous processes. To locate the transverse processes, keep

a thumb or finger on the spinous process and poke into the sulcus medial to the posterior superior iliac crest (figure 17.266). Due to the ample musculature in the area, finding the transverse process of L5 can be tricky. To ensure that you are firmly on the transverse process, keep a thumb or finger on the spinous process and monitor it for movement. Repeat on the opposite side.

Testing

Phase 1: Normally, I evaluate one side of the entire vertebral column and then start over on the other side, but for the sake of this exercise, once testing of one side of L5 is complete, move to the opposite side of the subject and repeat the same procedure for the other side of L5. With the subject prone, place one hand flat on the sacrum and the palm or thumb of the other hand between the ipsilateral (same side as you) spinous and transverse processes (on the laminae) of L5. In a combined movement, stabilize the sacrum and apply force into the bone medially and toward the table (figure 17.267).

This test is simple but efficient. The obliquity of the force application simultaneously tests the quality of the spinous process, laminae, transverse process, and pedicle on one side while at the same time testing the micromobility of the whole vertebra in relation to its neighbor below. Move to the other side of the subject and repeat the procedure for the other side of L5. After testing both sides, does one or both sets of segments feel like wood or like concrete? Does the connection between L5 and the sacrum have some healthy bounce or is it stuck? If all feels normal, move to the next bone to be tested. If one or both sides of L5 or the connection between the L5 and

the sacrum is compacted, move to phase 2 for further testing.

Phase 2 (for the vertebra): Start by testing the most rigid side of L5. Place one thumb on the *inside* of the spinous process of L5 and the other thumb on the transverse process of the same side. Apply a tensile force between your thumbs, spreading and twisting the bone to determine the most rigid torsional pattern of compaction (figure 17.268).

Phase 2 (for L5/sacrum): For the connection between L5 and the sacrum, place one hand on the sacrum and the other on L5. Spread and twist L5 from the sacrum to determine the most rigid torsional pattern of compaction (figure 17.269).

Local treatment

Treating the vertebrae is challenging. It requires a special combination of force and finesse to simultaneously contact the bone through the paravertebral muscles while not stifling the therapeutic cushion within the bone. This may take a little practice. The following treatment approach

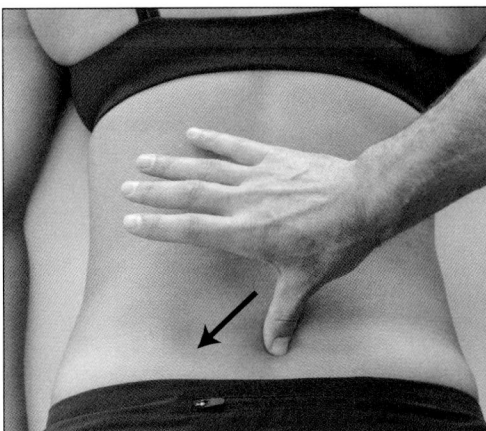

Figure 17.267. Phase 1: Testing the right side of L5 with the thumb (as well as the micromobility of L5 with the sacrum) by applying a force medially and toward the table. During the test, the other hand stabilizes the sacrum (not shown).

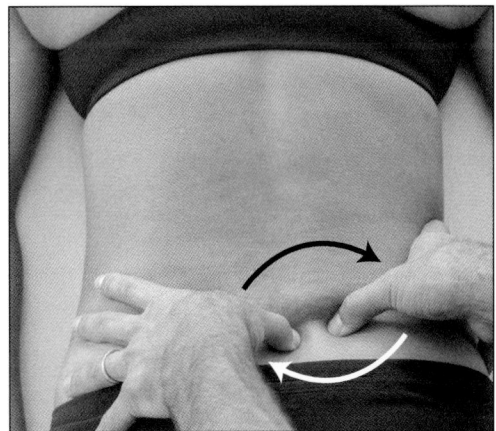

Figure 17.268. Phase 2 (for the vertebra): Spreading and twisting the right side of L5 by applying a tensile force between the thumbs.

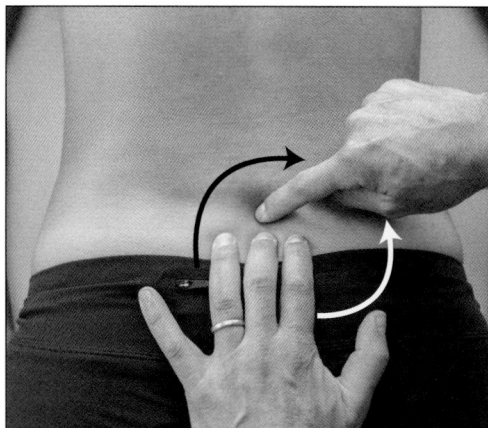

Figure 17.269. Phase 2 (for the connection between L5 and the sacrum): Place one hand on the sacrum and the other on L5 (it may be easier to use several fingers lined up along L5 instead of just one finger, as shown). Spread and twist L5 from the sacrum to determine the most rigid torsional pattern of compaction.

can be applied to all the vertebrae and their connections—from L5 all the way up to the first thoracic vertebra (T1). If only one side of L5 is compacted, treat that side. If both sides of L5 are compacted, start with the side that is more so, then proceed to the other side.

Grasp the vertebra and proceed with the six stages of BST treatment (see "Quick Guide to the Six Stages of BST Treatment"). Place one thumb on the *outside* of the spinous process and place the other thumb on the extremity of the transverse process on the *opposite* side of the vertebra (figure 17.270).

If you wish, for the final two stages, rotate your body and adjust your thumb positions to more efficiently apply a spreading force into the same side of L5 (figure 17.271).

Regional treatment

Integrate the local treatment of L5 into the region by using the lumbar gather technique (see "Regional Treatment").

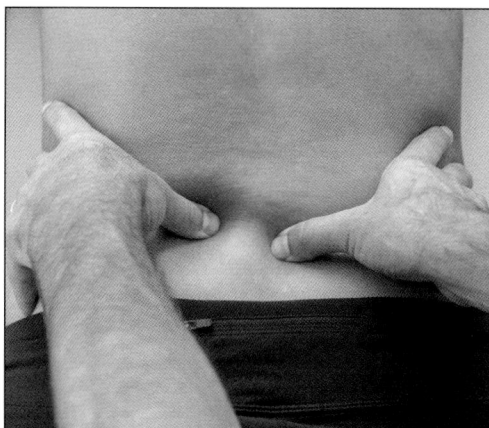

Figure 17.270. Hand position for the cocooning, compression, dialogue, and augmentation stages of local treatment of the left side of L5. The right thumb is placed on the right side of the spinous process, and the left thumb is placed on the left transverse process.

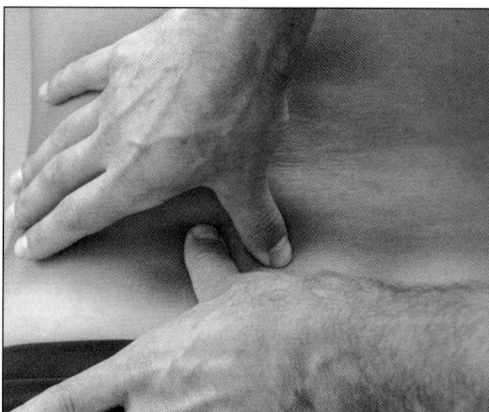

Figure 17.271. Hand positions for the spreading and integration stages for the local treatment of one side of L5. After rotating your body, the left thumb remains on the left transverse process, and the right thumb switches from the right side to the left side of the spinous process to more efficiently apply a spreading force into the bone.

Fourth to first lumbar vertebra

Palpation, testing, and local treatment

Move up the lumbar spine, from L4 to L1, using similar hand positions used for L5 and repeating the same palpatory, testing, and local treatment protocols. Test and treat both sides of the vertebra itself and the connections to the one below it.

Regional treatment

Integrate the local treatment of L4 to L1 into the region by using the lumbar gather technique (see "Regional Treatment").

THORAX

The thorax contains 37 bones: 12 vertebrae, 24 ribs, and the sternum (comprising manubrium, body, xiphoid process) (figure 17.272).

Thoracic Spine

Like the lumbars, each thoracic vertebra has similar anterior (body) and posterior (pedicles, transverse processes, laminae, spinous processes) segments. Unlike the lumbars, however, the thoracic vertebrae connect to ribs, which we'll discuss soon. The evaluation of the thoracic spine happens in series and is nearly identical from one vertebra to the next. Likewise, the local treatment of the vertebrae is very similar. To guide your palpation, testing, and treatment, we'll review some of the unique characteristics of a few of the thoracic

vertebrae in the series; namely, the twelfth thoracic vertebra (T12), the eleventh thoracic vertebra (T11), the tenth thoracic vertebra (T10), the ninth thoracic vertebra (T9), and the first thoracic vertebra (T1).

Twelfth and eleventh thoracic vertebrae

T12 (figure 17.273) sits between L1 below, T11 above, and the twelfth ribs on each side. The body forms the anterior segment and is marked on each side near the base of the pedicle by facets for the heads of the twelfth ribs. The pedicles connect the body to the transverse processes, and the laminae join the transverse processes to the spinous process. Compared with other thoracic vertebrae, the spinous process of T12 is smaller, and the transverse processes lack the facet for the tubercle of a rib. The superior articular

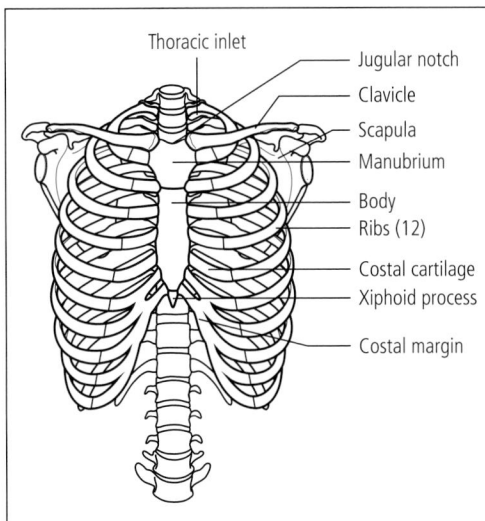

Figure 17.272. Thorax.

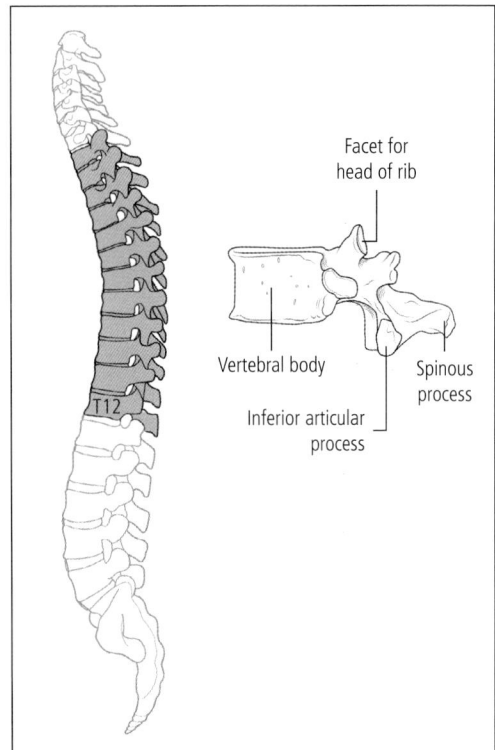

Figure 17.273. Thoracic vertebrae and (inset) T12 (lateral view).

processes articulate with the inferior articular processes of T11 above, and the inferior articular facets join the superior articular facets of L1 below.

T11 (figure 17.274) is similar in form to T12, and like the latter, contains no facet for the ribs on its transverse processes. Here, the eleventh ribs connect only to the pedicles. The superior articular processes articulate with the inferior articular processes of T10 above, and the inferior articular facets join the superior articular facets of T12 below.

Neighbors

T12:
L1
T11
Twelfth ribs

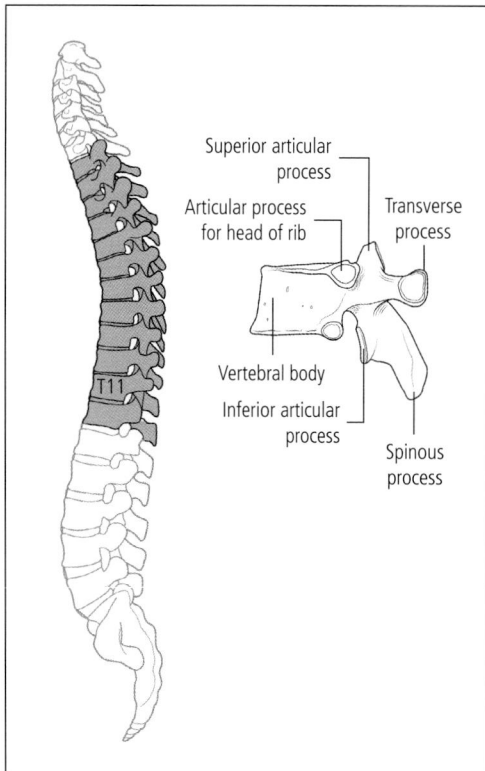

Figure 17.274. Thoracic vertebrae and (inset) T11 (lateral view).

Superior articular process

Articular process for head of rib

Transverse process

Vertebral body

Inferior articular process

Spinous process

T11

T11:
T12
T10
Eleventh ribs

Palpation

From the spinous process of L1, move up one level to the spinous process of T12 and then up another level to the spinous process of T11. For the transverse processes, contact the spinous process with one hand and the transverse process with the other. The transverse processes for the thoracic vertebrae are located roughly one half to one full level up from the corresponding spinous processes. Once you've found the transverse process, give it a push and make sure the movement is felt with your other hand on the spinous process.

Testing

Local treatment

As was the case with the lumbars, treating the thoracic vertebrae is challenging. It requires a special combination of force and finesse to simultaneously contact the bone through the musculature while not stifling the therapeutic cushion within the bone. The following treatment approach can be applied to all the thoracic vertebrae and their connections— from T12 all the way up to T1. If only one side of the vertebra is compacted, treat that side. If both sides are compacted, start with the side that is more so, then proceed to the other side.

Grasp the vertebra and proceed with the six stages of BST treatment (see "Quick Guide to the Six Stages of BST Treatment"). Place one thumb on the *outside* of the spinous process and place the other thumb on the extremity of the transverse process on the *opposite* side of the vertebra.

Regional treatment

Integrate the local treatment of all the thoracic vertebrae into the region by using the prone thoracic barrel technique (see "Regional Treatment").

Tenth thoracic vertebra

T10 sits between T11 below and T9 above, and the tenth ribs on each side. The body forms the anterior segment and is marked on each side near the base of the pedicle by a facet for the head of the tenth rib. Unlike T11 and T12 (but like all the other thoracic vertebrae), another articular facet exists on the lateral surface of the tip of the transverse process for articulation with the tubercle of the tenth rib. The inferior articular facets join the superior articular facets of T11 below and the superior articular processes articulate with the inferior articular processes of T9 above.

Neighbors

T11
T9
Tenth ribs

Palpation, testing, treatment, and regional treatment

Same for all the thoracic vertebrae.

Ninth thoracic vertebra

T9 sits between T10 below and T8 above, and the ninth ribs on each side. The body forms the anterior segment and is marked on each side near the base of the pedicle by a demifacet for the inferior part of the head of the ninth rib. Like the other thoracic vertebrae, another articular facet exists on the lateral surface of the tip of the transverse process for articulation with the tubercle of the ninth rib. The inferior articular facets join

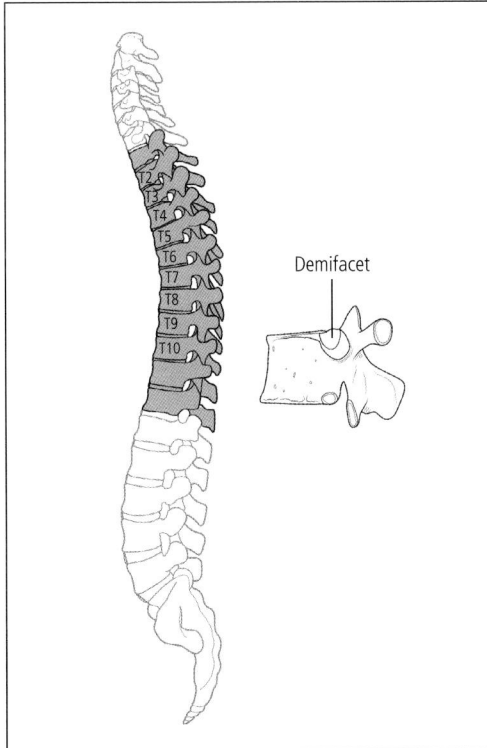

Figure 17.275. Thoracic vertebrae and (inset) typical thoracic vertebra (T2 to T10), lateral view.

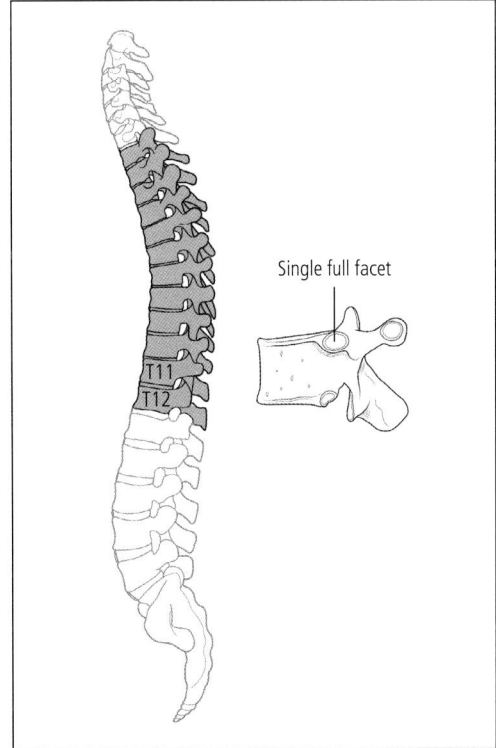

Figure 17.276. Thoracic vertebrae and (inset) T11, T12 (lateral view).

the superior articular facets of T10 below and the superior articular processes articulate with the inferior articular processes of T8 above.

Neighbors

T10
T8
Ninth ribs

Palpation, testing, treatment, and regional treatment

Same for all the thoracic vertebrae.

Eighth to second thoracic vertebra

From T8 to T2, besides the thoracic neighbors above and below, each vertebra articulates with both the head of the corresponding rib *and* the one below it.

For example, T6 articulates with both the sixth and seventh ribs (figure 17.277).

Neighbors

Thoracic vertebra above
Thoracic vertebra below
Corresponding ribs
Ribs of the vertebra below

Palpation, testing, treatment, and regional treatment

Same for all the thoracic vertebrae.

First thoracic vertebra

T1 (figure 17.278) sits between T2 below and C7 above, and the first ribs on each side. The body forms the anterior segment and is marked on each side near the base of the pedicle by a full facet for the head of the

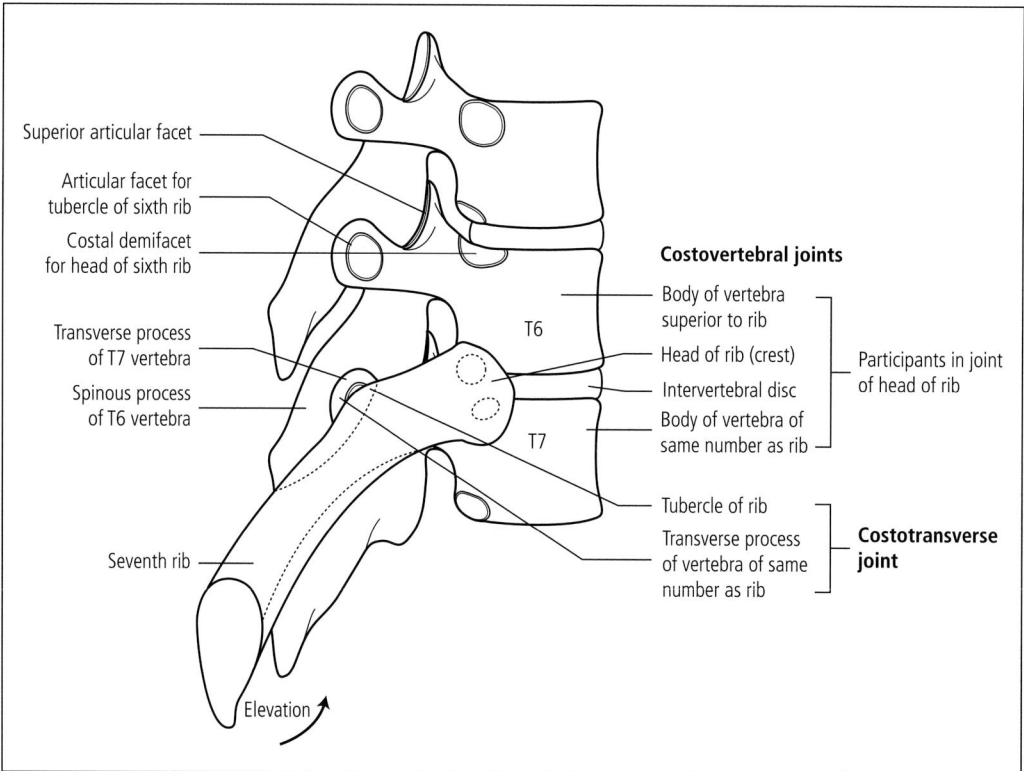

Figure 17.277. T6 showing facets for adjoining sixth and seventh ribs.

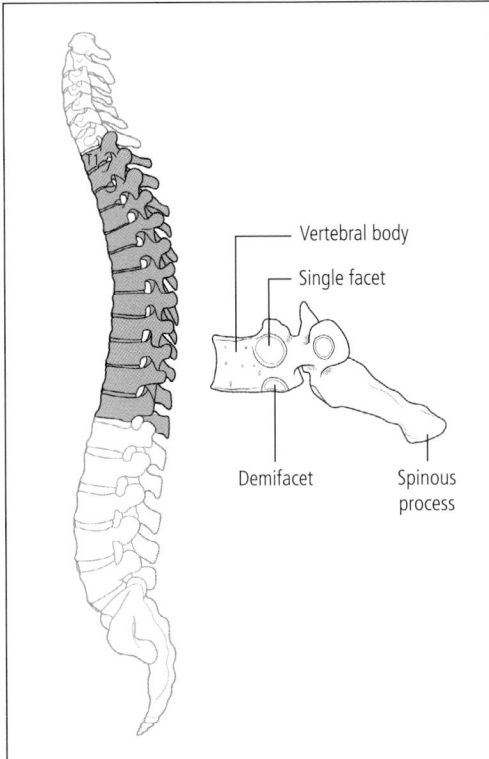

Figure 17.278. Thoracic vertebrae and (inset) T1 (lateral view).

first rib, and a demifacet for the upper half of the head of the second rib. Like the other thoracic vertebrae, another articular facet exists on the lateral surface of the tip of the transverse process for articulation with the tubercle of the first rib. The inferior articular facets join the superior articular facets of T2 below and the superior articular processes articulate with the inferior articular processes of C7 above.

Neighbors

T2
C7
First ribs

Palpation, testing, treatment, and regional treatment

Same for all the thoracic vertebrae.

Ribs and Costal Cartilages

Ribs

Ribs 1 through 10 are connected in the back to the spine and in front to the sternum via the costal cartilages. Owing to the complexities of evaluating and treating the first rib with BST, we will not spend much time discussing it here. Ribs 11 and 12, the "floating" ribs, are only connected to the spine, and their anterior extremities float freely. The upper ribs sit almost perpendicularly to the spine, whereas the lower ribs sit obliquely, where the anterior extremity is lower than the posterior (figure 17.279). The spaces between the ribs are called the intercostal spaces, and the width of the spaces is greater in front than in back. Each rib has two extremities, a posterior or vertebral and an anterior or sternal, and in between the extremities is the shaft. The posterior extremity has a head, neck, and tuberosity. Generally, the head articulates with the costal cavity formed by the junction of the

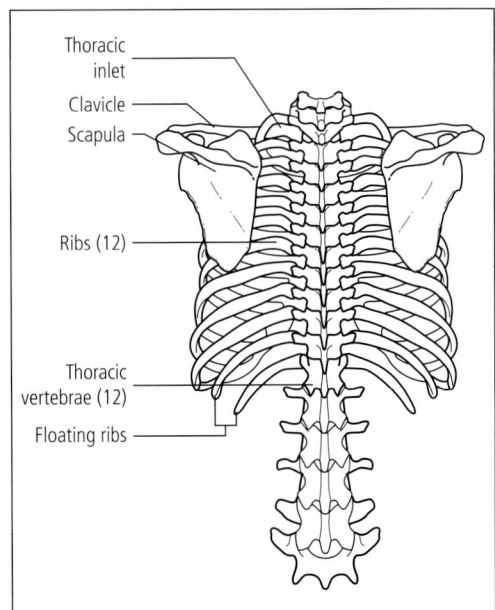

Figure 17.279. Ribs and costal cartilages.

bodies of two adjoining thoracic vertebrae. The neck of the rib extends from the head and articulates with the transverse process of the lower of the two vertebrae with which the head articulates. The anterior extremity of ribs 1 through 10 has a concave depression, which receives the corresponding costal cartilage. The eleventh, twelfth, and first ribs have a single posterior facet and connect only to the eleventh, twelfth, and first thoracic vertebrae, respectively.

Costal cartilages

The costal cartilages extend from the medial border of the ribs to the sternum. The first seven ribs each have their own cartilage, which is connected directly to the sternum. Ribs 8 through 10 are connected to the cartilage of the preceding rib. As do the ribs themselves, the cartilaginous extremities of the eleventh and twelfth ribs float freely.

Palpation, testing, and treatment of the ribs and costal cartilages can be divided into three sections: posterior (figure 17.280), lateral (figure 17.288), and anterior (figure 17.292). I'll describe the palpation, testing, and treatment protocols for each section separately.

Posterior section

Palpation

With the subject prone, start at the posterior superior iliac crest and move up along the lateral side of the posterior thorax to the posterior aspect of the twelfth rib, which will be the first bony eminence (figure 17.281). You can trace the twelfth rib along its posterior border to its pointed extremity (figure 17.282). Return to the

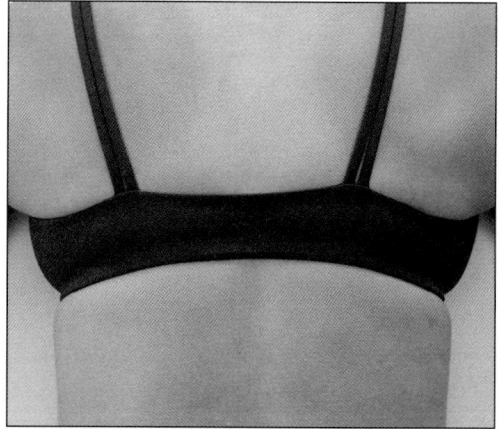

Figure 17.280. Posterior section of ribs.

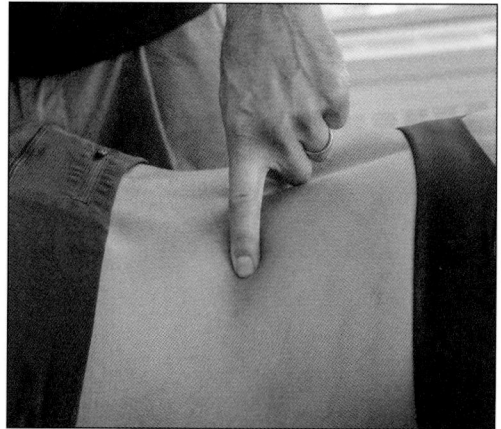

Figure 17.281. Palpating the posterior section of the right twelfth rib with the index finger.

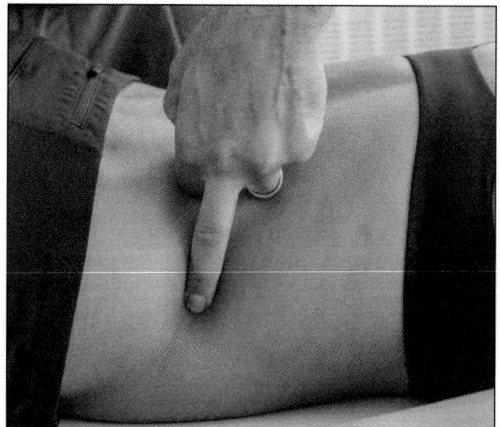

Figure 17.282. Palpating the extremity of the right twelfth rib with the index finger.

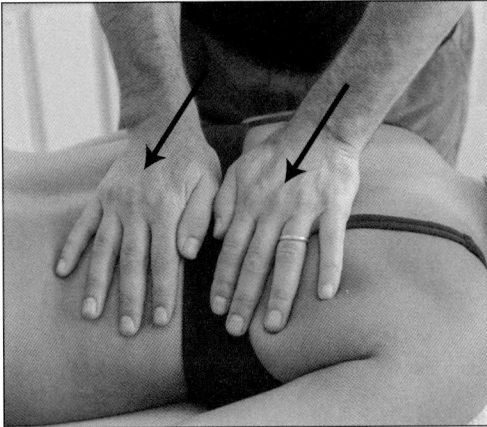

Figure 17.283. Phase 1: Testing the posterior section of the ribs.

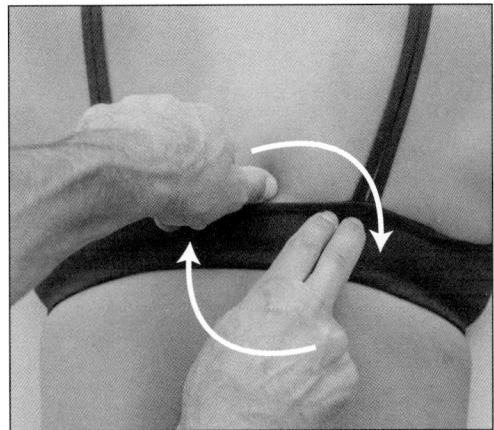

Figure 17.284. Phase 2: Spreading and twisting the posterior section of the seventh rib with the fingers.

posterior section and move up the thorax toward the head of the subject, counting the ribs as you go.

Testing

Phase 1: With the subject still prone, line up the fingers of both hands along one side of the posterior border of the ribs. Apply a tensile force toward the table and laterally, along the axis of the ribs (figure 17.283). Repeat on the other side. Evaluate the elasticity of the connections between the ribs and the thoracic spine and of the bone itself.

Do the posterior ribs and the connections possess elasticity? If so, move to the next section to be tested. If one or several of the posterior ribs or any of their connections are compacted, proceed to phase 2.

Phase 2: Using both hands, spread and twist the compacted rib (figure 17.284) or the connection between the rib and the spine (figures 17.285 and 17.286) to determine the specific torsional pattern of compaction.

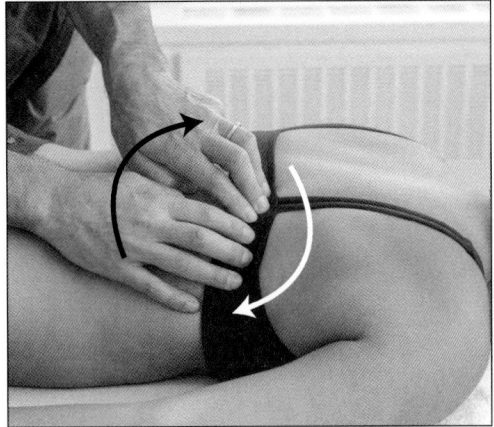

Figure 17.285. Phase 2: Spreading and twisting the connection between the posterior section of the right seventh rib and T6. The thumb of the left hand stabilizes T6, while the index and middle fingers of the right hand apply a lateral tensile force into the rib, spreading the joint.

Local treatment

Grasp the posterior section of the rib (figure 17.287) and proceed with the six stages of BST treatment (see "Quick Guide to the Six Stages of BST Treatment").

Regional treatment

Integrate the local treatment of all the posterior ribs into the region by using the prone thoracic barrel technique (see "Regional Treatment").

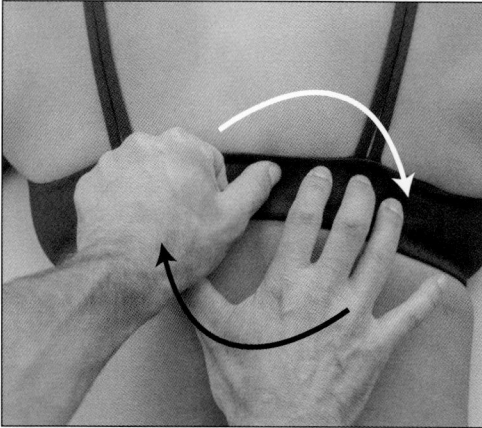

Figure 17.286. Phase 2: Spreading and twisting the connection between the posterior section of the right seventh rib and T7. The thumb of the left hand stabilizes T7, while the index and middle fingers of the right hand apply a lateral tensile force into the rib, spreading the joint.

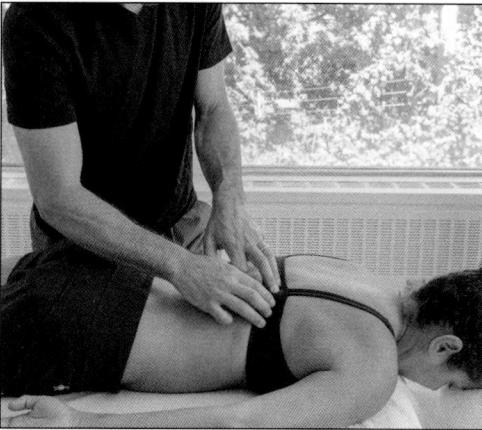

Figure 17.288. Lateral section of ribs.

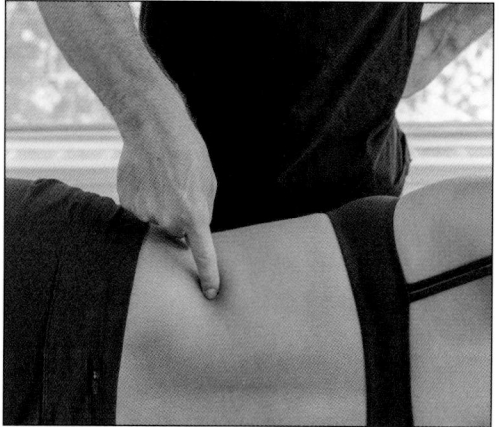

Figure 17.287. Hand and body position for the local treatment of the posterior section of the right seventh rib using the fingers.

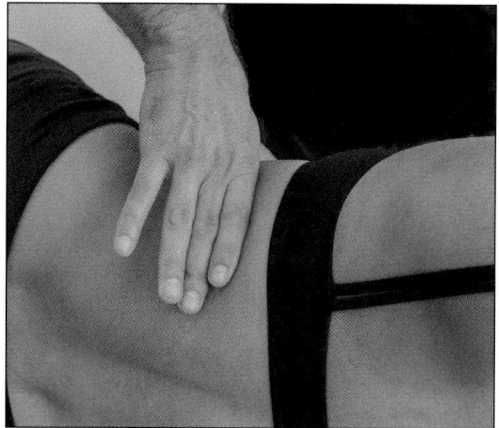

Figure 17.289. Palpating the lateral section of the left twelfth rib with the index finger.

Lateral section

Palpation

With the subject lying on the side opposite the one to be treated, start at the posterior superior iliac crest and move up along the lateral side of the trunk to the twelfth rib, which will be the first bony eminence (figures 17.288 and 17.289). Move up the thorax toward the head of the subject, counting the ribs as you go. Due to the location of the scapulae and associated musculature, the lateral section of the uppermost ribs is not easily accessed.

Testing

Phase 1: With the subject still side-lying, apply a compressive and spreading pressure down toward the table, moving up or down the thorax, in series, testing the elasticity of the lateral section of the ribs (figure 17.290). Repeat on the other side.

Do the lateral ribs possess elasticity?
If so, move to the next section. If one or several of the ribs are compacted, proceed to phase 2.

Phase 2: Using both hands, spread and twist the compacted bone to determine the specific torsional pattern of compaction (figure 17.291).

Local treatment

Same as for the posterior section.

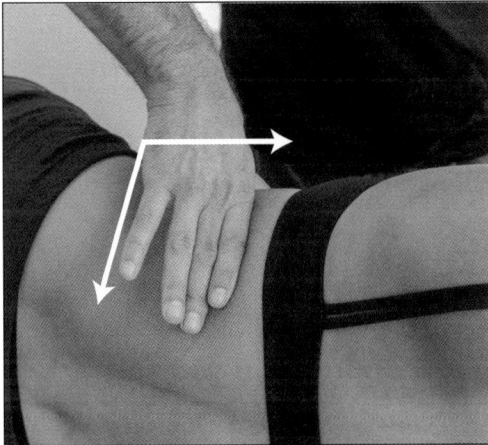

Figure 17.290. Phase 1: Testing the lateral section of a left rib by simultaneously applying a compressive and spreading force into the bone and toward the table.

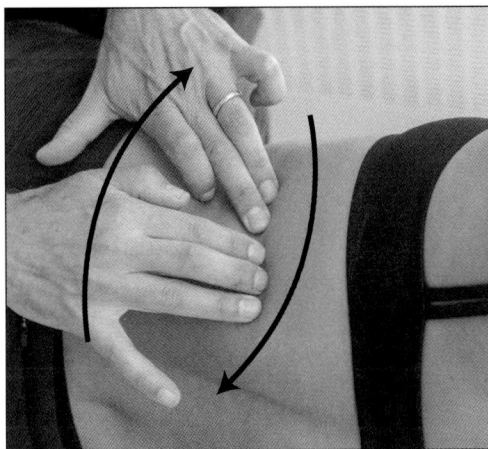

Figure 17.291. Phase 2: Spreading and twisting the lateral section of the left tenth rib with the fingers.

Regional treatment

Integrate the local treatment of all the posterior ribs into the region by using either the prone or the supine thoracic barrel technique (see "Regional Treatment").

Anterior section

Palpation

Have the subject lie supine. Start at the center of the sternum and move laterally onto the second costal cartilage, which is the next eminence just below the clavicle (figures 17.292 and 17.293). Move downward, counting the cartilages (figure 17.294). From each cartilage, move laterally onto the corresponding rib, which will have a more rigid texture (figure 17.295). From the lower segment of the sternum, palpate the lower border of the rib cage and the cartilages of the seventh through tenth ribs. Slide laterally across the border, and then down onto the pointed extremity of the eleventh rib (figure 17.296).

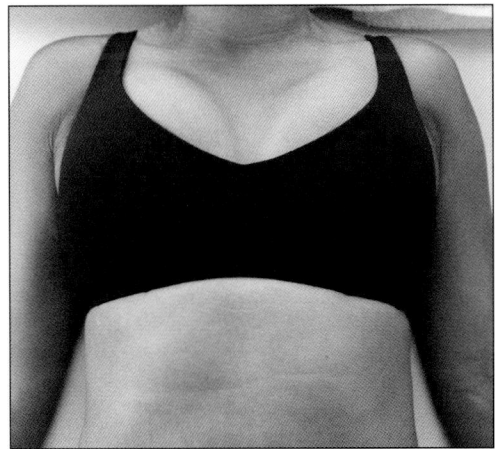

Figure 17.292. Anterior section of ribs.

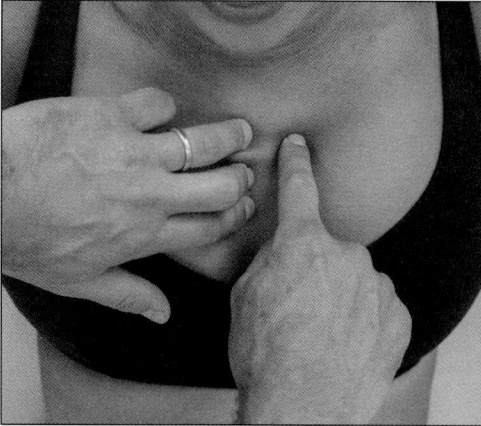

Figure 17.293. Palpating the second left costal cartilage with the index finger.

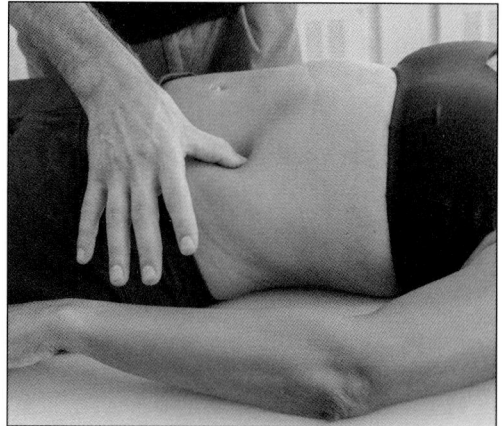

Figure 17.296. Palpating the extremity of the left eleventh rib with the right thumb.

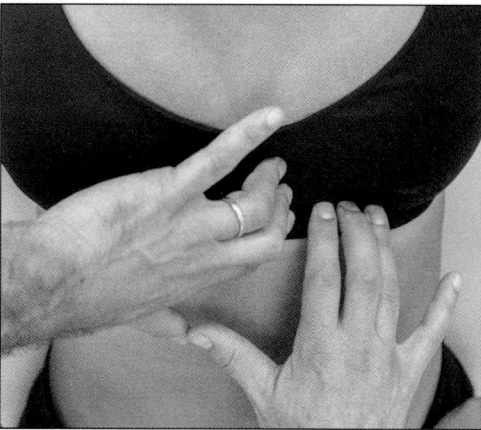

Figure 17.294. Palpating the middle right costal cartilages with the fingers of the right hand.

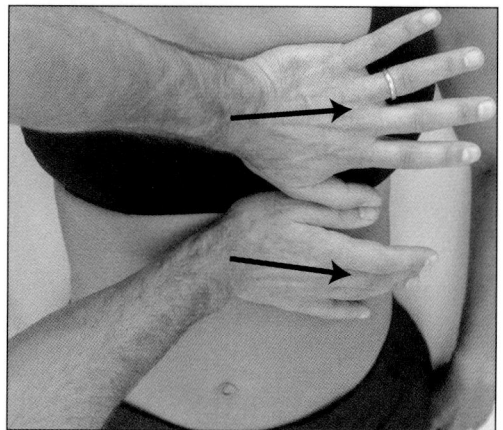

Figure 17.297. Phase 1: Testing the left costal cartilages and their connections with the sternum using the palms of both hands.

Testing

Phase 1: With the palms of the hands on the upper costal cartilages and fingers along the ribs, apply a tensile force toward the table and laterally, testing the elasticity of the cartilages and their connections with the sternum (figure 17.297). Then, move the palms laterally onto the ribs themselves, and repeat, testing the elasticity of the bone and of the connections with the lateral extremities of the cartilages (figure 17.298). Move down, in series, toward the tenth rib. Repeat on the other side.

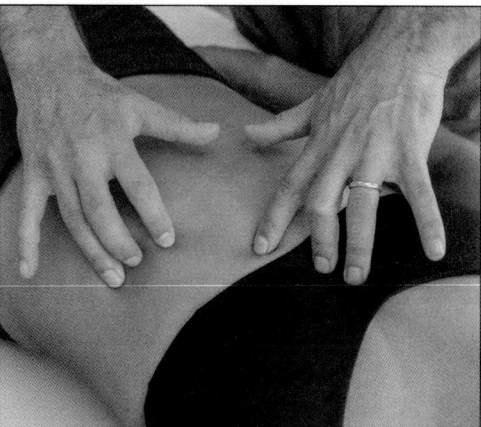

Figure 17.295. Palpating the lower anterior left ribs with the fingers of the right hand.

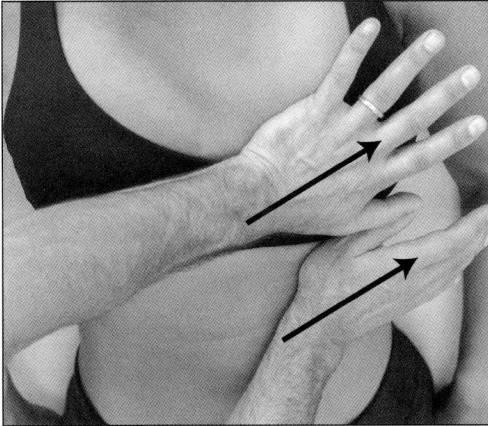

Figure 17.298. Phase 1: Testing the anterior left ribs and their connections with the costal cartilages. Be careful not to compress the breast tissue, as this can be invasive and/or painful for the subject.

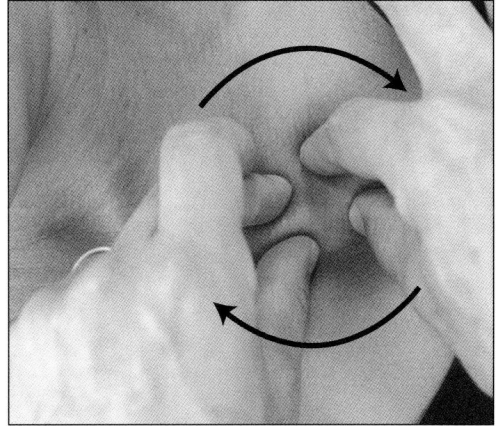

Figure 17.300. Phase 2: Spreading and twisting the left third rib with the thumbs and index fingers.

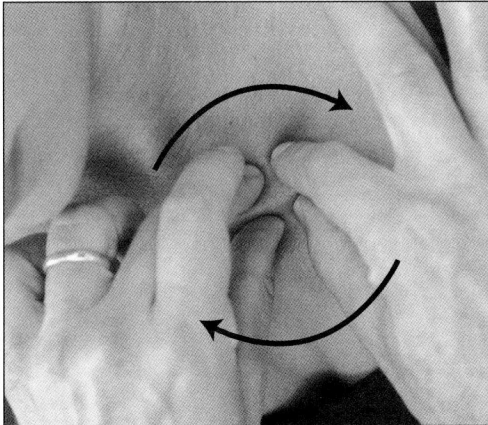

Figure 17.299. Phase 2: Spreading and twisting the left third costal cartilage with the thumbs and index fingers.

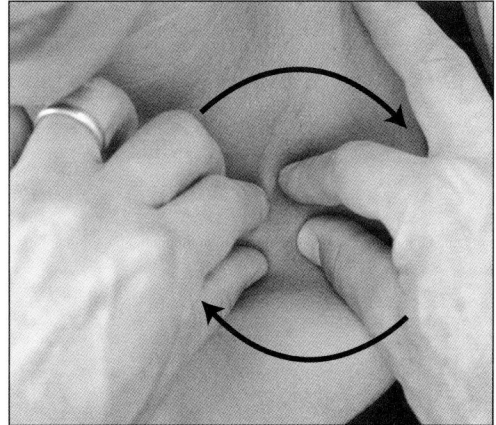

Figure 17.301. Phase 2: Spreading and twisting the connection between the left third costal cartilage and the left third rib.

Do the cartilages and anterior ribs possess elasticity? If so, move to the next bone to be tested. If one or several of the cartilages or ribs are compacted, proceed to phase 2.

Phase 2: Using both hands, spread and twist the compacted cartilage (figure 17.299) or bone (figure 17.300) or the connections between them (figure 17.301) to determine the specific torsional pattern of compaction.

Local treatment

Local treatment for the anterior ribs and cartilages is the same as for the other sections.

Regional treatment

Integrate the local treatment of all the anterior ribs and cartilages into the region by using the supine thoracic barrel technique (see "Regional Treatment").

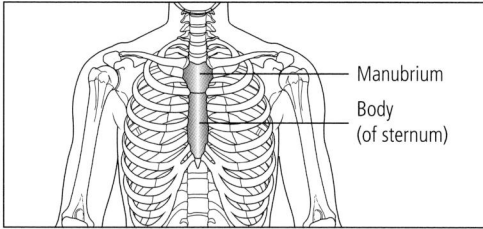

Figure 17.302. Sternum and manubrium.

Sternum

The sternum is a flat, narrow bone in the middle of the chest (figure 17.302), and like the sacrum, it's full of bumps and knobs. It technically has three parts: the manubrium, the gladiolus or body, and the xiphoid process. We will treat the manubrium and sternum as one bone, and the xiphoid process as another.

Sternum and manubrium

Neighbors

Clavicle
First through tenth costal cartilages
Xiphoid process

Palpation

From a distal approach, follow the inferior border of the rib cage up to where the seventh costal cartilage meets the distal extremity of the body of the sternum and base of the xiphoid process (figure 17.303). From either side of the chest, follow the ribs and costal cartilages medially to where they join the manubrium and sternum (figure 17.304). From a proximal approach, find the central space between the two sternoclavicular joints and descend onto the manubrium (figure 17.305).

Testing

Phase 1: Align the tips of the fingers of both hands along the body of the sternum and

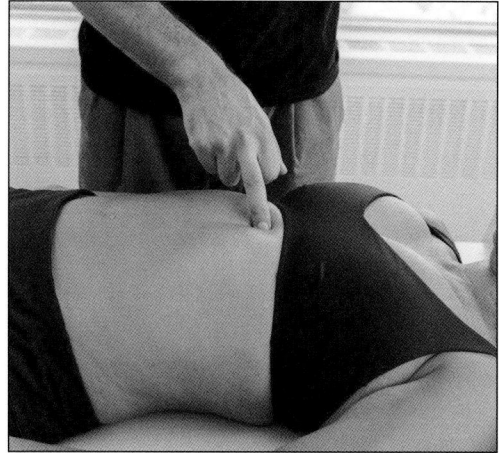

Figure 17.303. Palpating the sternum from the distal approach using the middle finger.

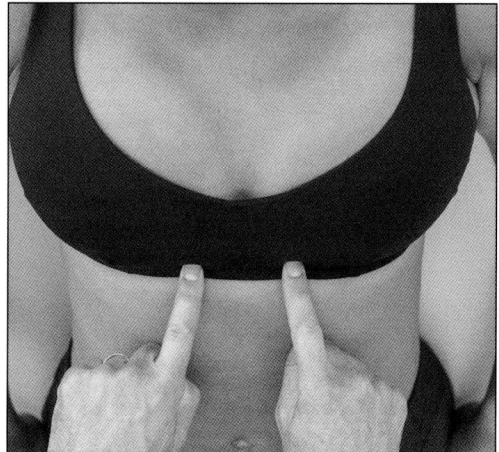

Figure 17.304. Palpating the sternum from the lateral approach using both index fingers.

manubrium. Apply light pressure toward the table while simultaneously spreading the whole bone (figure 17.306).

One at a time, hold each of the 14 costal cartilages and both clavicles with one hand and stabilize the sternum or manubrium with the other. Move from one to the next, testing each connection in series by spreading the sternocostal and sternoclavicular joints (figures 17.307 and 17.308).

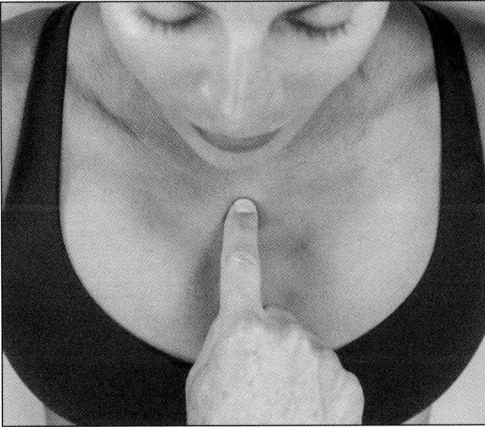

Figure 17.305. Palpating the manubrium from the proximal approach using the index finger.

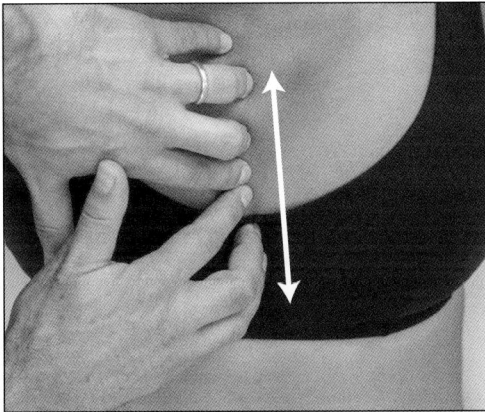

Figure 17.306. Phase 1: Testing the sternum and manubrium using the fingers of both hands.

Once complete, move to the distal end of the sternum and test the connection between the xiphoid process and the sternum (figure 17.309). As you did with the coccyx, use a delicate touch when testing the xiphoid process.

Does the sternum or manubrium or any of their connections feel compacted? If so, move to phase 2 of testing.

Phase 2: Using the same hand positions, spread and twist the bones and cartilages to

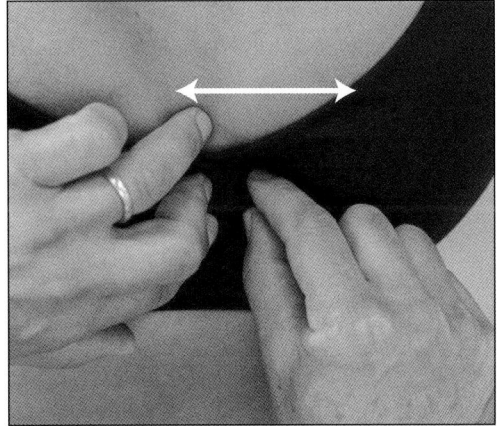

Figure 17.307. Phase 1: Testing the connection between the sternum and the left fifth costal cartilage. The fingers of the left hand stabilize the sternum while the index finger and thumb of the right hand grasp the costal cartilage and apply a lateral tensile force into the joint.

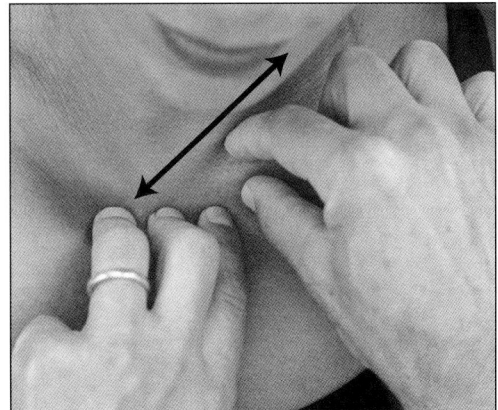

Figure 17.308. Phase 1: Testing the connection between the manubrium and the clavicle. The fingers of the left hand stabilize the manubrium while the index and thumb of the right hand grasp the left clavicle and apply a lateral tensile force into the joint.

find the most compacted torsional pattern within (figure 17.310) or between them (figures 17.311 to 17.313).

Local treatment

Local treatment of the sternum and manubrium resembles that of the sacrum. Both structures have large, relatively flat

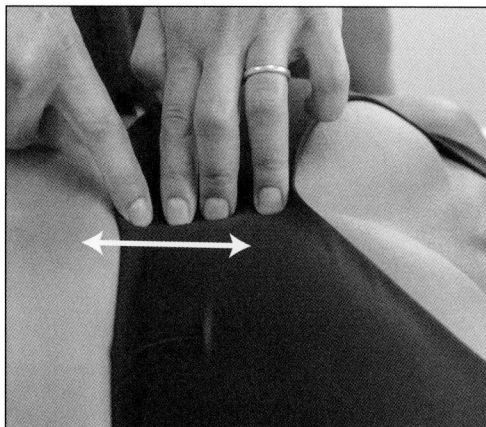

Figure 17.309. Phase 1: Testing the connection between the sternum and the xiphoid process. The fingers of the left hand stabilize the sternum while the index finger of the right hand contacts the xiphoid process and applies a tensile proximal-to-distal force into the joint.

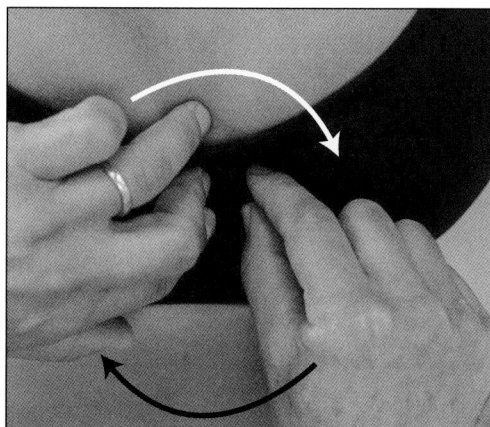

Figure 17.311. Phase 2: Spreading and twisting the connection between the sternum with the fifth costal cartilage. The fingers of the left hand stabilize the sternum while the index and thumb of the right hand grasp the costal cartilage and apply a spreading and twisting force into the joint.

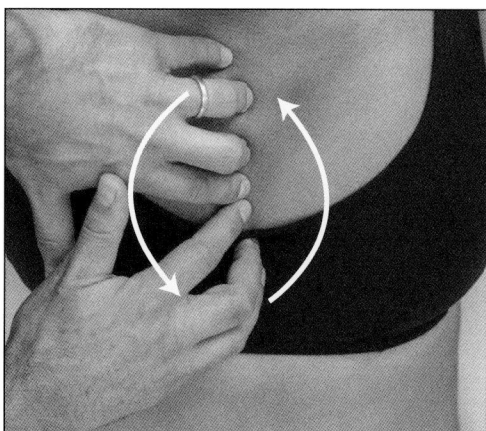

Figure 17.310. Phase 2: Spreading and twisting the sternum and manubrium using the fingers of both hands.

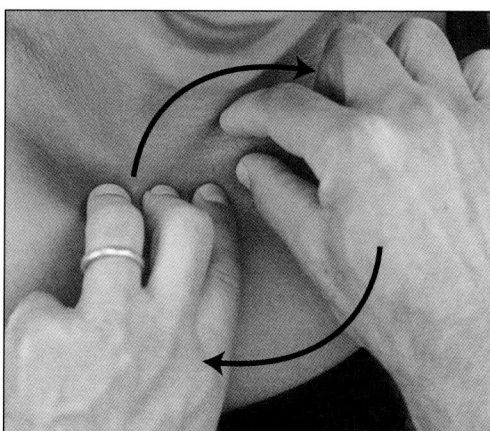

Figure 17.312. Phase 2: Spreading and twisting the connection between the manubrium and the clavicle. The fingers of the left hand stabilize the manubrium while the index finger and thumb of the right hand grasp the left clavicle and apply a spreading and twisting force into the joint.

surface areas with various options and angles for treatment. Line the fingers of both hands along the sternum (figure 17.314) and proceed with the six stages of BST treatment (see "Quick Guide to the Six Stages of BST Treatment").

Regional treatment

Integrate the local treatment of the sternum and manubrium into the region by using

the supine thoracic barrel technique (see "Regional Treatment").

Xiphoid process

The xiphoid process is the small, delicate, pointy bone at the distal extremity of the sternum (figure 17.315), and it can vary in

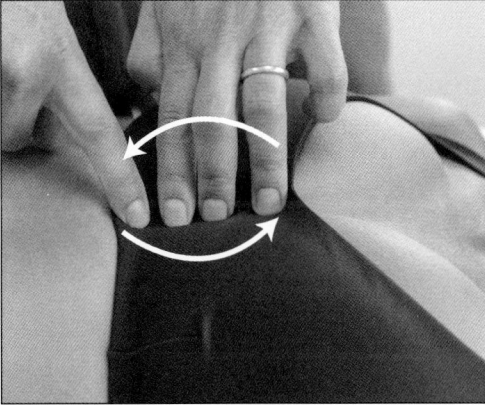

Figure 17.313. Phase 2: Spreading and twisting the connection between the sternum and the xiphoid process. The fingers of the left hand stabilize the sternum while the index finger of the right hand contacts the xiphoid process and applies a spreading and twisting force into the joint.

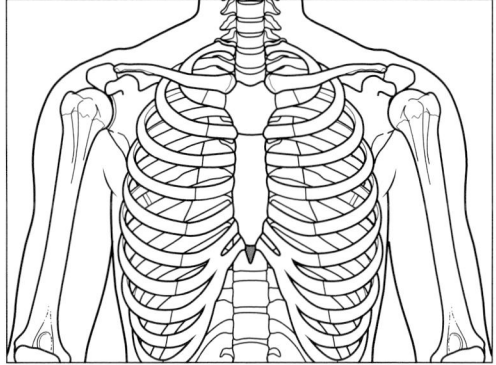

Figure 17.314. Hand and body position for the local treatment of the sternum and manubrium.

shape from one person to the next. I call it the "coccyx of the thorax."

Neighbors

Lower half of the seventh costal cartilage
Body of sternum

Palpation

Follow the body of the sternum down to the xiphoid process. Very gently continue along

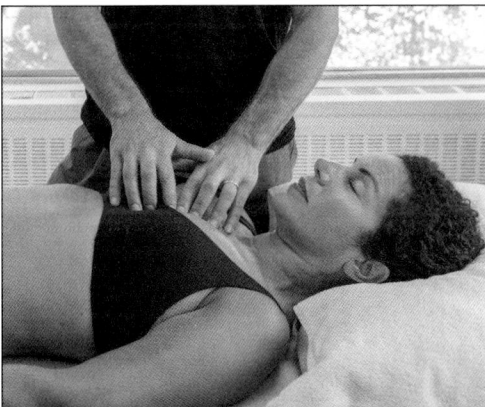

Figure 17.315. Xiphoid process.

the xiphoid process until you reach the distal end. As with the coccyx, you may have to gently dig a little into the soft tissue to locate the tip.

Testing

Using two fingers, spread (and gently twist, if possible) the xiphoid process to determine if the bone is compacted, and if so, the orientation of the pattern of compaction (figure 17.316). Then test the connection with the sternum (figure 17.317) and seventh costal cartilages (figure 17.318). As usual, if all feels good, move on to the next bone to be tested. If there exists a compaction within the xiphoid process or between it and any of its neighbors, proceed to local and then regional treatment.

Local treatment

Local treatment of xiphoid resembles that of the coccyx: both are small, delicate bones. Grasp the xiphoid process (figure 17.319) and proceed with the six stages of BST treatment (see "Quick Guide to the Six Stages of BST Treatment").

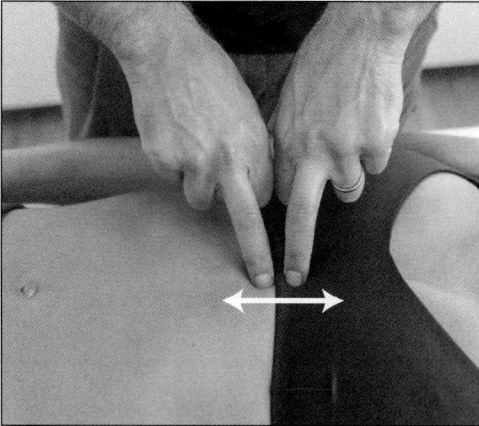

Figure 17.316. Testing the xiphoid process by spreading it with the middle fingers.

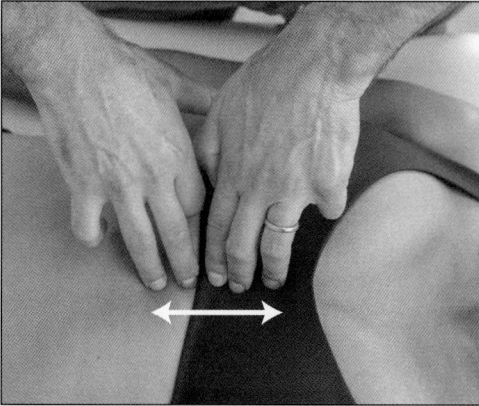

Figure 17.317. Testing the connection between the xiphoid process and the sternum. The fingers of the left hand stabilize the sternum while the middle finger of the right hand contacts the xiphoid process and applies a proximal-to-distal tensile force into the joint.

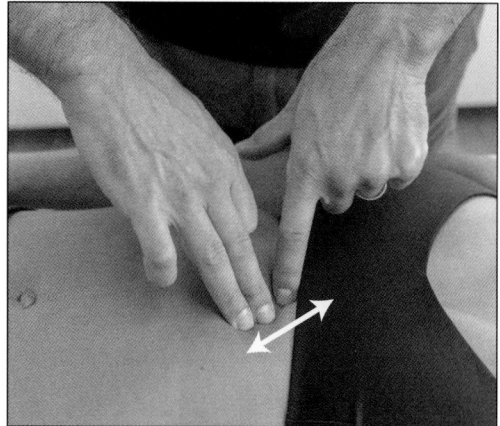

Figure 17.318. Testing the connection between the xiphoid process and the left seventh costal cartilage. The index finger of the left hand stabilizes the xiphoid process while the middle and ring fingers contact the costal cartilage and apply a tensile force into the joint.

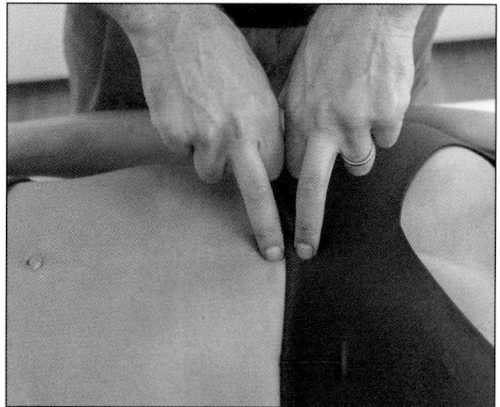

Figure 17.319. Hand position for the local treatment of the xiphoid process using the middle fingers.

Regional treatment

Integrate the local treatment of the xiphoid process into the region by using the supine thoracic barrel technique (see "Regional Treatment").

HAND AND WRIST

There are 27 bones in each hand and wrist: 14 phalanges, 5 metacarpals, and 8 carpals (figure 17.320). As I did for the foot, and especially for the phalanges and metacarpals, here I only describe the testing of the connections between neighboring bones *once*. For example, for the first proximal phalanx, even though its neighbors include both the first distal phalanx and the first metacarpal, I only describe testing the connection between it and the metacarpal, since its connection with the first distal phalanx had already been discussed in the "First distal phalanx" section.

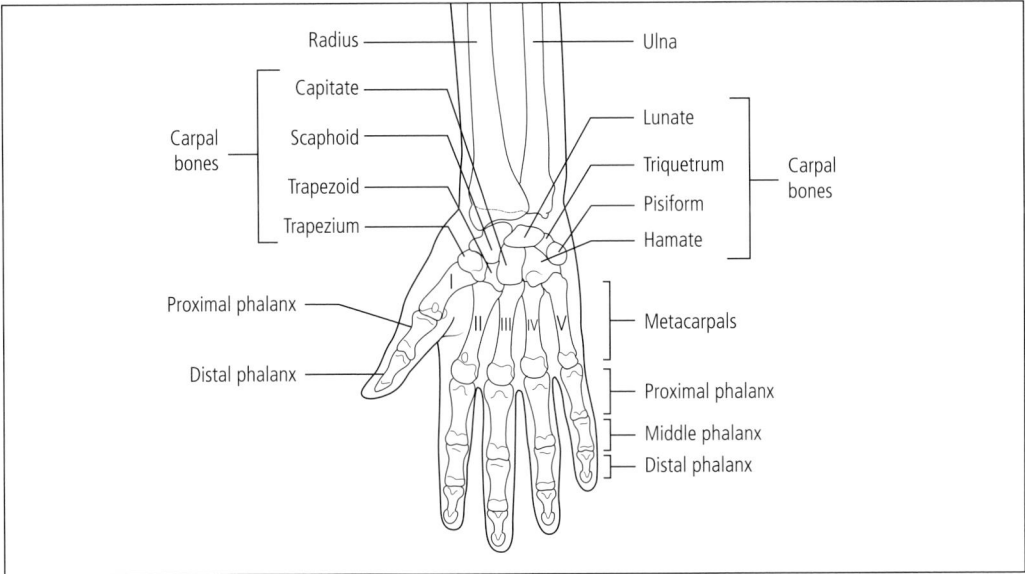

Figure 17.320. Hand and wrist.

Phalanges

Like the big toe, the thumb has only two phalanges, a distal phalanx and a proximal phalanx. The other four fingers each have three phalanges: distal, middle, and proximal. Below, testing and treatment of the first phalanges are described separately. Due to their similarities in shape and articulation, the second through fifth phalanges are described together but in three categories: distal, medial, and proximal.

First distal phalanx

Neighbor

First proximal phalanx

Palpation

The first distal phalanx is the tip of the thumb (figure 17.321). If you slide your fingers proximally over the thumb until you feel a bump just proximal to the base of the nail, you have reached the interphalangeal joint, the proximal limit of the distal phalanx.

Testing

Phase 1: Grasp the distal phalanx between your thumb and finger, with some overlap onto the proximal phalanx. Pinch and spread the distal phalanx (figure 17.322) and the interphalangeal joint (figure 17.323) between your thumb and finger, as if squeezing a gumdrop, squashing the bones and the connections between them from the center. Do the bones feel more like wood or like concrete? Does the connective tissue between the bones feel compliant or fibrotic?

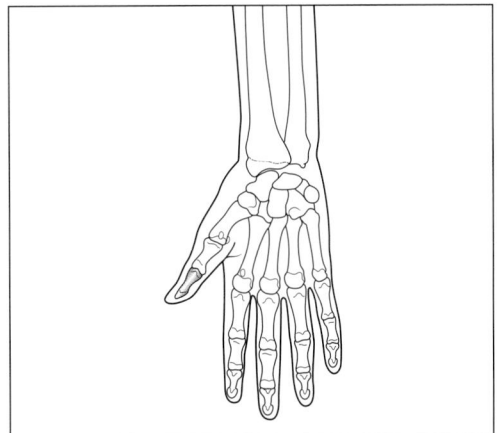

Figure 17.321. First distal phalanx.

191

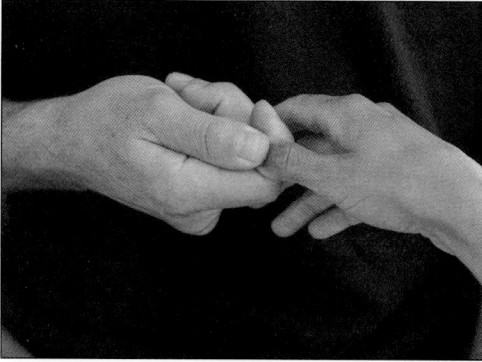

Figure 17.322. Phase 1: Testing the first distal phalanx by pinching and spreading the bone.

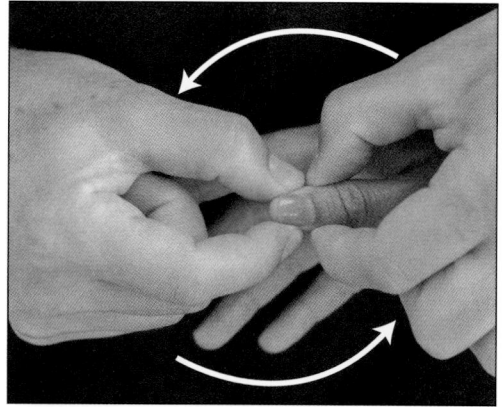

Figure 17.324. Phase 2: Spreading and twisting the first distal phalanx.

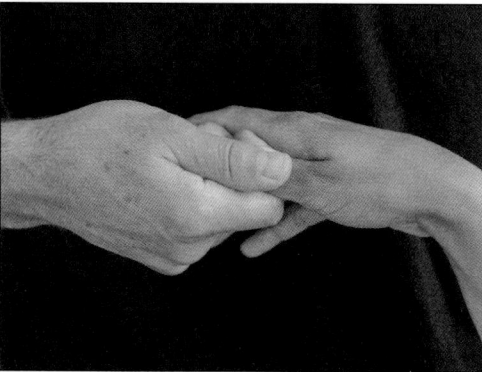

Figure 17.323. Phase 1: Testing the connection between the first distal phalanx and the first proximal phalanx by squeezing and spreading the joint line with the thumb and index finger.

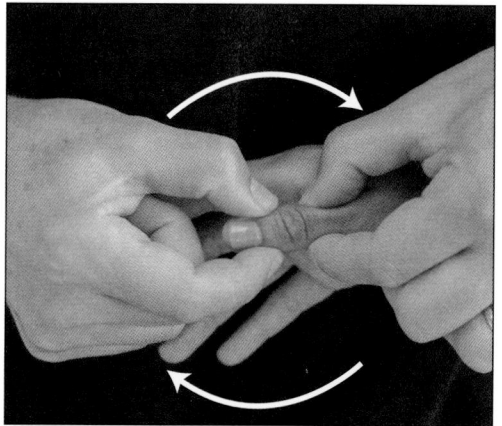

Figure 17.325. Phase 2: Spreading and twisting the connection between the first distal phalanx and the first proximal phalanx.

If both the bone and the connection with its neighbor possess elasticity, move to the next bone to be tested. If the bone itself feels compacted or the connective tissue between the distal and proximal phalanx feels fibrotic, move to phase 2 for further testing.

Phase 2: Spread and twist the bone(s) in different directions to determine the most rigid pattern within (figure 17.324) or between them (figure 17.325).

Local treatment

Grasp the phalanx (figure 17.326) and proceed with the six stages of BST treatment (see "Quick Guide to the Six Stages of BST Treatment").

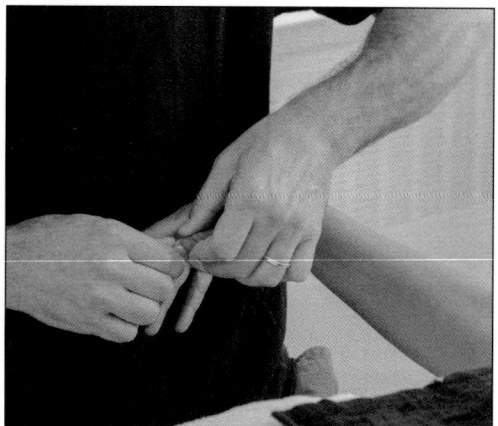

Figure 17.326. Hand and body position for the treatment of the first distal phalanx.

Regional treatment

Integrate the local treatment of the distal phalanx into the region by using the hand and wrist gather technique (see "Regional Treatment").

First proximal phalanx

Neighbors

First distal phalanx
First metacarpal

Palpation

The first proximal phalanx is located between the first distal phalanx and the first metacarpal (figure 17.327). If you slide your fingers proximally from the distal phalanx over the bump just proximal to the base of the thumbnail, you'll be on the first proximal phalanx.

Testing

Phase 1: Pinch and spread the proximal phalanx between your thumb and fingers, squashing the bone from the center (figure 17.328). Does it feel more like wood or like concrete? Adjust your fingers and test the micromobility between the bone and its neighbors by squeezing the joint line, spreading the bones apart (figure 17.329).

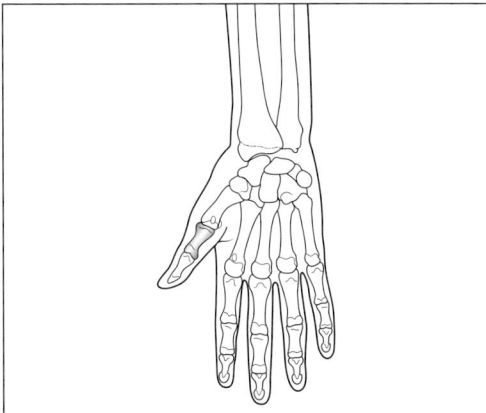

Figure 17.328. Phase 1: Testing the first proximal phalanx by pinching and spreading the bone.

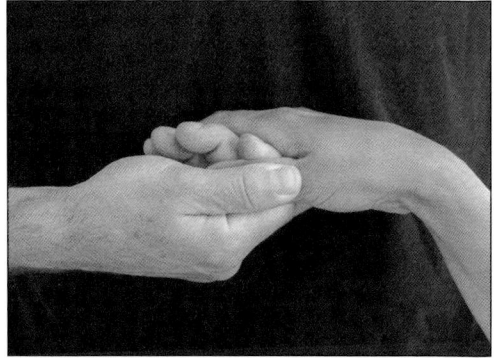

Figure 17.329. Phase 1: Testing the connection between the first proximal phalanx and the first metacarpal by squeezing and spreading the joint line with the thumb and index finger.

Does the connective tissue between the bones feel compliant or fibrotic?

If both the bone and the connections possess some bounce, move to the next bone to be tested. If the bone feels more like concrete or the connective tissue between the bones feels fibrotic, move to phase 2.

Phase 2: Spread and twist the bone(s) in different directions to determine the most rigid pattern within (figure 17.330) or between them (figure 17.331).

Local treatment

Grasp the bone (figure 17.332) and proceed with the six stages of BST treatment

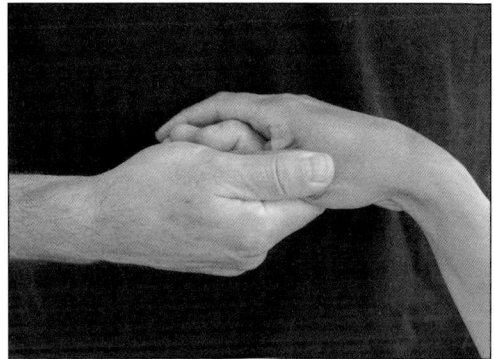

Figure 17.327. First proximal phalanx.

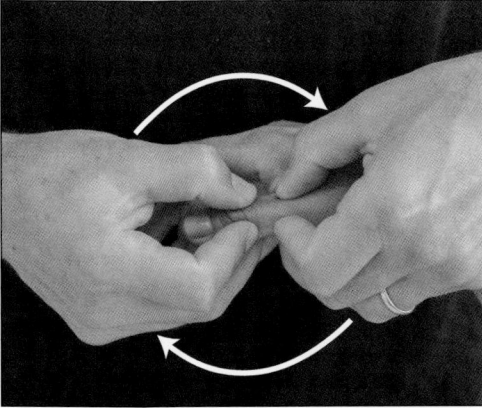

Figure 17.330. Phase 2: Spreading and twisting the first proximal phalanx.

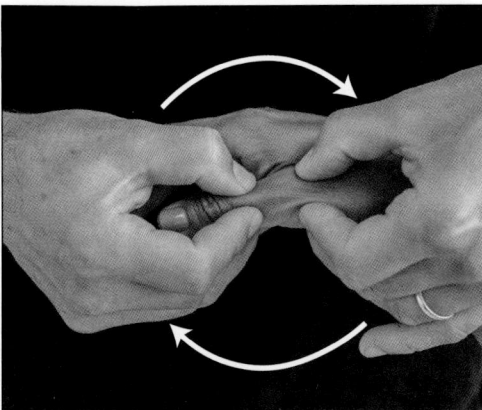

Figure 17.331. Phase 2: Spreading and twisting the first proximal phalanx and the first metacarpal. The fingers of the right hand of the therapist could be placed closer to the joint line than they are in the photo.

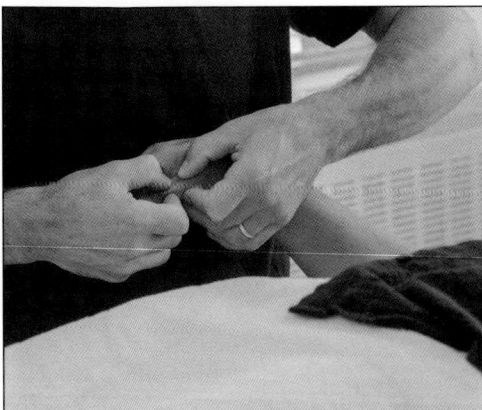

Figure 17.332. Hand and body position for treatment of the first proximal phalanx.

(see "Quick Guide to the Six Stages of BST Treatment").

Regional treatment

Integrate the local treatment of the proximal phalanx into the region by using the hand and wrist gather technique (see "Regional Treatment").

Second to fifth distal phalanges

Neighbors

Second to fifth middle phalanges

Palpation

The second to fifth distal phalanges are the tips of the other four fingers (figure 17.333). If you slide your fingers proximally over each finger until you feel a bump just proximal to the base of the nail, you have reached the distal interphalangeal joint, the proximal end of the distal phalanx.

Testing

Phase 1: Pinch and spread the distal phalanx (figure 17.334) and the connection with the corresponding middle phalanx (figure 17.335) between your thumb and fingers, as if

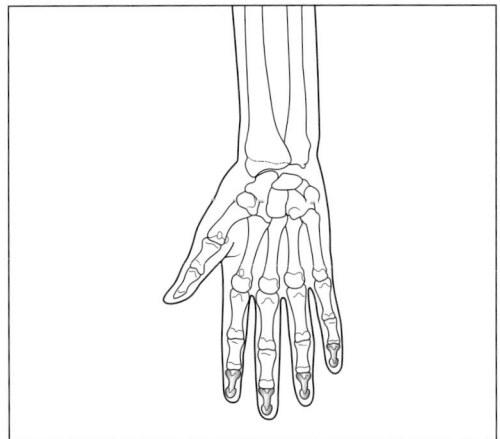

Figure 17.333. Second to fifth distal phalanges.

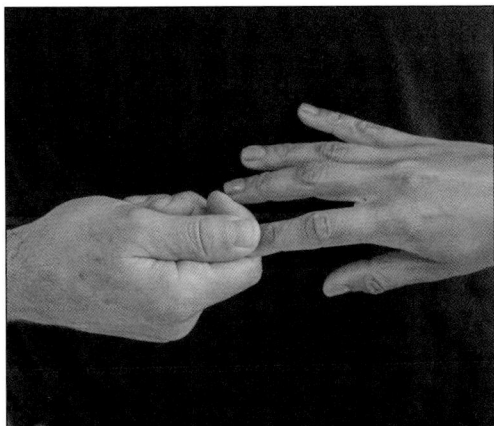

Figure 17.334. Phase 1: Testing the second distal phalanx by pinching and spreading the bone.

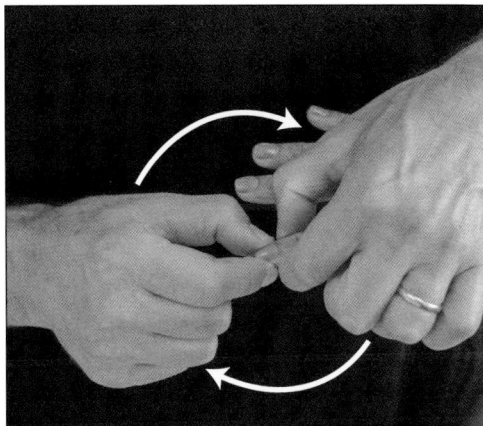

Figure 17.336. Phase 2: Spreading and twisting the second distal phalanx.

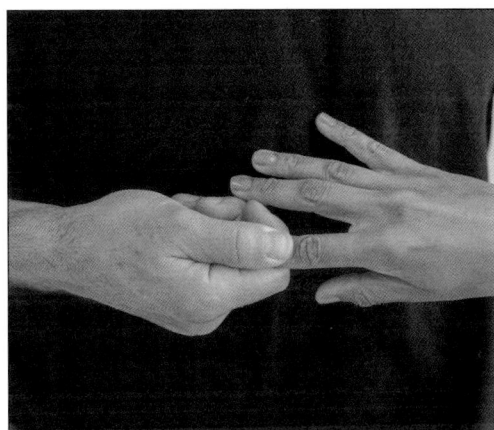

Figure 17.335. Phase 1: Testing the connection between the second distal and middle phalanges by squeezing and spreading the joint line with the thumb and index finger.

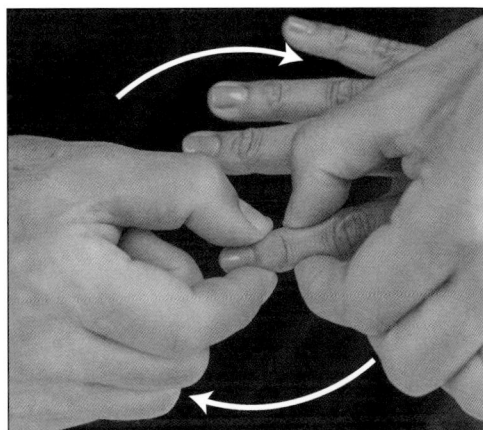

Figure 17.337. Phase 2: Spreading and twisting the connection between the second distal and middle phalanges.

squeezing a gumdrop, squashing the bone(s) from the center.

If both the bone and the connections possess elasticity, move to the next bone to be tested. If the bone itself feels like concrete or the connective tissue between the bones feels fibrotic, move to phase 2 for further testing.

Phase 2: Spread and twist the bone(s) in different directions to determine the most rigid pattern within (figure 17.336) or between them (figure 17.337).

Local treatment

Grasp the bone with both sets of fingers (figure 17.338) and proceed with the six stages of BST treatment (see "Quick Guide to the Six Stages of BST Treatment").

Regional treatment

Integrate the local treatment of the distal phalanx into the region by using the hand and wrist gather technique (see "Regional Treatment").

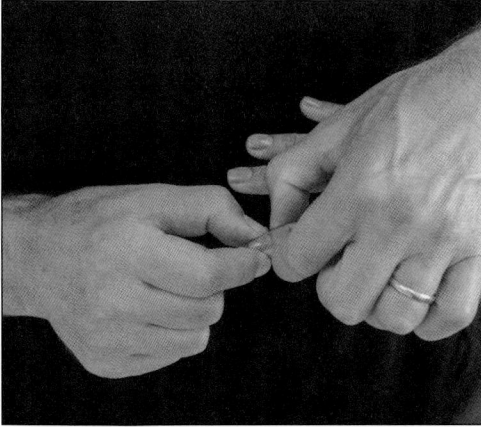

Figure 17.338. Hand position for treatment of the second distal phalanx.

Second to fifth middle phalanges

Neighbors

Second to fifth distal phalanges
Second to fifth proximal phalanges

Palpation

The second to fifth middle phalanges are located between their corresponding distal and proximal phalanges (figure 17.339). If you slide your fingers proximally from the distal interphalangeal joint to the next eminence on the finger, you will have reached the proximal interphalangeal joint, which joins the middle phalanx to the proximal phalanx.

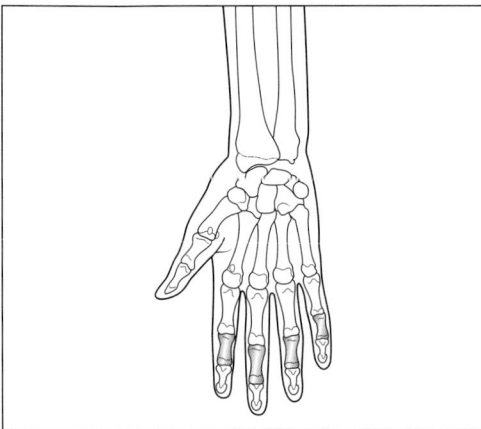

Figure 17.339. Second to fifth middle phalanges.

Testing

Phase 1: Pinch and spread the middle phalanx between your thumb and fingers, as if squeezing a gumdrop, squashing the bone from the center (figure 17.340). Does it feel more like wood or more like concrete? Now, adjust your fingers and test the micromobility between the bone and its neighbors by squeezing and spreading the joint lines (figure 17.341).

If both the bone and the connections possess elasticity, move to the next bone to be tested.

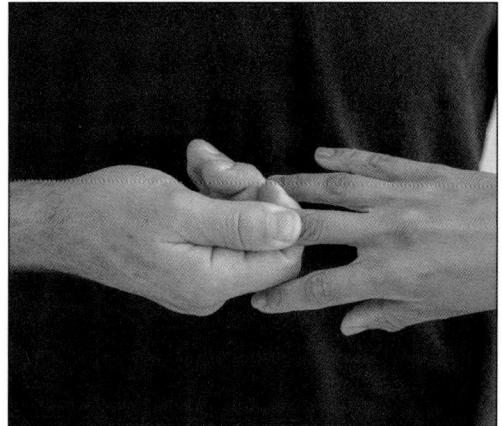

Figure 17.340. Phase 1: Testing the third middle phalanx by pinching and spreading the bone.

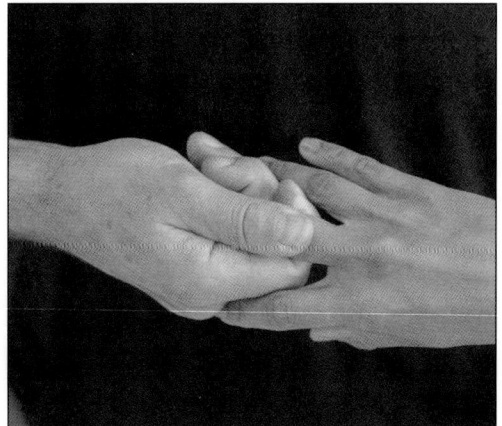

Figure 17.341. Phase 1: Testing the connection between the third middle and proximal phalanges by squeezing and spreading the joint line with the thumb and index finger.

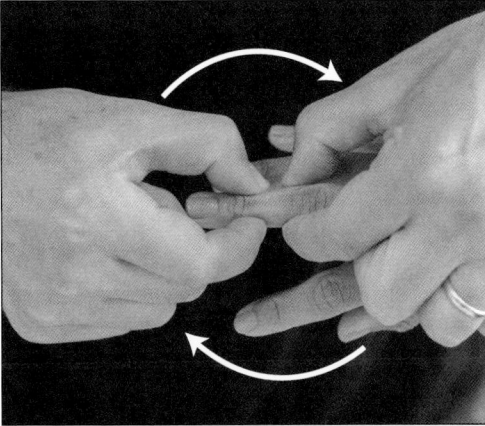

Figure 17.342. Phase 2: Spreading and twisting the third middle phalanx.

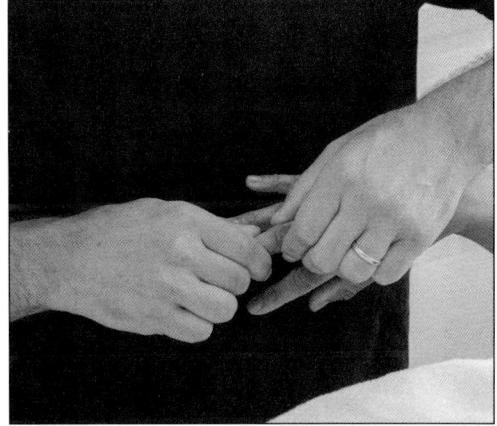

Figure 17.344. Hand and body position for local treatment of the third middle phalanx.

(see "Quick Guide to the Six Stages of BST Treatment").

Regional treatment

Integrate the local treatment of the middle phalanx into the region by using the hand and wrist gather technique (see "Regional Treatment").

Second to fifth proximal phalanges

Neighbors

Second to fifth middle phalanges
Second to fifth metacarpals

Palpation

The second to fifth proximal phalanges are located between the corresponding middle phalanges and metacarpals (figure 17.345). If you slide your fingers proximally from the proximal interphalangeal joint to the next eminence on the finger, you will have reached the metacarpophalangeal joint, which joins the proximal phalanx to the metacarpal.

Testing

Phase 1: Pinch and spread the proximal phalanx between your thumb and fingers,

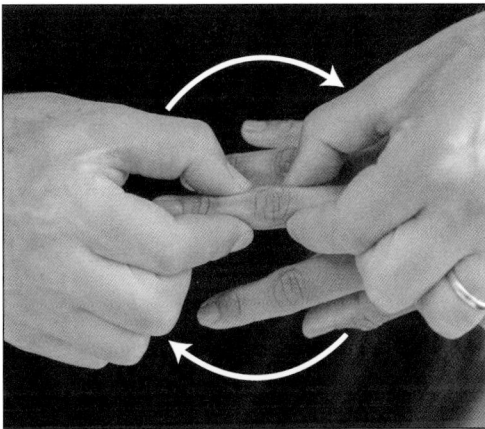

Figure 17.343. Phase 2: Spreading and twisting the connection between the third middle and proximal phalanges.

However, if the bone itself feels like concrete or the connective tissue between the bones feels fibrotic, move to phase 2 for further testing.

Phase 2: Spread and twist the bone(s) in different directions to determine the most rigid pattern within (figure 17.342) or between them (figure 17.343).

Local treatment

Grasp the bone (figure 17.344) and proceed with the six stages of BST treatment

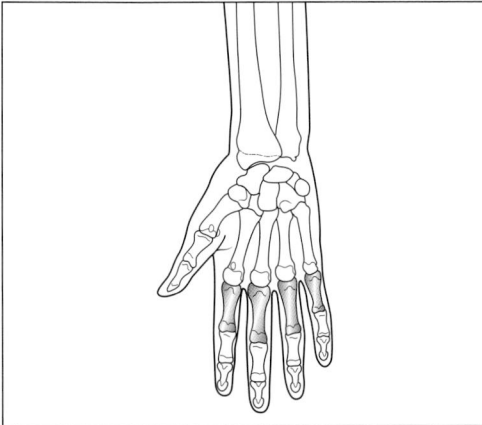

Figure 17.345. Second to fifth proximal phalanges.

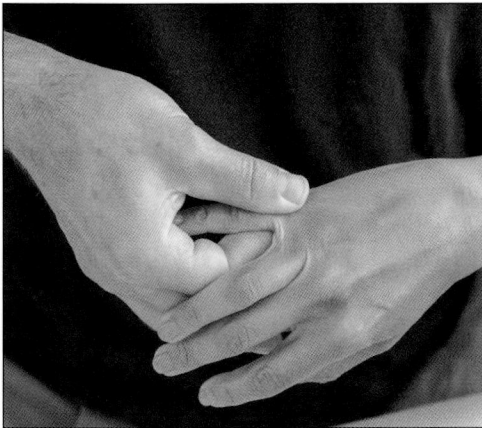

Figure 17.346. Phase 1: Testing the fifth proximal phalanx by pinching and spreading the bone.

squashing the bone from the center (figure 17.346). Does it feel like wood or concrete?

Adjust your fingers and test the micromobility between the bone and its neighbors by squeezing and spreading the joint lines (figure 17.347).

If both the bone and the connections with its neighbors possess elasticity, move to the next bone to be tested. However, if the bone feels like concrete or the connective tissue between the bones feels fibrotic, move to phase 2.

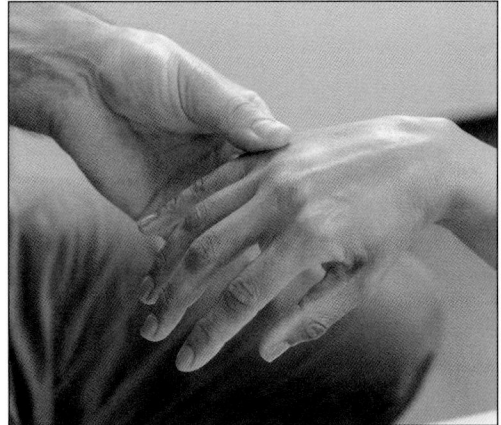

Figure 17.347. Phase 1: Testing the connection between the fifth proximal phalanx and the fifth metacarpal by squeezing and spreading the joint line with the thumb and index finger (palmar surface; not shown).

Phase 2: Spread and twist the bone(s) in different directions to determine the most rigid torsional pattern within (figure 17.348) or between them (figure 17.349).

Local treatment

Grasp the bone (figure 17.350) and proceed with the six stages of BST treatment (see "Quick Guide to the Six Stages of BST Treatment").

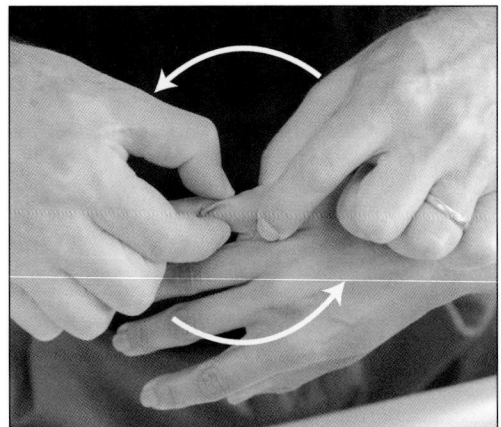

Figure 17.348. Phase 2: Spreading and twisting the fifth proximal phalanx.

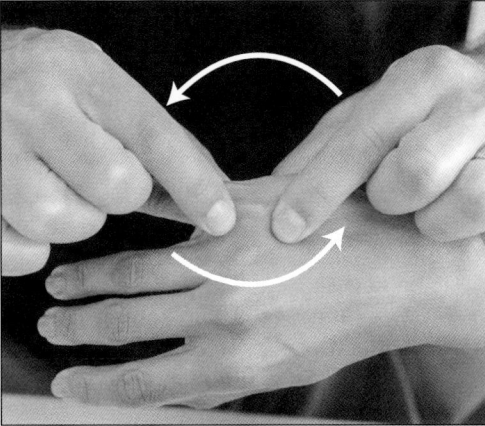

Figure 17.349. Phase 2: Spreading and twisting the connection between the fifth proximal phalanx and the fifth metacarpal with the thumbs (palmar surface) and index fingers.

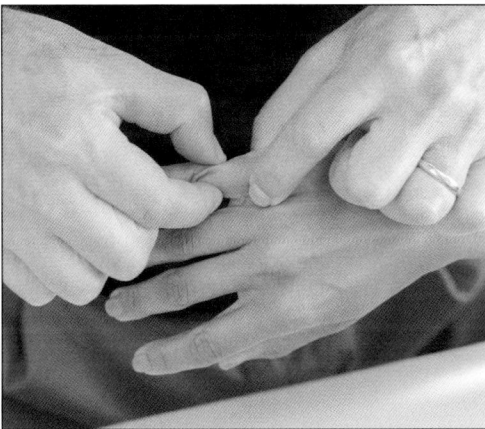

Figure 17.350. Hand position for the local treatment of the fifth proximal phalanx.

Regional treatment

Integrate the local treatment of the proximal phalanx into the region by using the hand and wrist gather technique (see "Regional Treatment").

Metacarpals

Since the five metacarpals are similar in shape but have varied proximal articulations, there are a few palpatory quirks that afford separate descriptions. Here we'll use the "wiggle test"

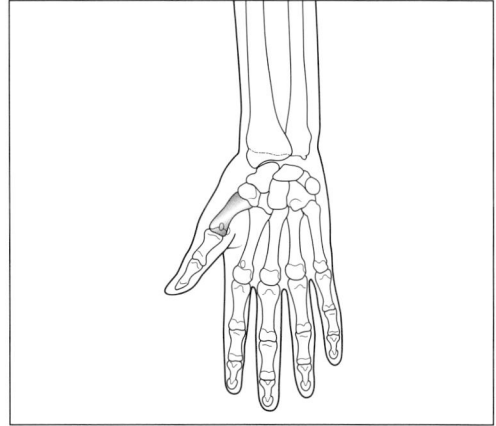

Figure 17.351. First metacarpal.

again—a useful exercise introduced earlier—for finding and palpating the metacarpals and their neighbors.

First metacarpal

The first metacarpal is the thickest and shortest of the five (figure 17.351).

Neighbors

First proximal phalanx
Trapezium

Palpation

When you move your fingers proximally over the first metacarpophalangeal joint, you will be on the head of the first metacarpal. Follow the bone down toward the base, which articulates with the trapezium. To be sure that you are on the base of the metacarpal and not on the trapezium, wiggle the first metacarpal. Move the other hand proximally along the bone until the wiggling stops.

Testing

Phase 1: Grasp the shaft of the first metacarpal between your thumb and fingers, covering as much of the bone as possible (figure 17.352). Simultaneously squash

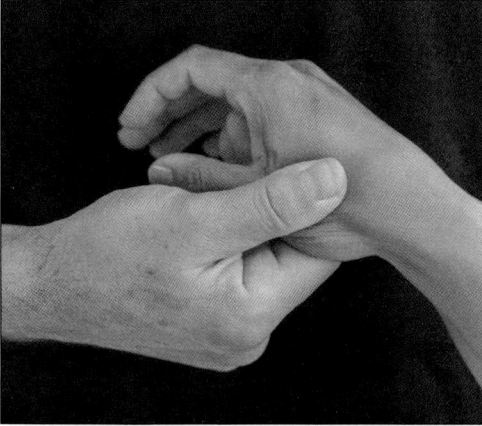

Figure 17.352. Phase 1: Testing the first metacarpal by squeezing and spreading the bone with the index finger (plantar surface) and thumb.

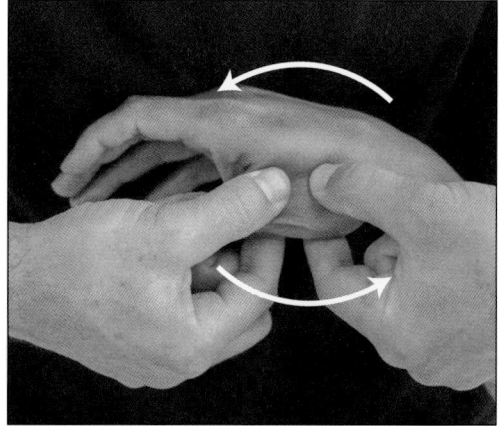

Figure 17.354. Phase 2: Spreading and twisting the first metacarpal.

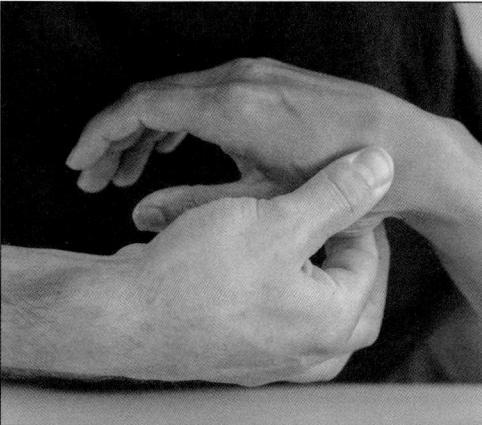

Figure 17.353. Phase 1: Testing the connections between the first metacarpal and the trapezium by squeezing and spreading the joint line with the index finger (plantar surface) and thumb.

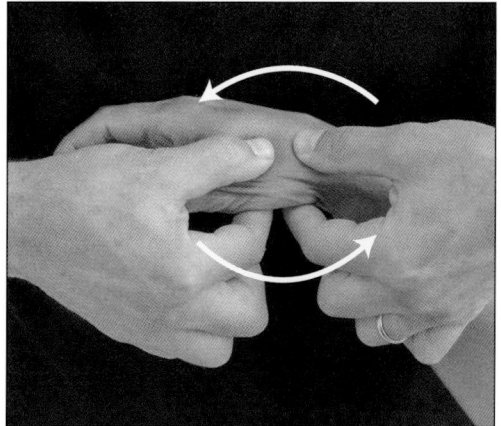

Figure 17.355. Phase 2: Spreading and twisting the connection between the first metacarpal and the trapezium.

the bone and spread it with your fingers. Does it feel like wood or concrete?

Now, adjust your fingers and test the micromobility between the first metacarpal and the trapezium by squeezing and spreading the joint line (figure 17.353).

If both the bone and the connection possess elasticity, move to the next bone to be tested. If either the bone or the connection feels compacted, move to phase 2.

Phase 2: Spread and twist the bone(s) in different directions to determine the most rigid torsional pattern within (figure 17.354) or between them (figure 17.355).

Local treatment

Grasp the bone (figure 17.356) and proceed with the six stages of BST treatment (see "Quick Guide to the Six Stages of BST Treatment").

Regional treatment

Integrate the local treatment of the metacarpal into the region by using the hand

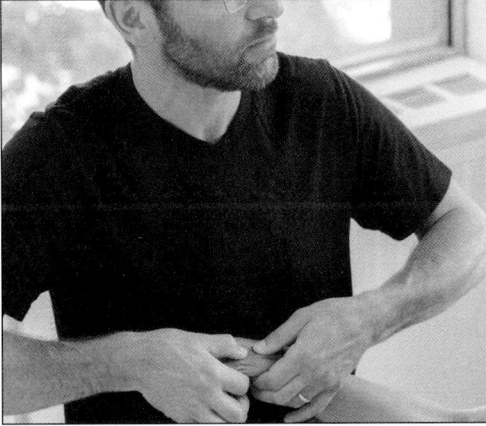

Figure 17.356. Hand and body position for the local treatment of the first metacarpal.

and wrist gather technique (see "Regional Treatment").

Second metacarpal

The second metacarpal is the longest of the five (figure 17.357).

Neighbors

Second proximal phalanx
Third metacarpal
Trapezium
Trapezoid
Capitate

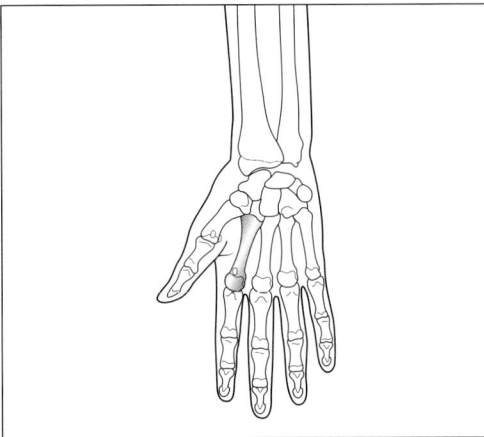

Figure 17.357. Second metacarpal.

Palpation

When you move your fingers proximally over the second metacarpophalangeal joint, you will be on the head of the second metacarpal, the base of which articulates with four other bones: the base of the third metacarpal, the trapezium, the trapezoid, and the capitate. As you did for the first metacarpal, and to be sure that you are on the base of the second metacarpal and not on any of the neighbors, wiggle the second metacarpal. Slide down the shaft of the bone with the other hand until the wiggling stops.

Testing

Phase 1: Grasp the shaft of the second metacarpal between your thumb and fingers, covering as much of the bone as possible (figure 17.358). Simultaneously squash the bone and spread it with your fingers. Does it feel like wood or concrete?

Now, adjust your fingers and test the micromobility between the second metacarpal and its neighbors by squeezing and spreading the joint lines (figures 17.359 to 17.362).

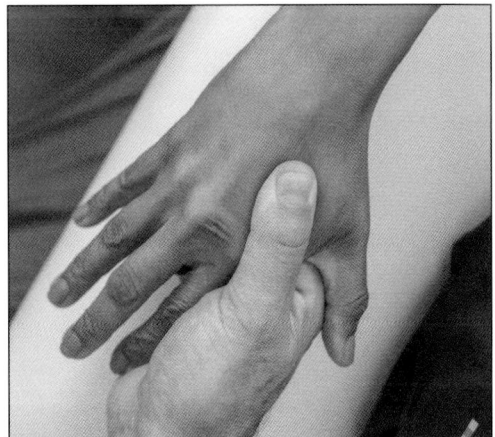

Figure 17.358. Phase 1: Testing the second metacarpal by squeezing and spreading the bone.

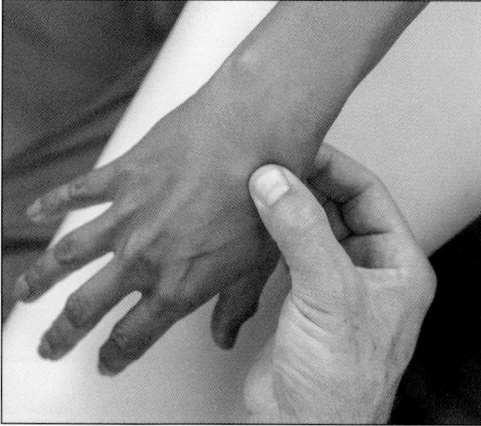

Figure 17.359. Phase 1: Testing the connection between the second metacarpal and the trapezium by squeezing and spreading the joint line with the thumb and index finger (palmar surface).

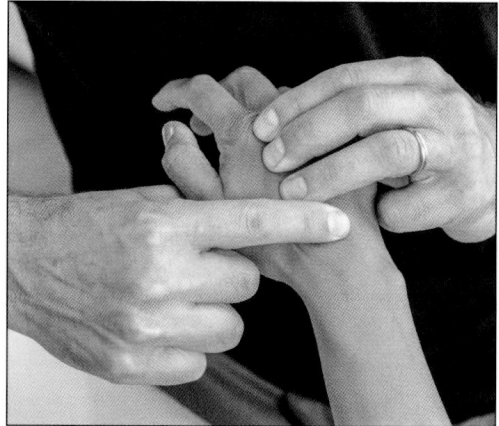

Figure 17.361. Phase 1: Testing the connection between the second metacarpal and capitate by squeezing and spreading the joint line.

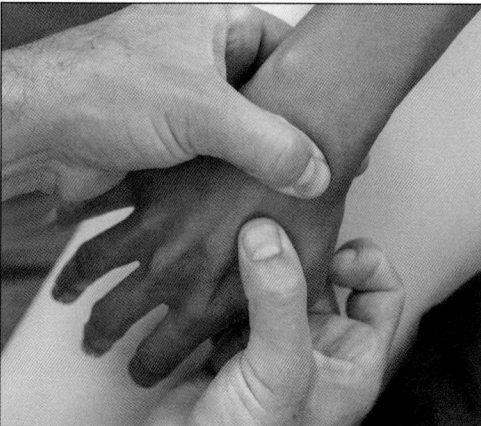

Figure 17.360. Phase 1: Testing the connection between the second metacarpal and trapezoid by pinching and spreading the joint line with the index finger (palmar surface) and thumb of the left hand.

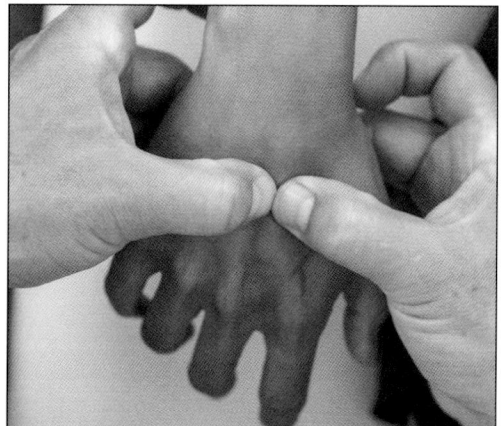

Figure 17.362. Phase 1: Testing the connection between the second and third metacarpals by squeezing and spreading the joint line with the left middle finger (palmar surface; not shown) and thumb of the left hand.

If both the bone and the connections possess elasticity, move to the next bone(s) to be tested. If either the bone or the connections feel compacted, move to phase 2.

Phase 2: Spread and twist the bone(s) in different directions to determine the most rigid torsional pattern of compaction within (figure 17.363) or between them (figures 17.364 to 17.367).

Local treatment

Grasp the second metacarpal with both sets of fingers (figure 17.368) and proceed with the six stages of BST treatment (see "Quick Guide to the Six Stages of BST Treatment").

Regional treatment

Integrate the local treatment of the metacarpal into the region by using the hand

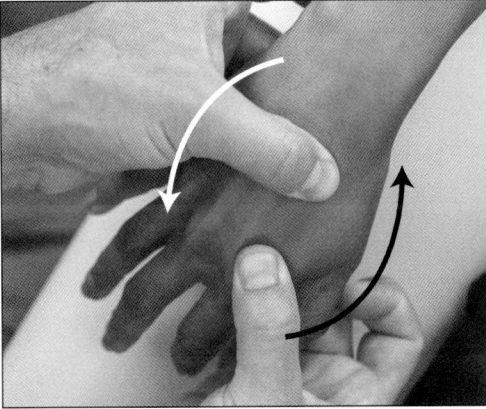

Figure 17.363. Phase 2: Spreading and twisting the second metacarpal with the thumbs and fingers (palmar surface).

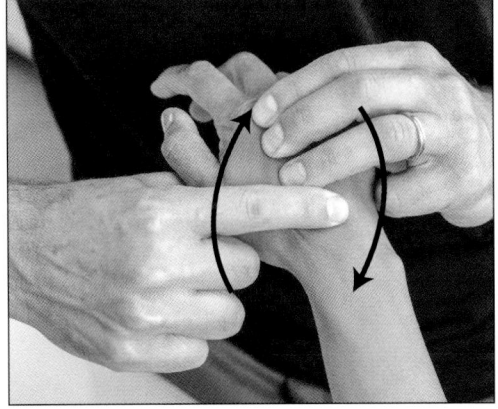

Figure 17.366. Phase 2: Spreading and twisting the connection between the second metacarpal and capitate.

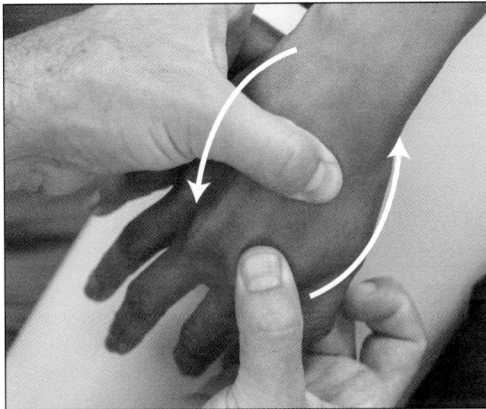

Figure 17.364. Phase 2: Spreading and twisting the connection between the second metacarpal and the trapezium with the thumbs and fingers (palmar surface).

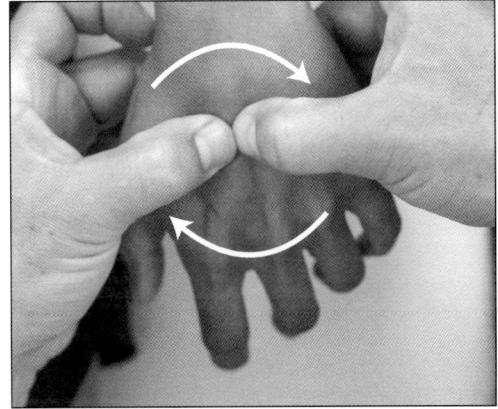

Figure 17.367. Phase 2: Spreading and twisting the connection between the second and third metacarpals with the thumbs and index fingers (palmar surface).

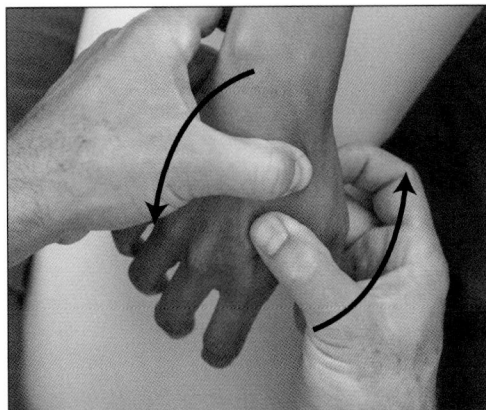

Figure 17.365. Phase 2: Spreading and twisting the connection between the second metacarpal and trapezoid with the thumbs and fingers (palmar surface).

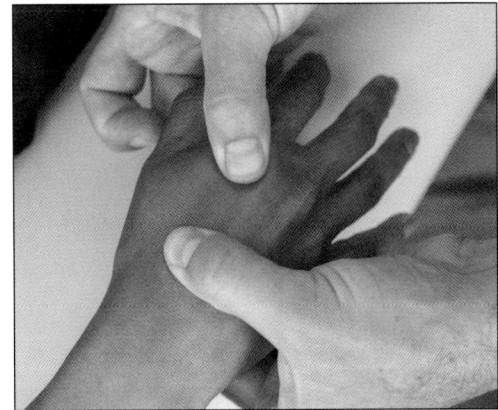

Figure 17.368. Hand position for the local treatment of the second metacarpal using the thumbs and fingers (palmar surface).

and wrist gather technique (see "Regional Treatment").

Third metacarpal

Neighbors

Third proximal phalanx
Second and fourth metacarpals
Capitate

Palpation

When you move your fingers proximally over the third metacarpophalangeal joint, you will be on the head of the third metacarpal (figure 17.369), the base of which articulates with three other bones: the bases of the second and fourth metacarpals and the capitate. To be sure that you are on the base of the third metacarpal and not on any of the neighbors, wiggle the third metacarpal, then move the other hand proximally along the bone until the wiggling stops.

Testing

Phase 1: Grasp the shaft of the third metacarpal between your thumb and fingers, covering as much of the bone as possible (figure 17.370). Simultaneously squash

the bone and spread it with your fingers. Does it feel like wood or concrete?

Now, adjust your fingers and test the micromobility between the third metacarpal and its neighbors by squeezing and spreading the joint lines (figures 17.371 and 17.372).

If both the bone and the connections possess elasticity, move to the next bone to be tested. If either the bone or the connections feel compacted, move to phase 2.

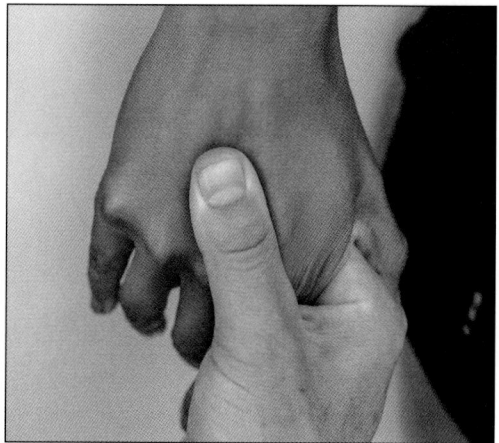

Figure 17.370. Phase 1: Testing the third metacarpal by squeezing and spreading the bone with the thumb and index finger (palmar surface).

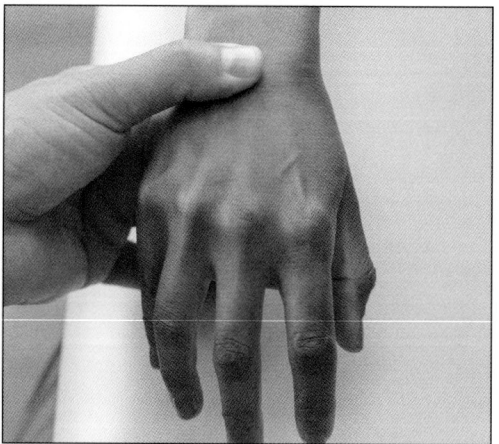

Figure 17.371. Phase 1: Testing the third metacarpal with capitate by squeezing and spreading the joint line with the thumb and index finger (palmar surface).

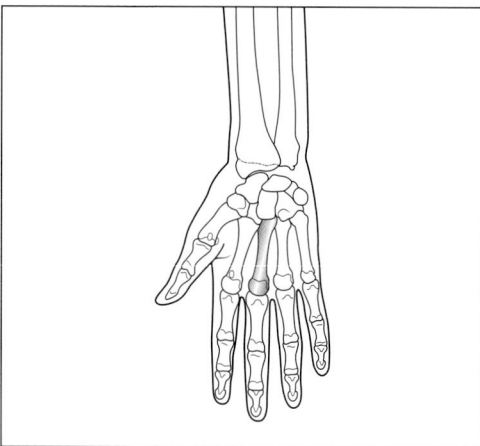

Figure 17.369. Third metacarpal.

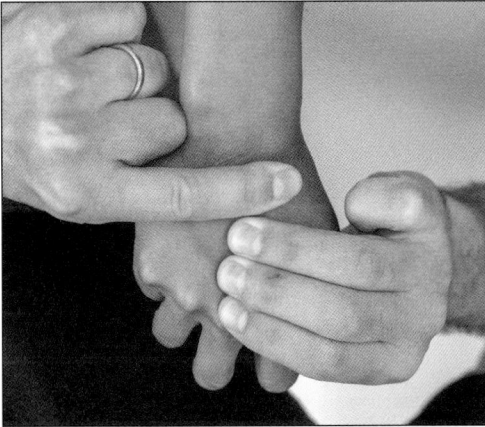

Figure 17.372. Phase 1: Testing the third metacarpal with the bases of the second and fourth metacarpals by squeezing and spreading the joint lines with the thumb (palmar surface) and index finger of the left hand.

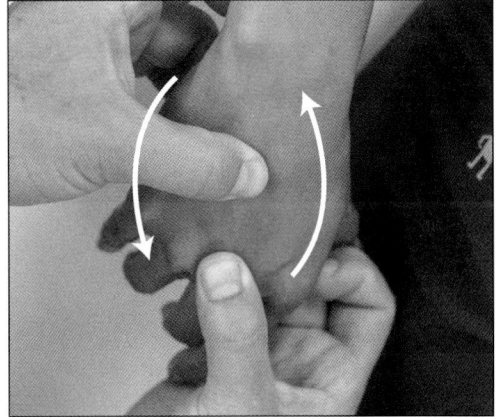

Figure 17.374. Phase 2: Spreading and twisting the third metacarpal with capitate using the thumbs and fingers (palmar surface).

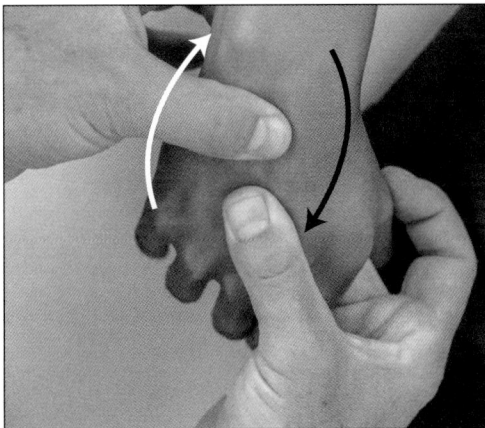

Figure 17.373. Phase 2: Spreading and twisting the third metacarpal with the thumbs and fingers (palmar surface).

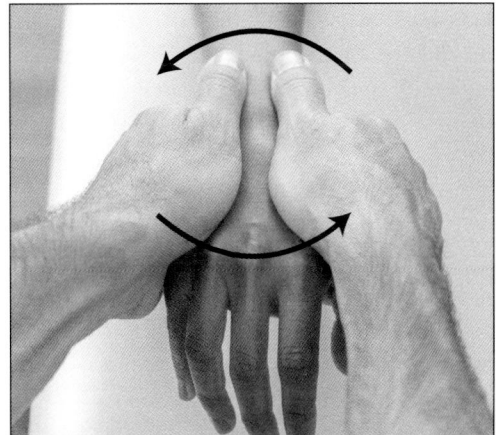

Figure 17.375. Phase 2: Spreading and twisting the third metacarpal with the bases of the second and fourth metacarpals.

Phase 2: Spread and twist the bone(s) in different directions to determine the most rigid pattern of compaction within (figure 17.373) and/or between them (figures 17.374 and 17.375).

Local treatment

Grasp the third metacarpal with both sets of fingers (figure 17.376) and proceed with the six stages of BST treatment (see "Quick Guide to the Six Stages of BST Treatment").

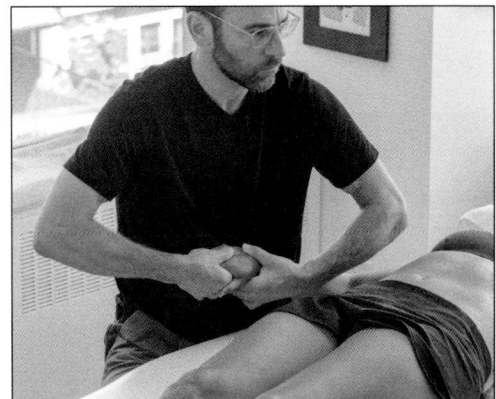

Figure 17.376. Hand and body position for the local treatment of the third metacarpal.

Regional treatment

Integrate the local treatment of the third metacarpal into the region by using the hand and wrist gather technique (see "Regional Treatment").

Fourth metacarpal

Neighbors

Fourth proximal phalanx
Third and fifth metacarpals
Capitate
Hamate

Palpation

When you move your fingers proximally over the fourth metacarpophalangeal joint, you will be on the head of the fourth metacarpal (figure 17.377), the base of which articulates with four other bones: the bases of the third and fifth metacarpals, the capitate, and the hamate. To be sure that you are on the base of the fourth metacarpal and not on any of the neighbors, wiggle the fourth metacarpal, then move the other hand proximally along the bone until the wiggling stops.

Testing

Phase 1: Grasp the shaft of the fourth metacarpal between your thumb and fingers,

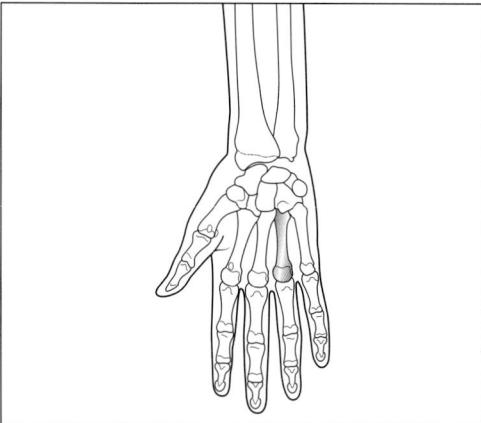

Figure 17.377. Fourth metacarpal.

covering as much of the bone as possible (figure 17.378). Simultaneously squash the bone and spread it with your fingers. Does it feel like wood or concrete?

Now, adjust your fingers and test the micromobility between the fourth metacarpal and its neighbors by squeezing and spreading the joint lines (figures 17.379 to 17.381).

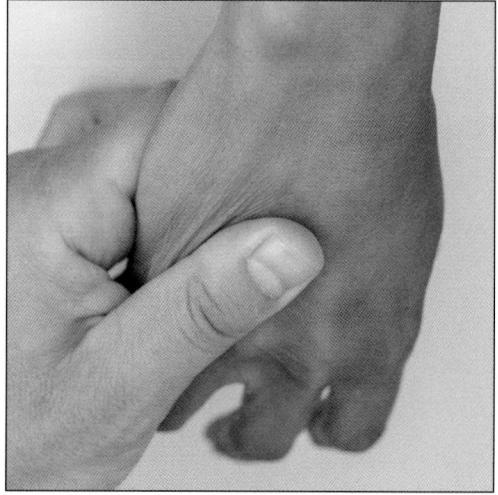

Figure 17.378. Phase 1: Testing the fourth metacarpal by squeezing and spreading the bone with the thumb and index finger (palmar surface).

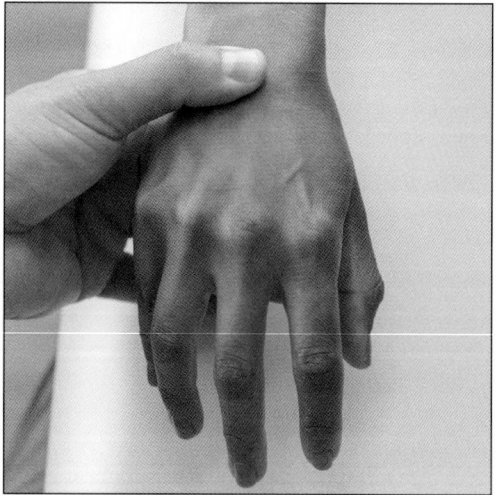

Figure 17.379. Phase 1: Testing the connection between the fourth metacarpal and capitate by squeezing and spreading the joint line with the thumb and index finger (palmar surface).

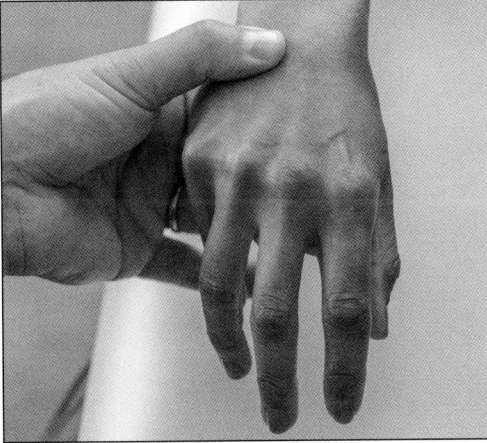

Figure 17.380. Phase 1: Testing the connection between the fourth metacarpal and hamate by squeezing and spreading the joint line with the thumb and index finger (palmar surface).

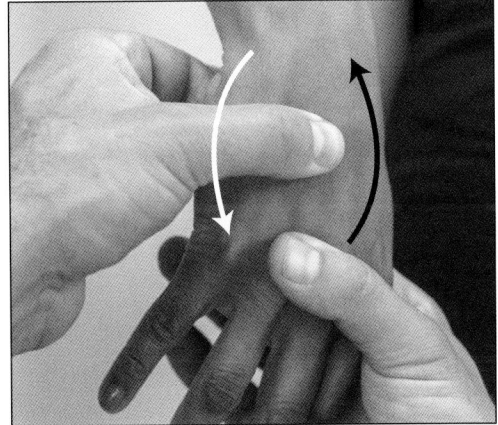

Figure 17.382. Phase 2: Spreading and twisting the fourth metacarpal with the thumbs and index fingers (palmar surface).

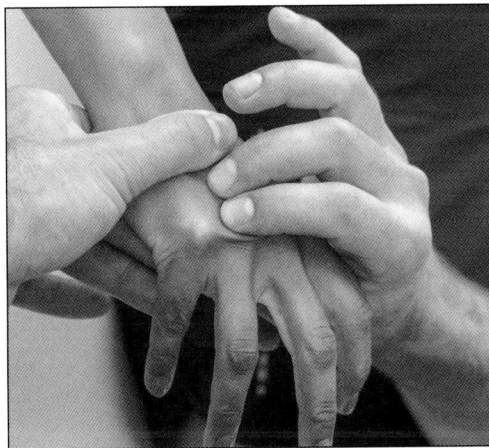

Figure 17.381. Phase 1: Testing the connection between the fourth metacarpal and the bases of the third and fifth metacarpals by squeezing and spreading the joint lines with the thumb and fingers (palmar surface) of the left hand.

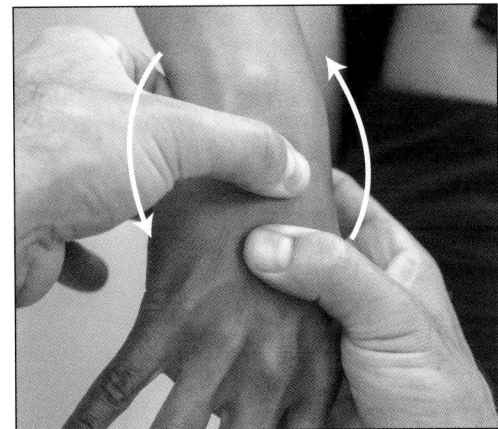

Figure 17.383. Phase 2: Spreading and twisting the connection between the fourth metacarpal and capitate with the thumbs and index fingers (palmar surface).

If both the bone and the connections possess elasticity, move to the next bone to be tested. If either the bone or the connections feel compacted, move to phase 2.

Phase 2: Spread and twist the bone(s) in different directions to determine the most rigid pattern of compaction within (figure 17.382) or between them (figures 17.383 to 17.385).

Local treatment

Grasp the fourth metacarpal with both sets of fingers (figure 17.386) and proceed with the six stages of BST treatment (see "Quick Guide to the Six Stages of BST Treatment").

Regional treatment

Integrate the local treatment of the metacarpal into the region by using the hand and wrist gather technique (see "Regional Treatment").

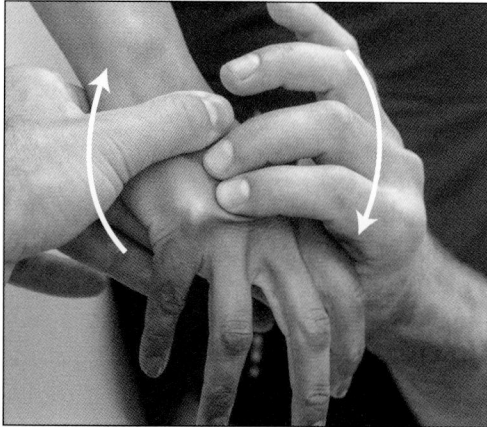

Figure 17.384. Phase 2: Spreading and twisting the connection between the fourth metacarpal and hamate with the left thumb and index finger and the right index and middle fingers.

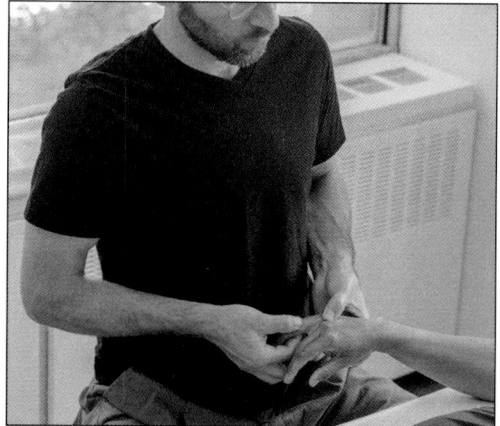

Figure 17.386. Hand and body position for the local treatment of the fourth metacarpal.

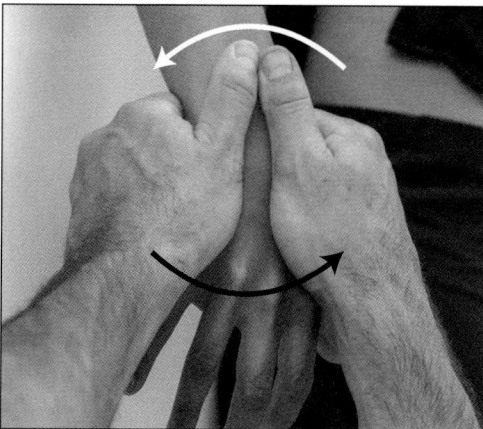

Figure 17.385. Phase 2: Spreading and twisting the connection between the fourth metacarpal and the bases of the third and fifth metacarpals using the thenar eminences and fingers (palmar surface).

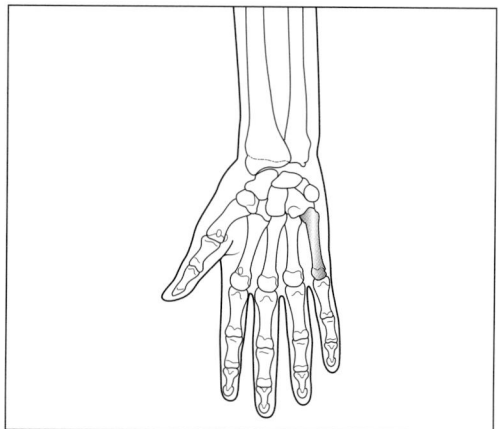

Figure 17.387. Fifth metacarpal.

Fifth metacarpal

Neighbors

Fifth proximal phalanx
Fourth metacarpal
Hamate

Palpation

When you move your fingers proximally over the fifth metacarpophalangeal joint, you will be on the head of the fifth metacarpal (figure 17.387), the base of which articulates with two other bones: the base of the fourth metacarpal and the hamate. To be sure that you are on the base of the fifth metacarpal and not on any of the neighbors, wiggle the fifth metacarpal, then move the other hand proximally along the bone until the wiggling stops.

Testing

Phase 1: Grasp the shaft of the fifth metacarpal between your thumb and fingers, covering as much of the bone as possible (figure 17.388). Simultaneously squash the bone and spread it with your fingers. Does it feel like wood or concrete?

Now, adjust your fingers and test the micromobility between the fifth metacarpal and its neighbors by squeezing and spreading the joint lines (figures 17.389 and 17.390).

If both the bone and the connections possess elasticity, move to the next bone to be tested. If either the bone or the connections feel compacted, move to phase 2.

Phase 2: Spread and twist the bone(s) in different directions to determine the most rigid pattern of compaction within (figure 17.391) or between them (figures 17.392 and 17.393).

Local treatment

Grasp the fifth metacarpal (figure 17.394) and proceed with the six stages of BST treatment (see "Quick Guide to the Six Stages of BST Treatment").

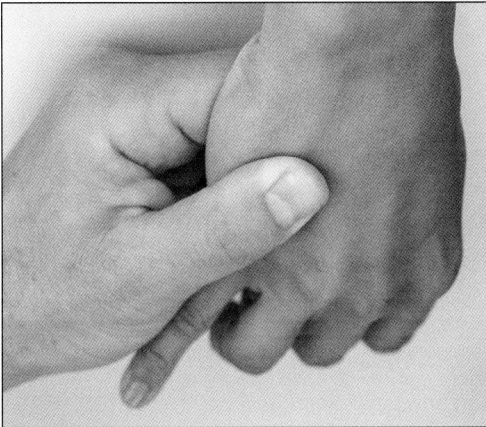

Figure 17.388. Phase 1: Testing the fifth metacarpal by squeezing and spreading the bone with the thumb and index finger (palmar surface).

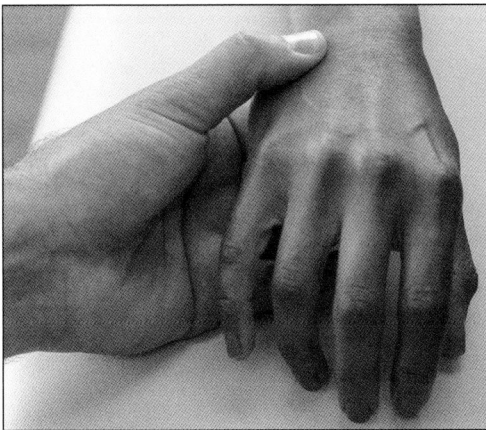

Figure 17.390. Phase 1: Testing the connection between the fifth and fourth metacarpals by squeezing and spreading the joint line with the thumb and index finger (palmar surface).

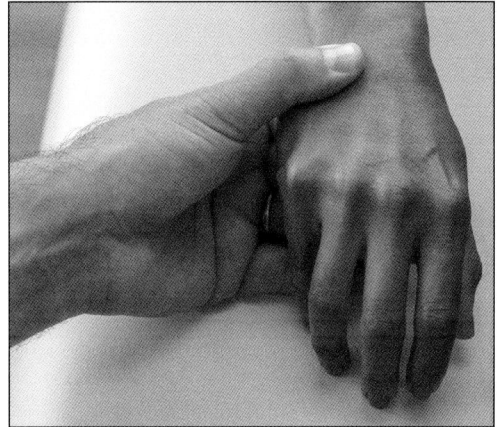

Figure 17.389. Phase 1: Testing the connection between the fifth metacarpal and hamate by squeezing and spreading the joint line with the thumb and index finger (palmar surface).

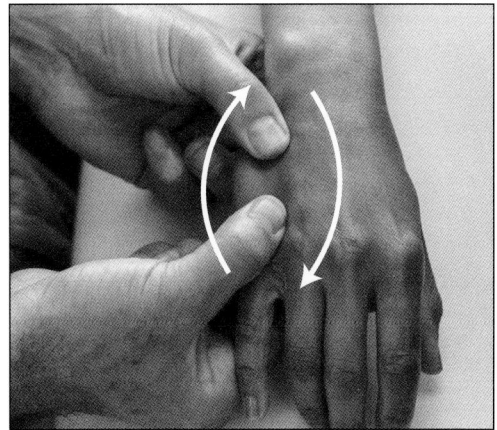

Figure 17.391. Phase 2: Spreading and twisting the fifth metacarpal with the thumbs and index fingers (palmar surface).

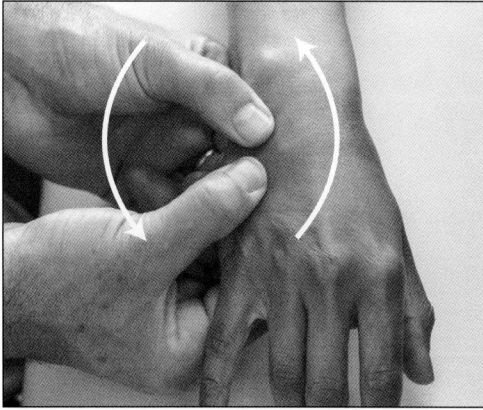

Figure 17.392. Phase 2: Spreading and twisting the connection between the fifth metacarpal and hamate using the thumbs and index fingers (palmar surface).

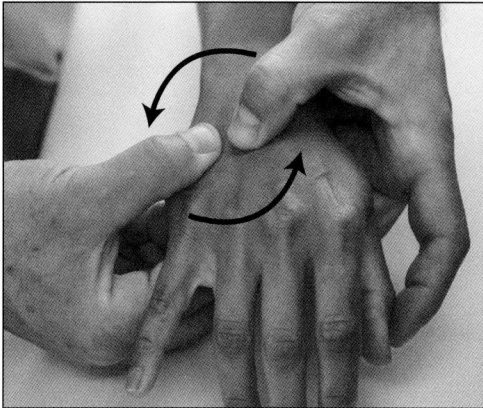

Figure 17.393. Phase 2: Spreading and twisting the connection between the fifth and fourth metacarpals using the thumbs and fingers (palmar surface).

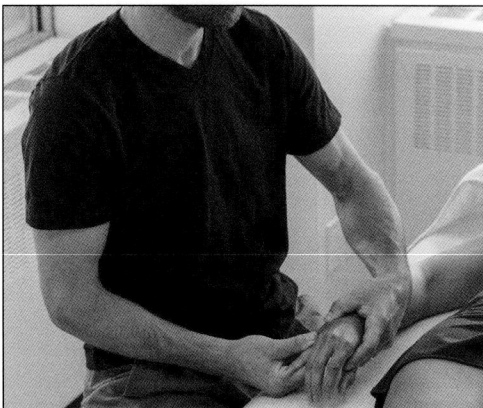

Figure 17.394. Hand and body position for the local treatment of the fifth metacarpal.

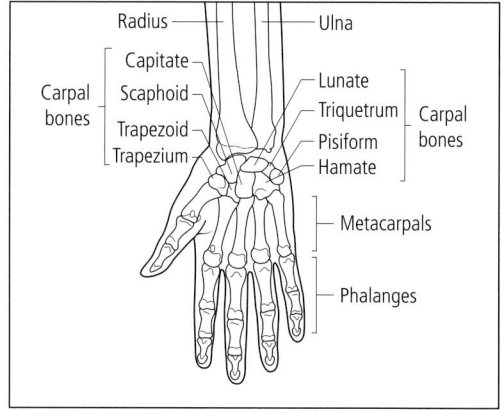

Figure 17.395. Carpal bones.

Regional treatment

Integrate the local treatment of the fifth metacarpal into the region by using the hand and wrist gather technique (see "Regional Treatment").

Carpals

The eight carpal bones form the wrist (figure 17.395). Due to both their proximity and small size, we'll test and treat them collectively, as if all eight bones were parts of the same "wrist bone." We'll still list the neighbors and review palpation tips for each individual carpal bone, so you can find and name them if you have to.

Trapezium

Neighbors

First and second metacarpals
Trapezoid
Scaphoid

Palpation

Follow the first proximal metacarpal down past the base, onto trapezium (figure 17.396). To make sure you are contacting the right bone, have the subject wiggle their thumb.

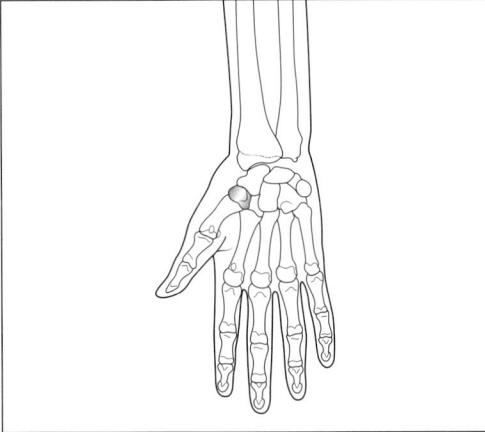

Figure 17.396. Trapezium.

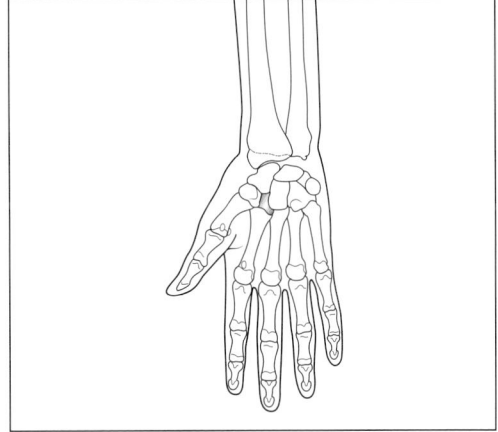

Figure 17.398. Trapezoid.

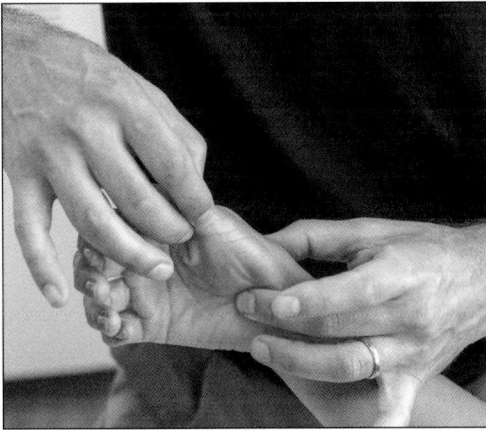

Figure 17.397. Palpating trapezium.

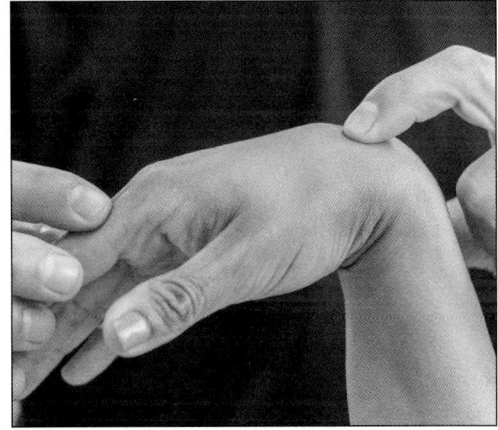

Figure 17.399. Palpating trapezoid.

The metacarpal will move, but trapezium will remain still (figure 17.397).

Trapezoid

Neighbors

Second metacarpal
Trapezium
Hamate
Scaphoid

Palpation

On the dorsal side of the hand, follow the second metacarpal down past the base into a small depression. Just proximal to the depression is the dorsal surface of trapezoid (figures 17.398 and 17.399).

Capitate

Capitate is the largest of the carpals and sits in the center of the wrist (figure 17.400).

Neighbors

Second, third, and fourth metacarpals
Scaphoid
Lunate
Hamate
Trapezoid

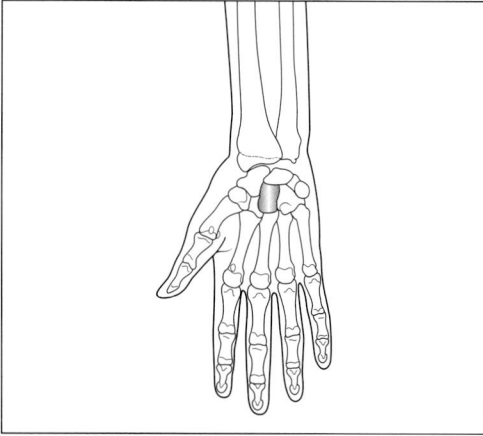

Figure 17.400. Capitate.

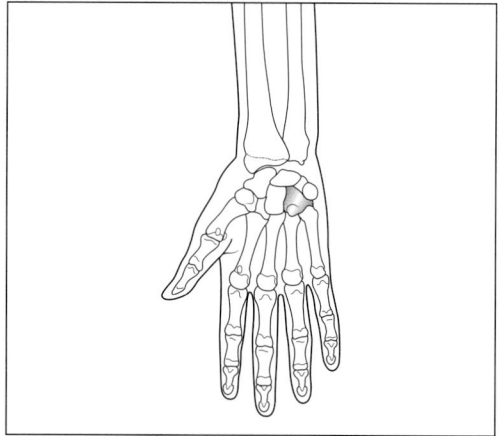

Figure 17.402. Hamate.

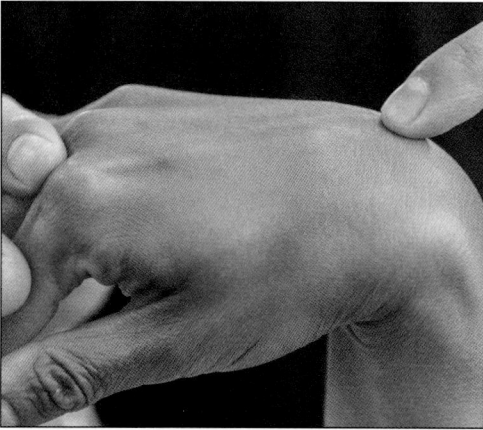

Figure 17.401. Palpating the capitate.

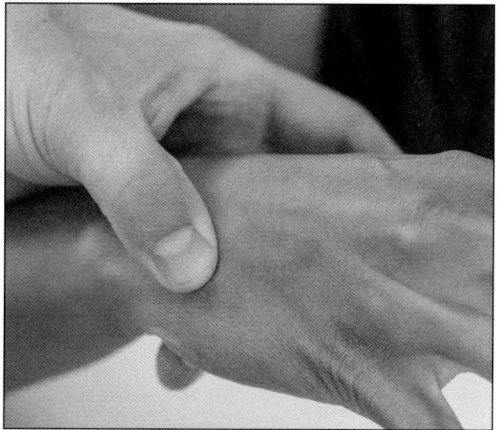

Figure 17.403. Palpating hamate (using the thumb).

Palpation

On the dorsal side of the hand, follow the third metacarpal down past the base into a small depression. Just proximal to the depression is the dorsal surface of capitate (figure 17.401).

Hamate

Neighbors

Fourth and fifth metacarpals
Capitate
Lunate
Triquetrum

Palpation

On the dorsal side of the hand, follow the fourth and fifth metacarpals down past their bases onto the dorsal surface of hamate (figures 17.402 and 17.403).

Scaphoid

Neighbors

Trapezium
Trapezoid
Capitate
Lunate
Radius

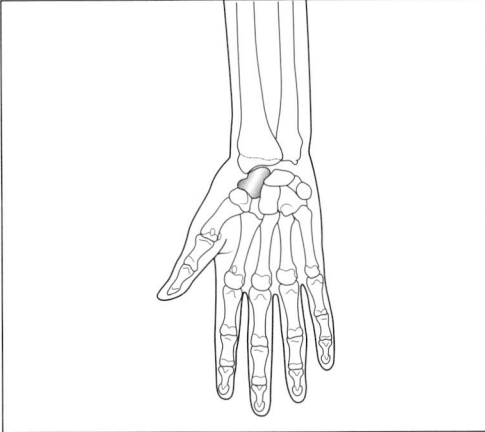

Figure 17.404. Scaphoid.

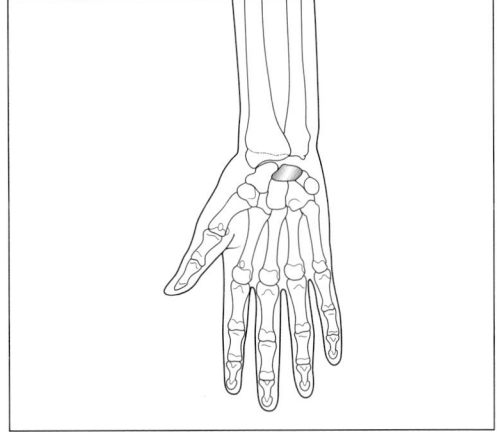

Figure 17.406. Lunate.

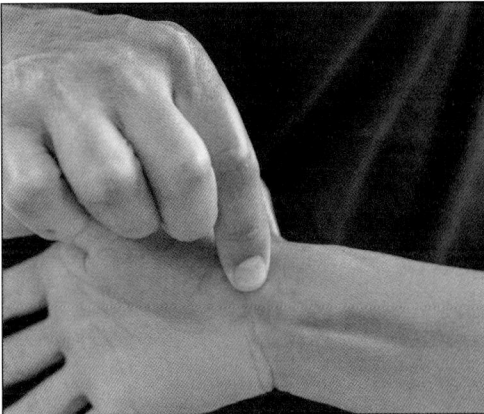

Figure 17.405. Palpating scaphoid.

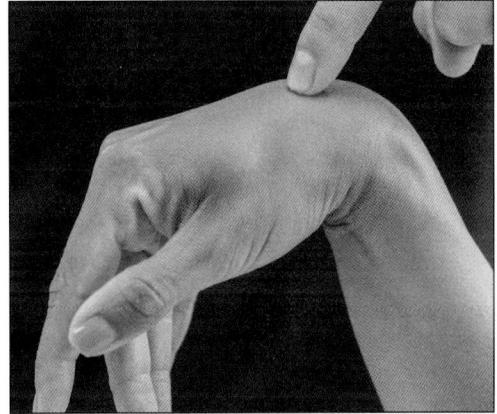

Figure 17.407. Palpating lunate.

Palpation

Move distally along the radius, over the styloid process at its distal extremity, and onto scaphoid (figures 17.404 and 17.405). For easier access to the bone, have the subject extend and perform an ulnar deviation of the hand.

Lunate

Neighbors

Scaphoid
Triquetrum
Hamate
Capitate
Radius

Palpation

Move distally along the radius, over the posterior tubercle at its distal extremity. Move the finger to the medial border of the tubercle, onto the radiocarpal joint line. Have the subject flex their hand. The dorsal surface of the lunate should poke into your finger (figures 17.406 and 17.407).

Triquetrum

Neighbors

Lunate
Pisiform
Hamate
Ulna

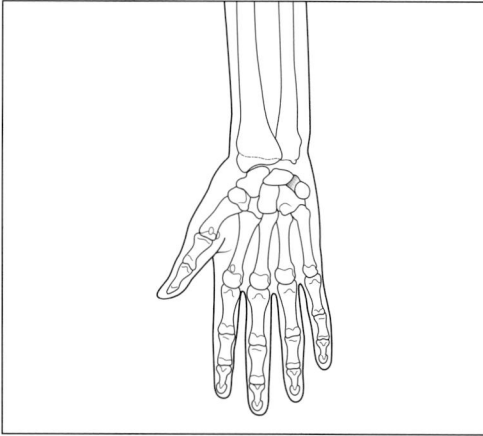

Figure 17.408. Triquetrum.

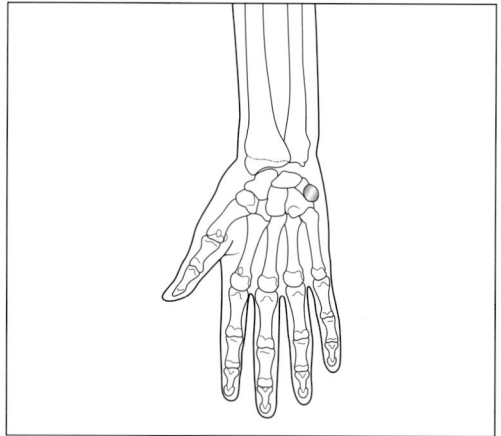

Figure 17.410. Pisiform.

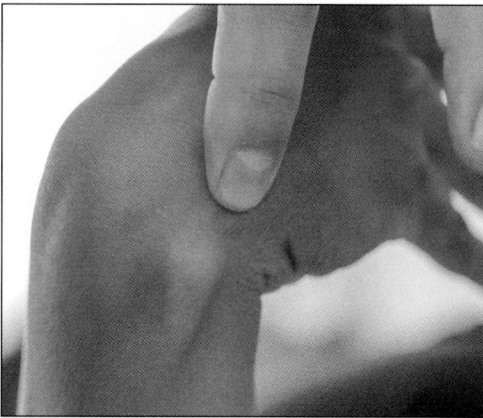

Figure 17.409. Palpating triquetrum.

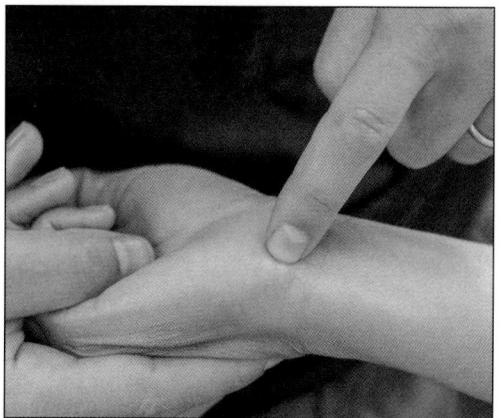

Figure 17.411. Palpating the pisiform (using the index finger).

Palpation

Move distally along the ulna, over the styloid process at its distal extremity, and onto the triquetrum (figure 17.408). Have the subject flex their hand and supinate the forearm to better expose the bone (figure 17.409).

Pisiform

Neighbor

Triquetrum

Palpation

The tendon of the flexor carpi ulnaris muscle connects directly to the pisiform at the base of the hypothenar eminence (figures 17.410 and 17.411).

Testing and treatment of the wrist

Testing

Grasp all eight carpal bones in both hands (figure 17.412). Squeeze and spread the bones collectively and see if any compacted zones emerge. If any specific zones within the wrist feel more like concrete than like wood, see if you can identify which carpal bones are compacted, and proceed with local treatment.

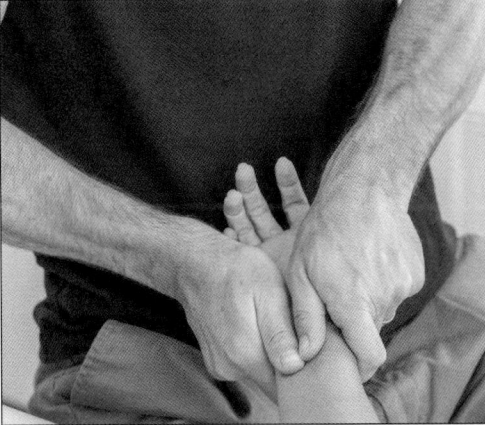

Figure 17.412. Testing the carpal bones.

Local treatment

Grasp the compacted carpal bone(s) (hamate, for example, figure 17.413) with both sets of fingers and proceed with the six stages of BST treatment (see "Quick Guide to the Six Stages of BST Treatment").

Regional treatment

Integrate the local treatment of the wrist into the region by using the hand and wrist gather technique (see "Regional Treatment").

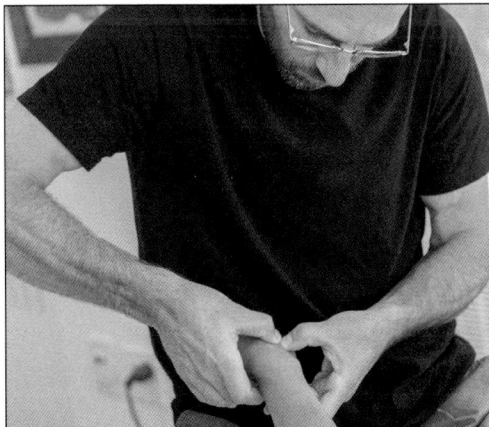

Figure 17.413. Hand and body position for the local treatment of hamate.

UPPER EXTREMITY

Excluding the bones of the hand and wrist, each upper extremity contains five bones: the radius, ulna, humerus, clavicle and scapula (figure 17.414).

Radius

The radius forms the lateral side of the forearm, and is shorter than the ulna, to which it sits parallel. Like other long bones, it has a shaft and two extremities (figure 17.415). The proximal extremity has a head, neck, and tuberosity. The distal extremity is larger and has two articulating surfaces: one for the ulna and one for the scaphoid and lunate.

Neighbors

Scaphoid
Lunate
Ulna
Humerus

Palpation

Sit at the side of the arm to be tested. To locate the head of the radius, have the patient flex

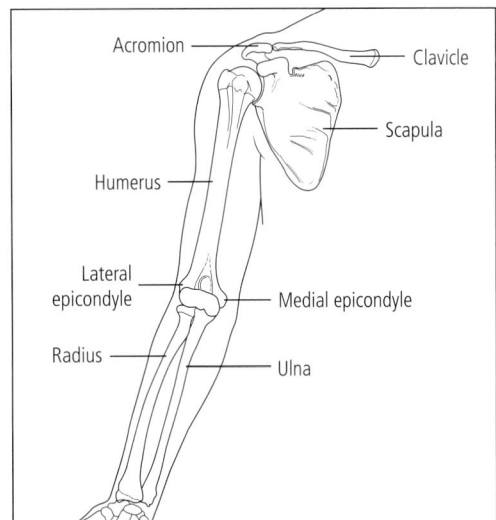

Figure 17.414. The upper extremity.

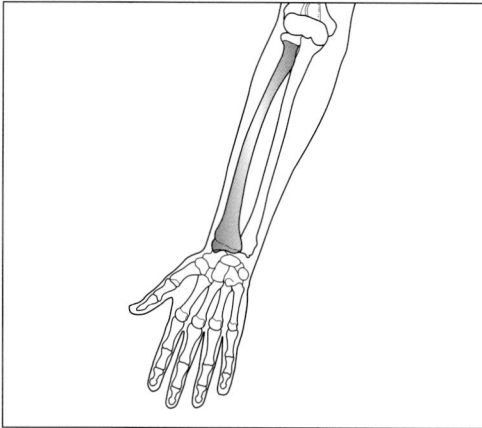

Figure 17.415. Radius.

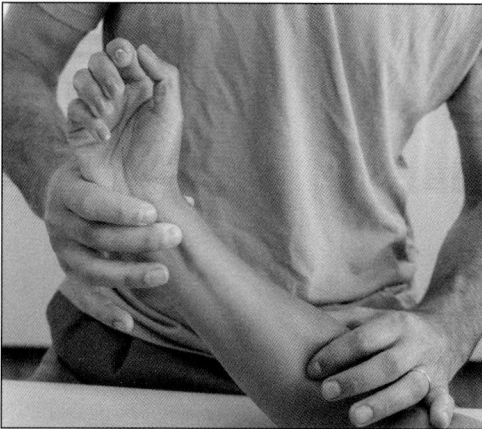

Figure 17.416. Palpating the head and neck (left hand) and the distal extremity (right hand) of the radius.

their arm. Locate the condyle of the humerus, then slide your finger distally over the joint line of the elbow onto the head of the radius. If the subject pronates and supinates the forearm, the radial head will move, but the humerus will remain still. Once you have located the head, slide distally down the radius an inch or so to the neck (figure 17.416) and then to its distal extremity where it meets the wrist.

Testing

As with other larger bones, global testing usually precedes more specific testing, and can be done in phases, if necessary.

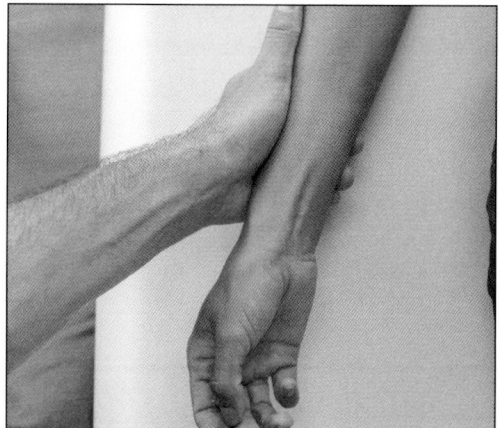

Figure 17.417. Phase 1: Transverse scan of the radius by applying firm pressure into and along the shaft of the bone.

Phase 1: Perform a transverse scan of the radius. Starting at the distal end, apply firm pressure transversely into the radius by pinching the forearm and moving up the bone in series toward the proximal end (figure 17.417). The scan is a quick way to test the bone's ability to flex. Take note of any specific compacted areas, including within the distal end, shaft, and proximal end.

Phase 2: Perform a global longitudinal test of the radius. With one hand, grasp the proximal end, and with the other hand, hold the distal end. Apply a longitudinal tensile force into the bone, twisting it in both directions (figure 17.418). Again, take note of any compacted areas.

Now, test the connections between the radius and its neighbors by applying a spreading and twisting force between them (figures 17.419 to 17.422).

If the whole bone and its connections possess elasticity, move to the next bone to be tested. If the entire radius, any segments, or any of the connections between the radius and its neighbors feel more like concrete than like wood or are fibrotic, proceed to local treatment.

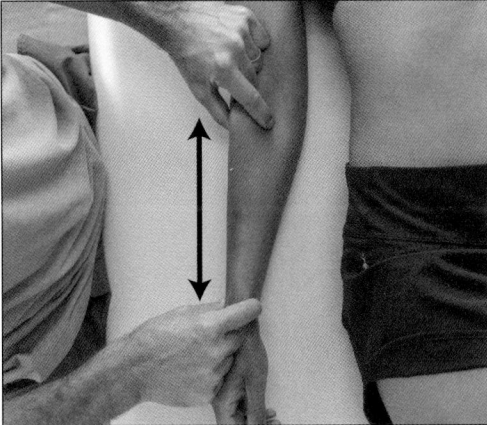

Figure 17.418. Phase 2: Longitudinal test of the radius.

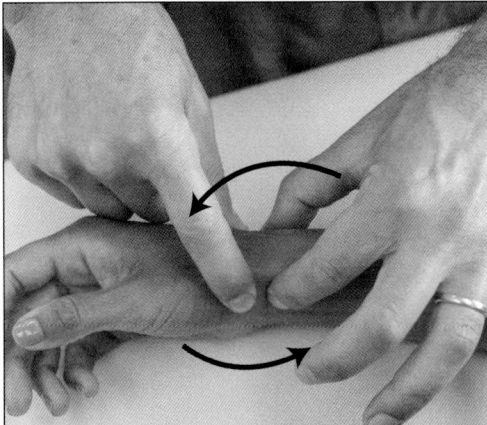

Figure 17.419. Spreading and twisting the connection between the radius and the scaphoid.

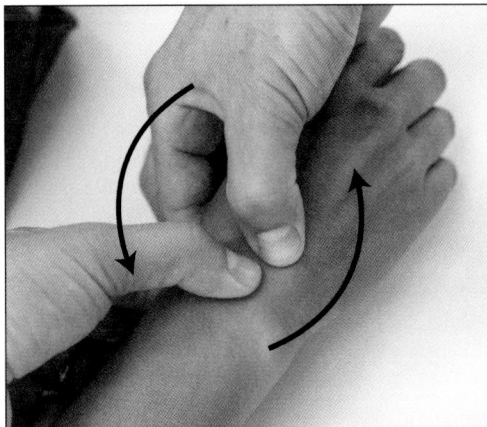

Figure 17.420. Spreading and twisting the connection between the radius and lunate with the thumbs and index fingers (palmar surface).

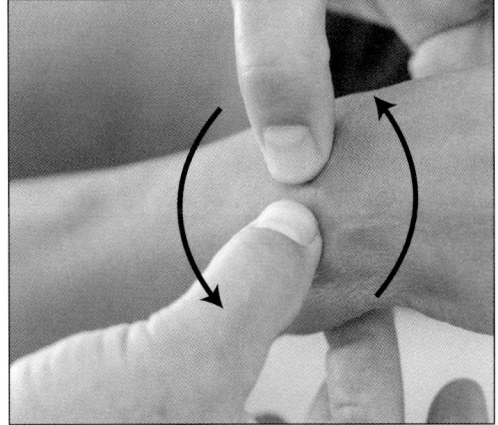

Figure 17.421. Spreading and twisting the connection between the radius and the ulna with the thumbs and middle fingers (palmar surface).

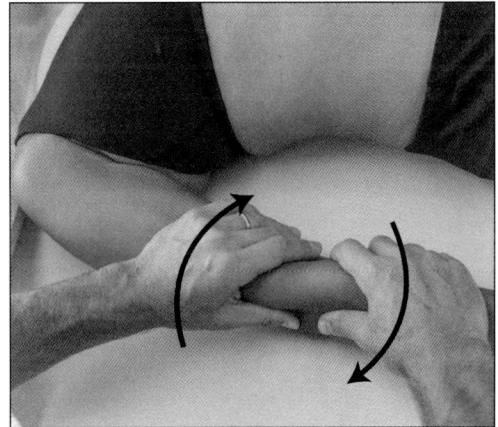

Figure 17.422. Spreading and twisting the connection between the radius and the humerus.

Local treatment

As with most of the larger bones, local treatment can be applied from either the global hold or from more specific holds to any of the segments or connections.

Global: Grasp the radius (figure 17.423) and proceed with the six stages of BST treatment (see "Quick Guide to the Six Stages of BST Treatment").

217

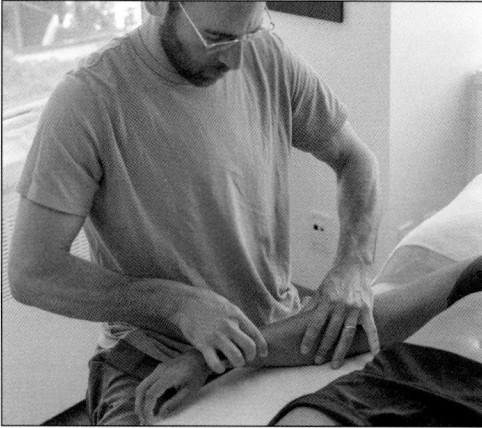

Figure 17.423. Hand and body position for the local treatment of the radius.

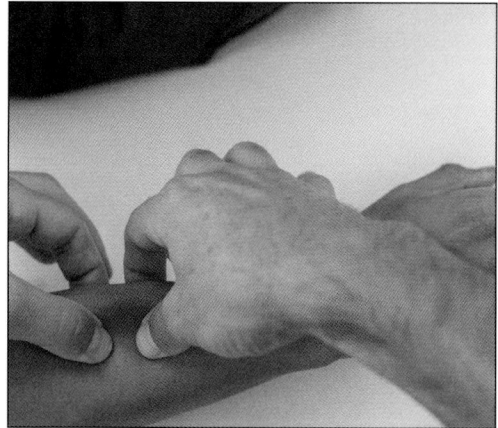

Figure 17.425. Specific treatment of a part of the shaft of the radius.

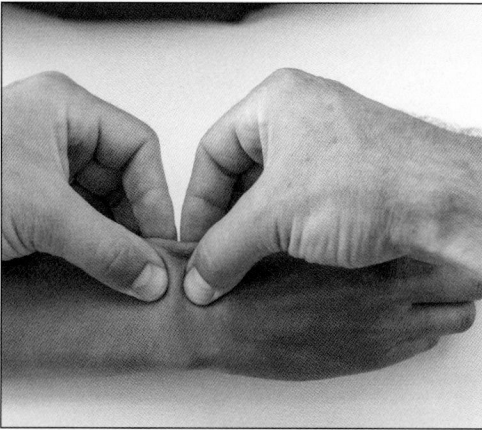

Figure 17.424. Specific treatment of the distal end of the radius.

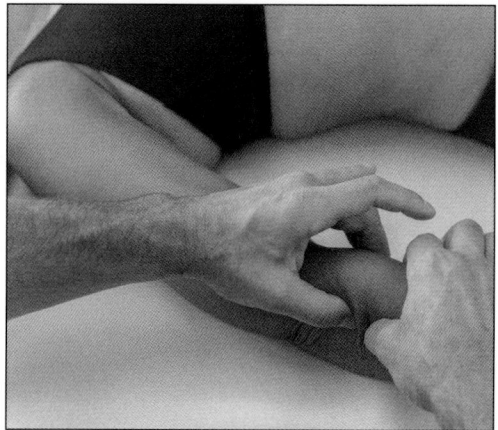

Figure 17.426. Specific treatment of the proximal end of the radius.

Specific segments: If one or more of the segments of the radius is compacted, and if the global approach is insufficient, change positions to apply the six stages of treatment with corresponding hand positions to the distal extremity (figure 17.424), specific parts of the shaft (figure 17.425), or proximal extremity (figure 17.426).

Regional treatment

Integrate the local treatment of the radius into the region by using the upper extremity gather technique (see "Regional Treatment").

Ulna

The ulna forms the medial side of the forearm, sits parallel to the radius, and is the largest of the two bones (figure 17.427). Like other long bones, it has a shaft and two extremities. Its distal end, or head, is small and connects to the carpals via an intra-articular fibrocartilage. The proximal end is more massive, forms the greater part of the elbow joint, and has two distinct processes. The olecranon process is a curved eminence at the proximal and posterior extremity of the ulna, forming the posterior part of the sigmoid cup. The second process at the proximal extremity

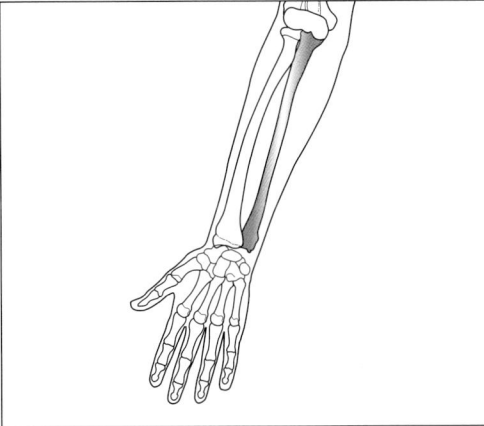

Figure 17.427. Ulna.

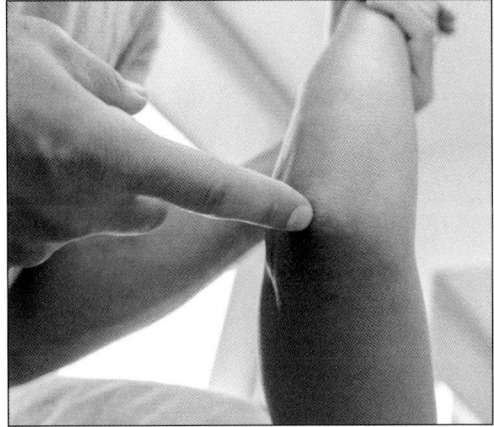

Figure 17.428. Palpating the olecranon process of the ulna with the index finger.

is called the coronoid process and forms the base of the cup. When the arm is flexed, the coronoid process is received by the coronoid depression of the humerus. The sigmoid cavity has two articulating surfaces; the larger of the two articulates with the trochlea of the humerus, and the lesser of the two joins the head of the radius. The head of the ulna is small, with a styloid process extending distally toward the wrist.

Neighbors

Radius
Humerus
Triquetral

Palpation

With the subject's arm flexed, palpate the olecranon process, which is the bony prominence between the medial and lateral condyles of the humerus (figure 17.428). Follow the shaft of the ulna distally to the head, where it articulates with the triquetral (figure 17.429).

Testing

As with other larger bones, global testing usually precedes more specific testing, and can be done in phases, if necessary.

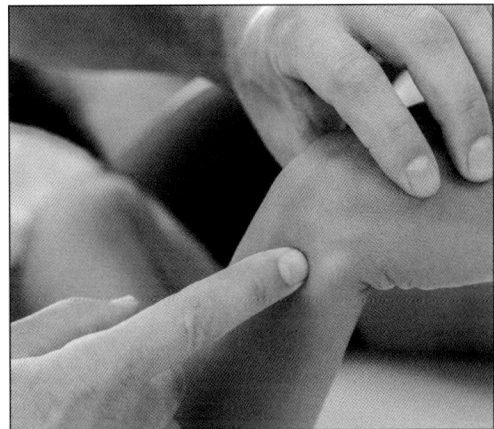

Figure 17.429. Palpating the head of the ulna (using the right index finger).

Phase 1: Perform a transverse scan of the ulna. Starting at the distal end, apply firm pressure transversely into the ulna by pinching the forearm and moving up the bone in series toward the proximal end (figure 17.430). The scan is a quick way to test the bone's ability to flex. Take note of any specific compacted areas, including within the distal end, shaft, and olecranon process.

Phase 2: Perform a global longitudinal test of the ulna. With one hand, grasp the proximal end and olecranon process, and with the other hand, hold the distal end. Apply a

219

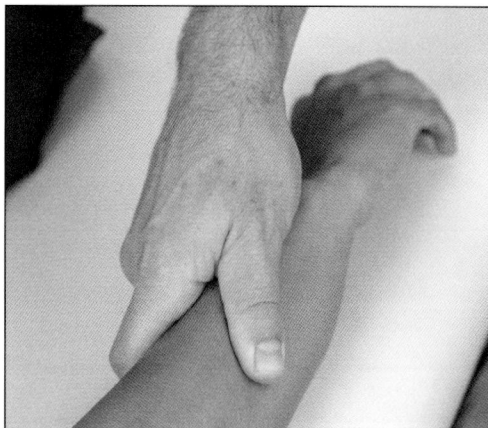

Figure 17.430. Transverse scan of the ulna by applying firm pressure into and along the shaft of the bone by pinching it with the thumb and index finger.

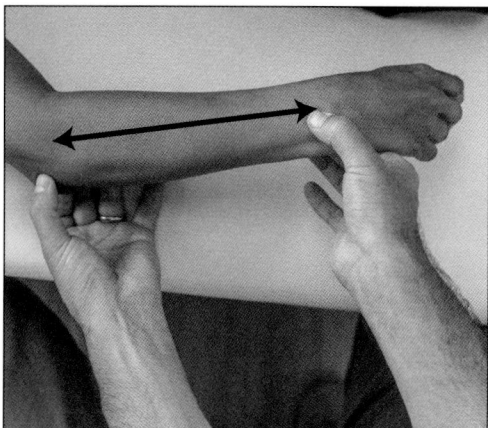

Figure 17.432. Spreading and twisting the connection between the ulna and the triquetral with the thumbs and fingers (palmar surface).

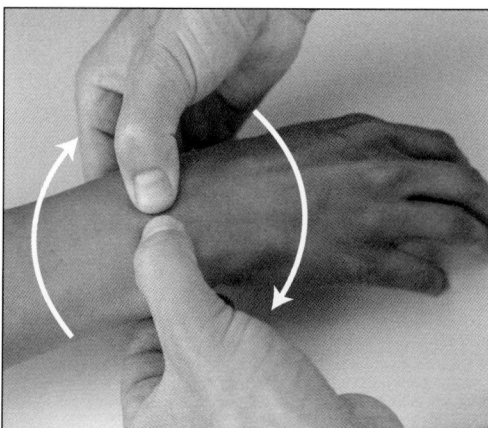

Figure 17.431. Longitudinal test of the ulna.

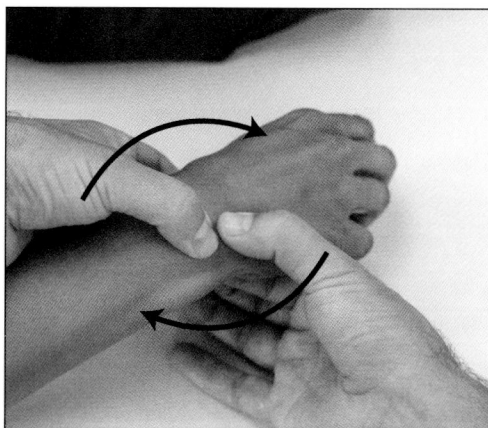

Figure 17.433. Spreading and twisting the connection between the ulna and the radius using the thumbs and fingers.

longitudinal tensile force into the bone, twisting it in both directions (figure 17.431). Again, take note of any compacted patterns or zones.

Now, test the connections between the ulna and its neighbors by applying a spreading and twisting force between them (figures 17.432 to 17.434).

If the whole bone and its connections possess elasticity, move to the next bone to be tested. If the entire ulna, any segments, or any of the connections with the ulna and its neighbors feel more like concrete than like wood or are fibrotic, proceed to local treatment.

Local treatment

As with most of the larger bones, local treatment can be applied from either the global hold or from more specific holds to any of the segments or connections.

Global: Flex the subject's arm 130 to 140 degrees to relax the triceps tendon and gap the olecranon process from the

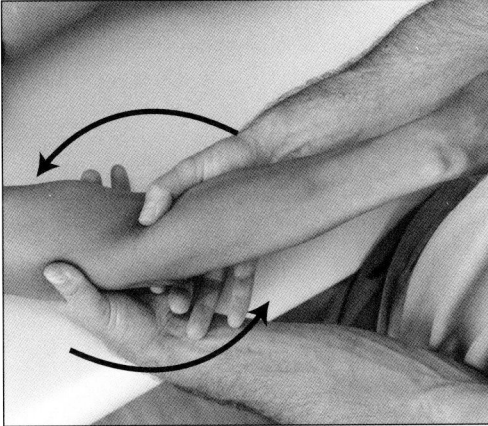

Figure 17.434. Spreading and twisting the connection between the ulna and humerus.

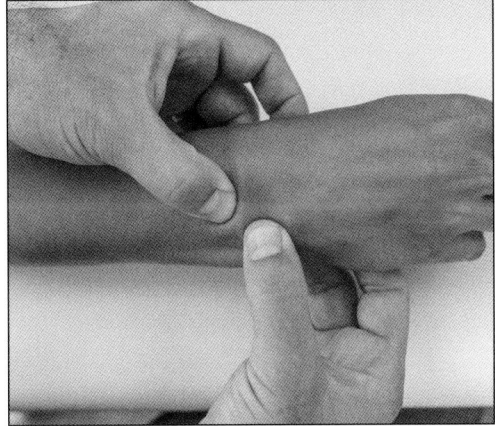

Figure 17.436. Specific treatment of the head of the ulna.

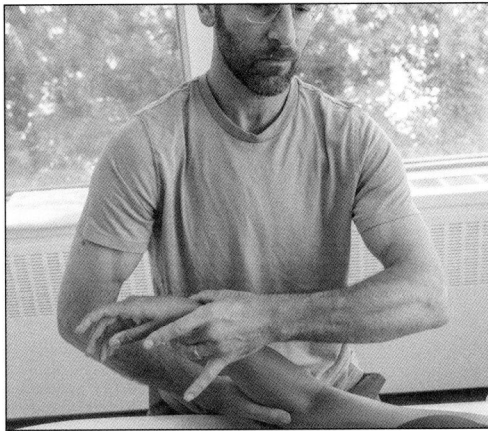

Figure 17.435. Hand and body position for the local treatment of the ulna.

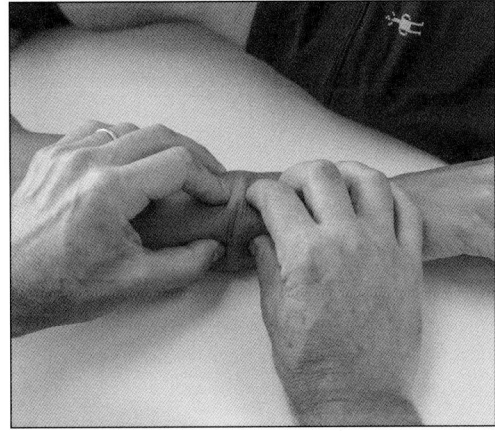

Figure 17.437. Specific treatment of a part of the shaft of the ulna.

olecranon fossa. Cross your arms and grasp the ulna at each end (figure 17.435) and proceed with the six stages of BST treatment (see "Quick Guide to the Six Stages of BST Treatment").

Specific segments: If one or more of the segments of the ulna is compacted, and if the global approach is insufficient, change positions to apply the six stages of treatment with corresponding hand positions specifically to the head (figure 17.436), specific parts of the shaft (figure 17.437), or the olecranon process (figure 17.438).

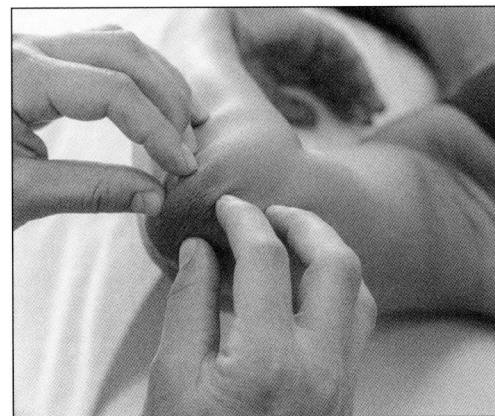

Figure 17.438. Specific treatment of the olecranon process of the ulna.

Regional treatment

Integrate the local treatment of the ulna into the region by using the upper extremity gather technique (see "Regional Treatment").

Humerus

The humerus is the longest bone of the upper extremity (figure 17.439). Like other long bones, it has a shaft and two extremities. The proximal end has a large, rounded head, a narrower neck, and two eminences: the greater and lesser tuberosities. The head articulates with the glenoid fossa of the scapula. The neck separates the head from the two tuberosities and sits at an oblique angle with the shaft. Between the tuberosities sits the bicipital groove, which guides the tendon of the long head of the biceps muscle. Along with the olecranon process of the ulna, the distal extremity forms the elbow joint. The articular surface of the distal extremity is made up of lateral and medial condyles separated by the trochlea, a central groove with two deep depressions. During elbow extension, the olecranon process of the ulna is received by the olecranon depression on the posterior surface of the distal extremity. During full flexion, the coronoid process of the ulna is received by the coronoid

depression on the anterior surface of the distal extremity. The lateral, or radial, head of the distal extremity articulates with the head of the radius.

Neighbors

Radius
Ulna
Scapula

Palpation

To palpate the proximal end of the humerus, follow the clavicle to its lateral extremity where it meets the acromion process of the scapula. Have the subject internally and externally rotate the arm. From the acromioclavicular joint, move down onto the head of the humerus, which will be moving under your fingers (figure 17.440). To palpate the lateral condyle at the distal end, find the olecranon process of the ulna, and move laterally onto the next bony eminence (figure 17.441). To palpate the olecranon fossa, flex the subject's arm approximately 130–140 degrees to simultaneously expose the fossa and relax the triceps tendon. Start on the lateral side of the humerus and then slide into the fossa, moving aside the tendon (figure 17.442). To palpate the medial

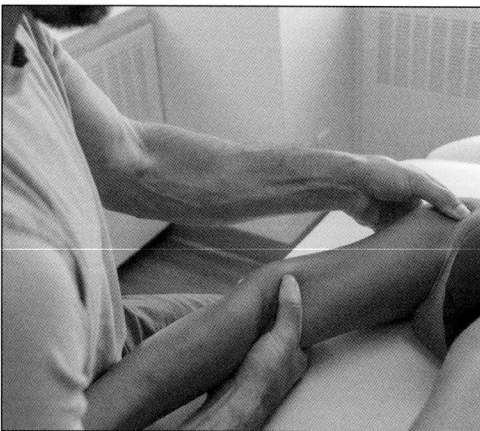

Figure 17.439. Humerus.

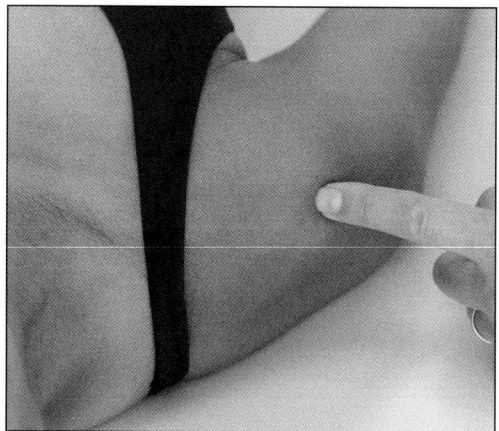

Figure 17.440. Palpating the head of the humerus.

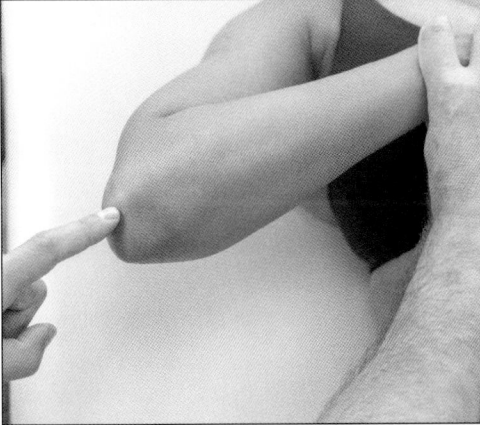

Figure 17.441. Palpating the lateral condyle of the humerus with the left index finger.

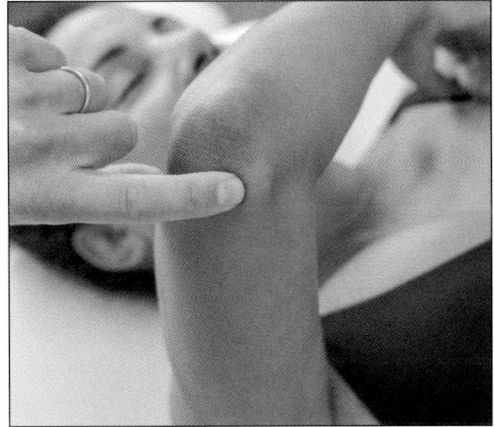

Figure 17.443. Palpating the medial condyle of the humerus.

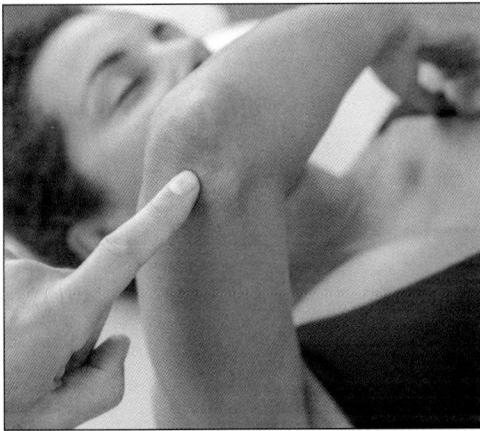

Figure 17.442. Palpating the olecranon fossa of the humerus.

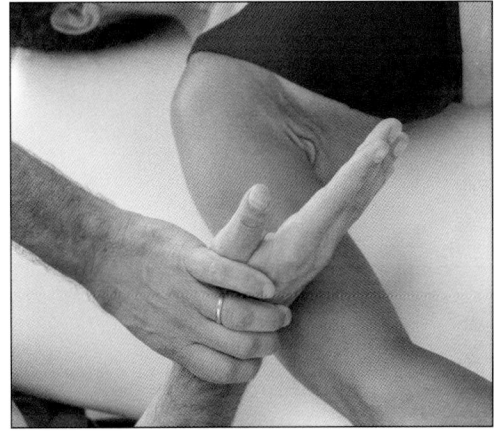

Figure 17.444. Transverse scan of the internally rotated humerus. Apply pressure in series into and along the length of the bone.

condyle, find the olecranon process of the ulna and move medially onto the next bony eminence (figure 17.443).

Testing

As with other larger bones, global testing usually precedes more specific testing, and can be done in phases, if necessary.

Phase 1: Perform a transverse scan of the humerus. Starting at the distal end, apply firm pressure transversely into the humerus moving up the bone in series toward the proximal end (figure 17.444). The scan is a

quick way to test the bone's ability to flex. This test may be more effective and more comfortable if the subject internally rotates their arm, exposing the lateral surface of the humerus where there is less muscle mass. If this isn't practical, stabilize the humerus with your medial hand and test from the lateral side (figure 17.445). Take note of any specific compacted areas, including within the distal end, shaft, and head.

Phase 2: Perform a global longitudinal test of the humerus. With one hand, grasp the

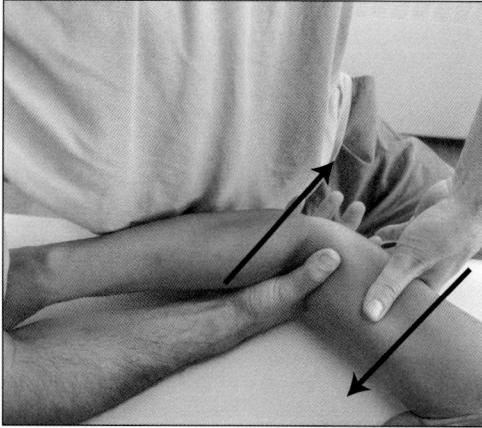

Figure 17.445. Transverse scan the left humerus by stabilizing it with the right hand while applying pressure in series into and along the length of the bone with the other hand.

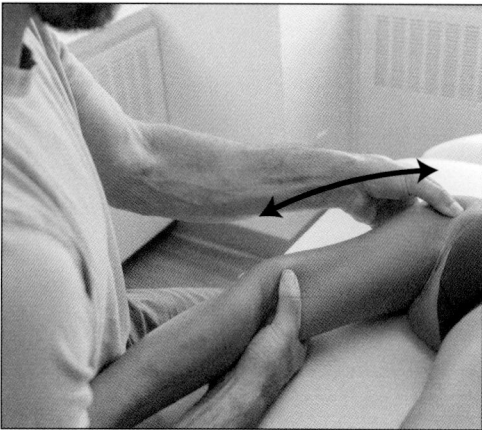

Figure 17.446. Longitudinal test of the humerus. Apply a longitudinal tensile force into the bone, twisting it in both directions.

head, and with the other hand, hold the distal end. Apply a longitudinal tensile force into the bone, twisting it in both directions (figure 17.446). Again, take note of any compacted patterns or zones.

Now, test the connections between the humerus and its neighbor by applying a spreading and twisting force between them (figure 17.447).

If the whole bone and its connections possesses elasticity, move to the next bone(s)

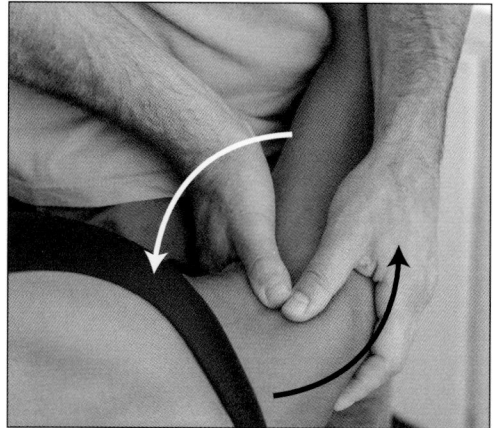

Figure 17.447. Spreading and twisting the connection between the humerus and the scapula.

to be tested. If the entire humerus, any segments, or any of the connections with the humerus and its neighbors feel more like concrete than like wood or are fibrotic, proceed to local treatment.

Local treatment

As with most of the larger bones, local treatment can be applied from either the global hold or from more specific holds to any of the segments or connections.

Global: Grasp the humerus at each end (figure 17.448) and proceed with the six

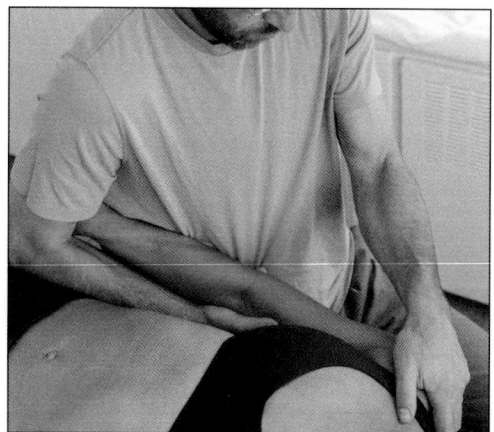

Figure 17.448. Hand and body position for the global local treatment of the humerus.

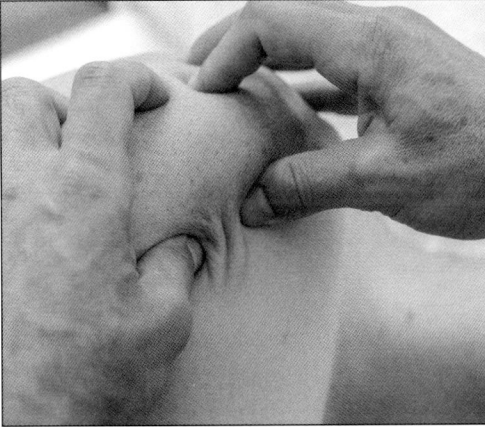

Figure 17.449. Specific treatment of the head of the humerus with the patient lying on the opposite side.

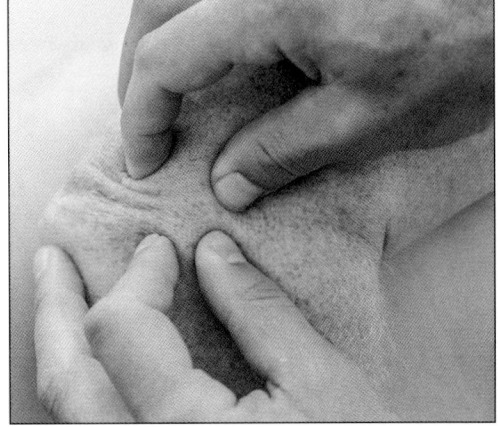

Figure 17.451. Specific treatment of the lateral condyle of the humerus.

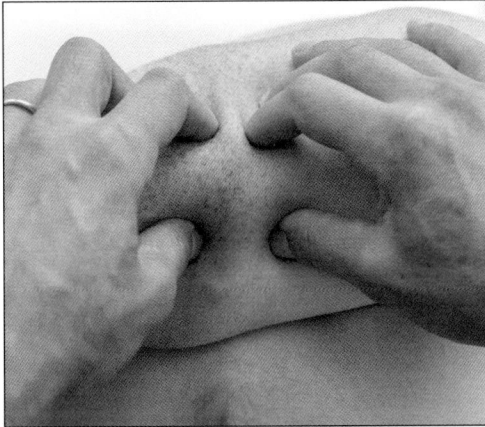

Figure 17.450. Specific treatment of a part of the shaft of the humerus.

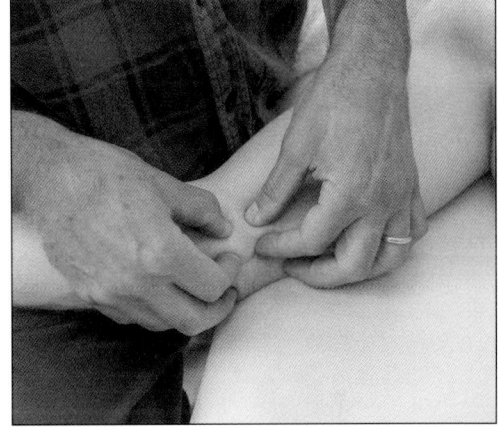

Figure 17.452. Specific treatment of the medial condyle of the humerus.

stages of BST treatment (see "Quick Guide to the Six Stages of BST Treatment").

Specific segments: If one or more of the segments of the humerus are compacted, and if the global approach is insufficient, change positions to apply the six stages of treatment with corresponding hand positions specifically to the head (figure 17.449), specific parts of the shaft (figure 17.450), the lateral condyle (figure 17.451), or the medial condyle (figure 17.452).

Regional treatment

Integrate the local treatment of the ulna into the region by using the upper extremity gather technique (see "Regional Treatment").

Scapula

The scapula, or shoulder blade, is a triangle-shaped bone that forms the posterior part of the shoulder (figure 17.453). It glides over the back of the thorax, and at rest is situated between the first and eighth ribs. The posterior surface of the scapula is divided

225

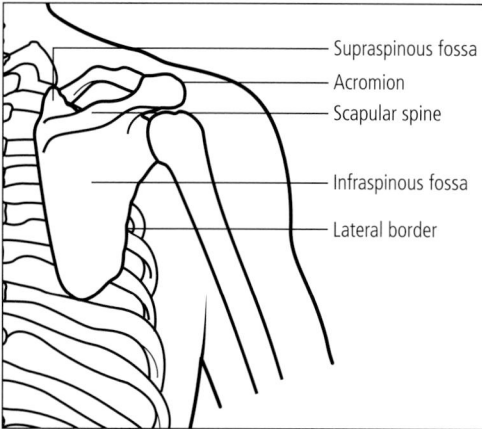

Figure 17.453. Scapula.

Labels: Supraspinous fossa, Acromion, Scapular spine, Infraspinous fossa, Lateral border

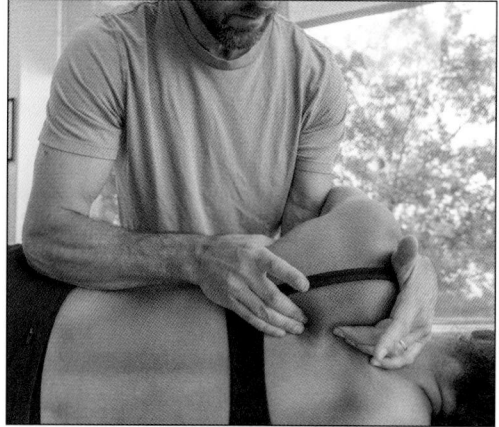

Figure 17.454. Palpating the borders of the posterior and anterior surfaces (anterior with the right thumb; not shown) of the scapula.

into two parts by the scapular spine: the supraspinous fossa above and the infraspinous process below. The spine is an oblique plate of bone, which narrows into the acromion process at the lateral end. The acromion process forms the summit of the shoulder, overhanging the glenoid cavity. The head of the scapula, otherwise known as the anterior border, is the thickest part of the bone and contains the glenoid fossa, which receives the head of the humerus. Surrounding the head of the scapula is the neck, and arising from the anterior aspect of the neck is another bony eminence, the coracoid process.

Neighbors

Humerus
Clavicle

Palpation

From the back and side, palpate the borders of the posterior and anterior surfaces of the scapula (figure 17.454). Locate the superior border and descend onto the spine (figure 17.455). From the top of the shoulder, follow the clavicle to its lateral extremity, and move posteriorly onto the acromion process (figure 17.456). From the upper arm, find the head of the humerus, then move your

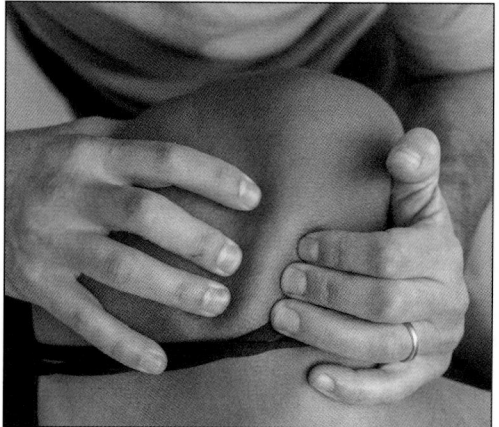

Figure 17.455. Palpating the spine of the scapula.

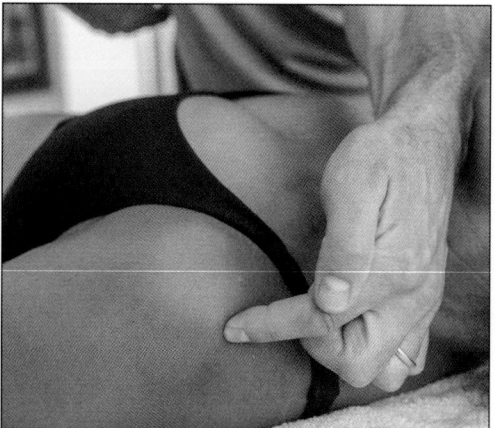

Figure 17.456. Palpating the acromion process of the scapula with the index finger.

226

finger medially onto the coracoid process (figure 17.457).

Testing

Phase 1: Sitting at the side of the subject, who is either in supine or side-lying, line the fingers along the medial (figure 17.458) and lateral (figure 17.459) borders of the scapula and spread the fingers to test the bone. Move to the head of the subject and spread the fingers along the superior border (figure 17.460) and spine (figure 17.461) to test the bone. Bunch the fingers up on the acromion (figure 17.462) and coracoid processes (figure 17.463), and

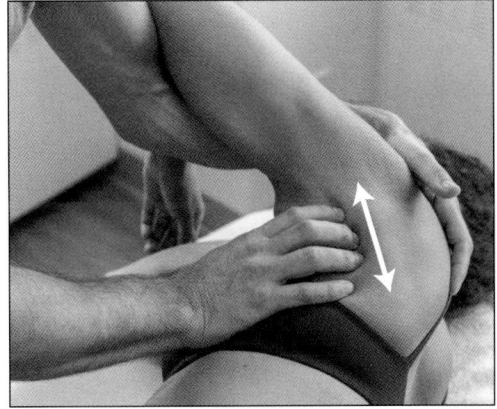

Figure 17.459. Phase 1: Testing the lateral border of the scapula by spreading the bone with the fingers of the right hand.

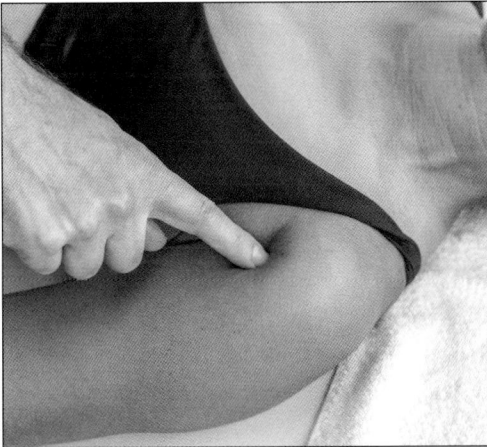

Figure 17.457. Palpating the coracoid process of the scapula.

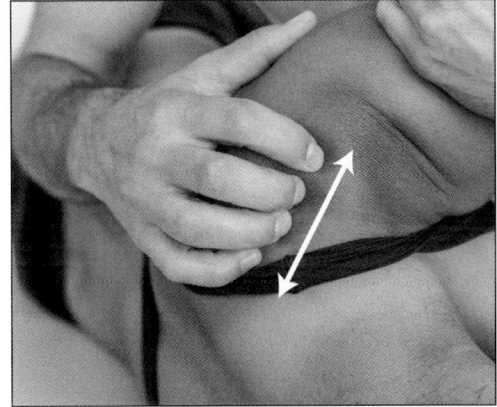

Figure 17.460. Phase 1: Testing the superior border of the scapula by spreading the bone with the fingers of the right hand.

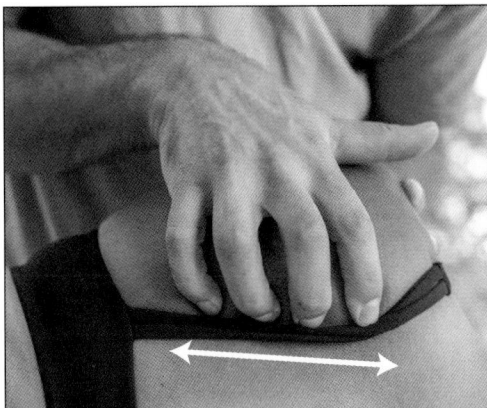

Figure 17.458. Phase 1: Testing the medial border of the scapula by spreading the bone with the fingers of the left hand.

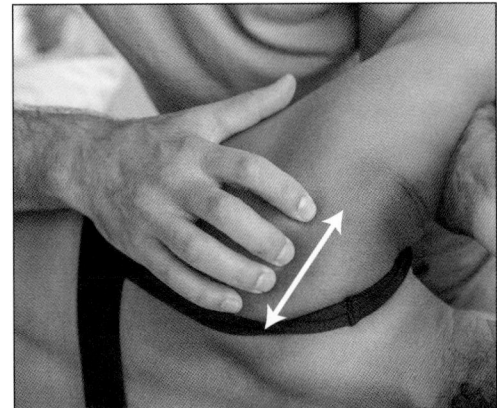

Figure 17.461. Phase 1: Testing the spine of the scapula by spreading the bone.

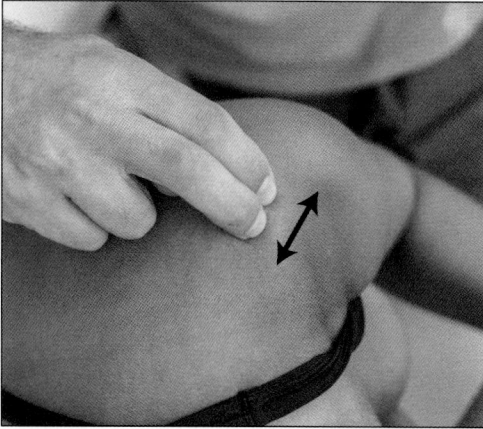

Figure 17.462. Phase 1: Testing the acromion process of the scapula by spreading the bone.

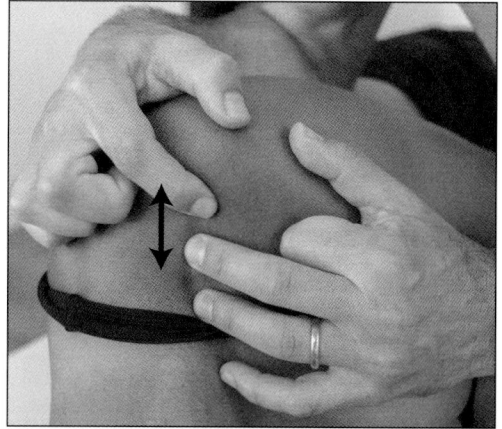

Figure 17.464. Phase 1: Testing the acromioclavicular joint with the right index finger and left middle finger by spreading the joint line.

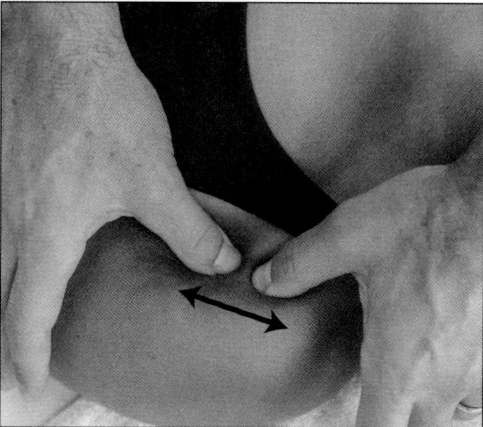

Figure 17.463. Phase 1: Testing the coracoid process of the scapula by spreading the bone.

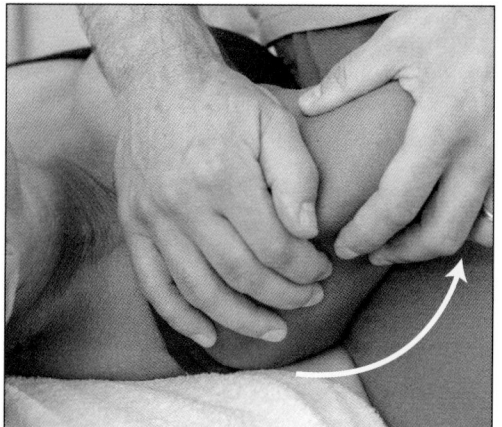

Figure 17.465. Phase 1: Testing the glenohumeral joint applying traction to the humeral head away from the glenohumeral fossa to spread the joint line. It helps to stabilize the axillae using the upper thigh, and then use the thigh to help spread the joint.

again, touch and spread the fingers to test the bone. Finally, test the quality of the acromioclavicular (figure 17.464) and glenohumeral joints (figure 17.465) by spreading the connection between the acromion and the clavicle and between the humerus and glenoid fossa, respectively. Does the bone or any segments of the bone or any of the connections feel normal or compacted?

If all is normal, move to the next bone to be tested. If a compaction exists within the scapula or within any of the connections, proceed to phase 2.

Phase 2: Spread and twist the compacted segments to determine the most rigid torsional pattern of compaction (figures 17.466 to 17.473).

Local treatment

With the subject supine, line the fingers up along the compacted section (figure 17.474)

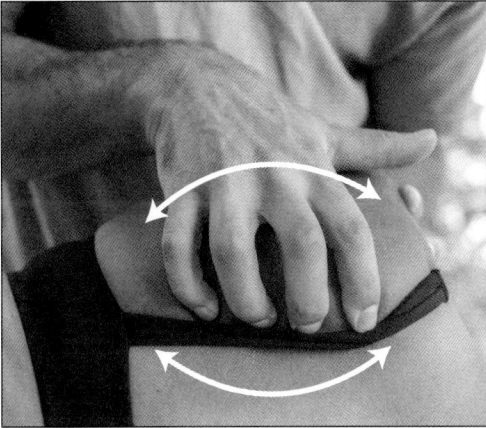

Figure 17.466. Phase 2: Spreading and twisting the medial border of the scapula.

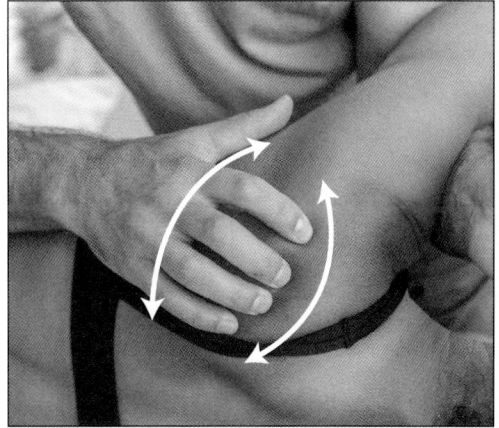

Figure 17.469. Phase 2: Spreading and twisting the superior border of the scapula.

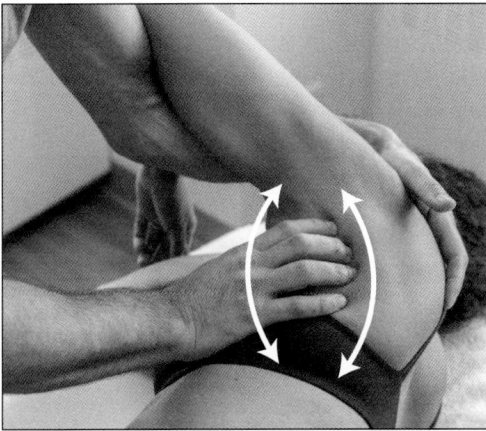

Figure 17.467. Phase 2: Spreading and twisting the lateral border of the scapula.

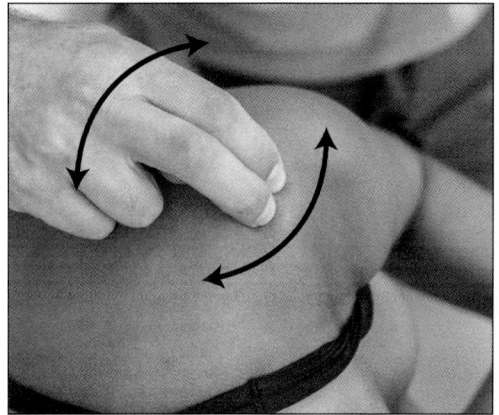

Figure 17.470. Phase 2: Spreading and twisting the acromion process of the scapula with the index and middle fingers.

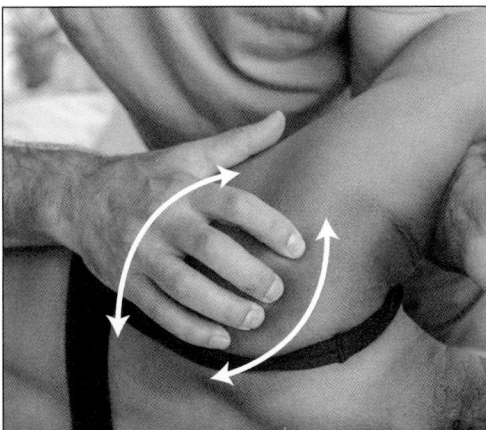

Figure 17.468. Phase 2: Spreading and twisting the spine of the scapula.

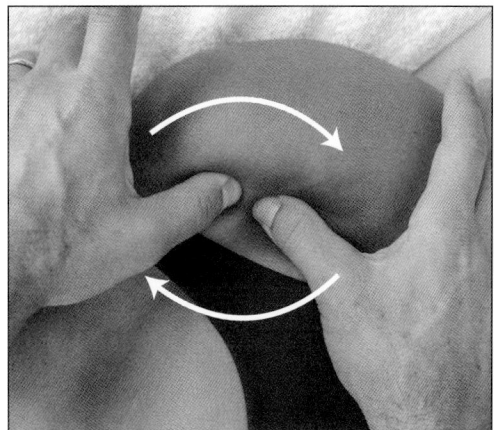

Figure 17.471. Phase 2: Spreading and twisting the coracoid process of the scapula.

229

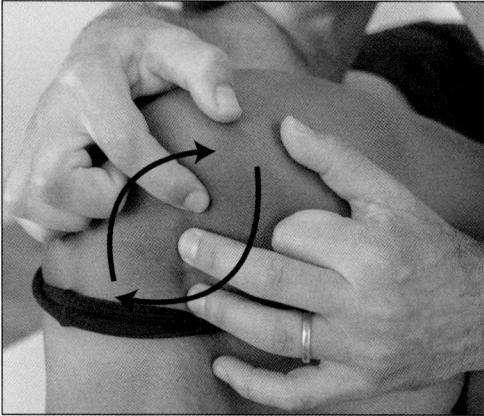

Figure 17.472. Phase 2: Spreading and twisting the acromioclavicular joint with the right index finger and left middle finger.

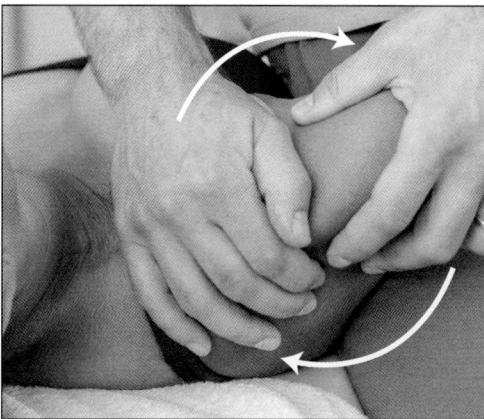

Figure 17.473. Phase 2: Spreading and twisting the glenohumeral joint.

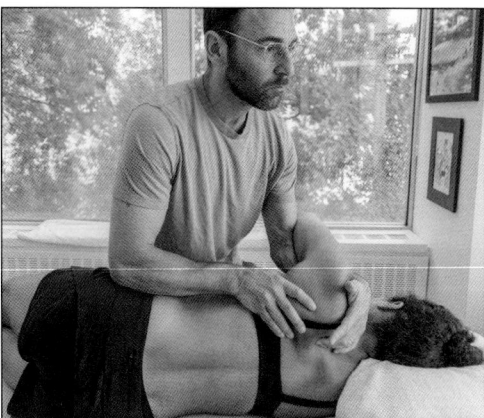

Figure 17.474. Hand and body position for the global treatment of the scapula.

and proceed with the six stages of BST treatment (see "Quick Guide to the Six Stages of BST Treatment").

Processes: If either the processes is compacted, apply the six stages of treatment with corresponding hand positions for the acromion (figure 17.475) or coracoid process (figure 17.476).

Regional treatment

Integrate the local treatment of the scapula into the region by using the shoulder gather technique (see "Regional Treatment").

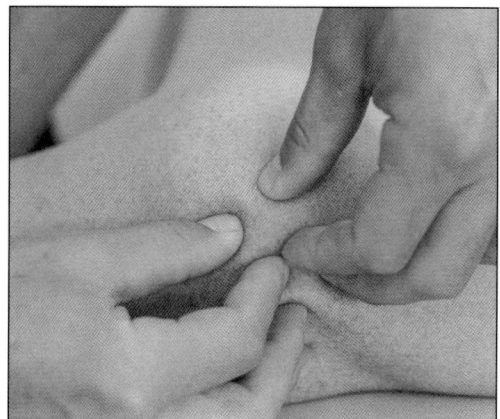

Figure 17.475. Specific treatment of the acromion process using the thumbs and index fingers.

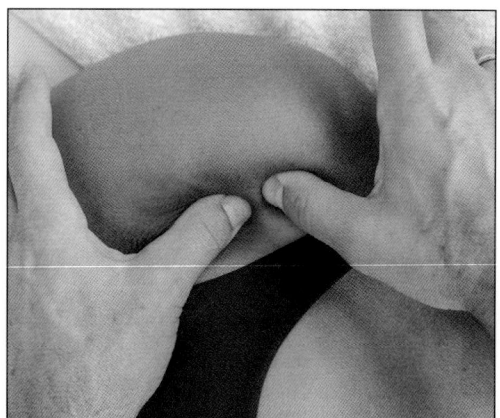

Figure 17.476. Specific treatment of the coracoid process.

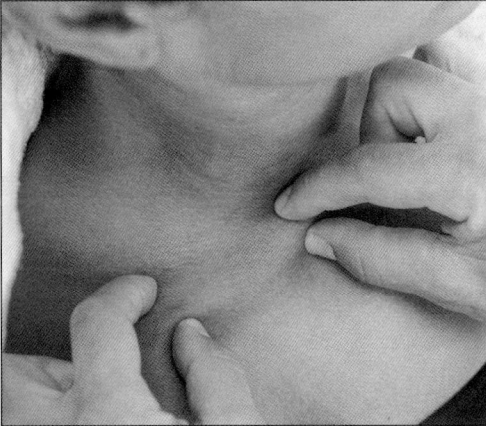

Figure 17.477. Clavicle.

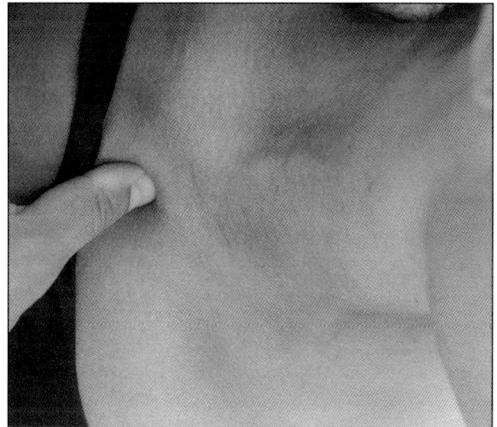

Figure 17.478. Palpating the sternal end of the clavicle.

Clavicle

The clavicle forms the anterior part of the shoulder (figure 17.477). It is a long, curved bone, and sits just above the first rib on the anterior surface of the upper thorax. It has a lateral, or acromial, extremity and a medial, or sternal, extremity, separated by the shaft. The lateral end articulates with the acromion process of the scapula, and the medial end articulates with the sternum and first rib.

Neighbors

Sternum
First rib
Scapula

Palpation

To palpate the sternal end, move proximally along the sternum to the manubrium, and then laterally onto the sternal extremity of the clavicle (figure 17.478). To palpate the acromial end, move laterally along the clavicle to the acromioclavicular joint (figure 17.479).

Testing

As with some other bones, global testing usually precedes more specific testing, and can be done in phases, if necessary.

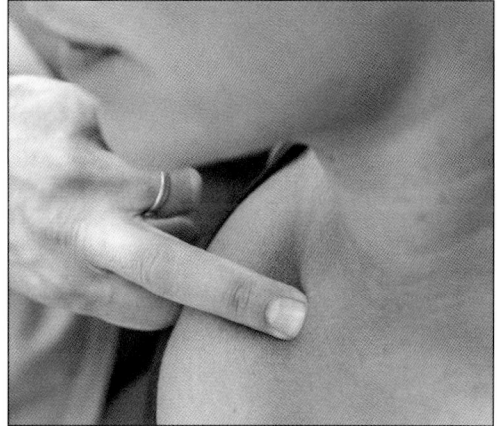

Figure 17.479. Palpating the acromial end of the clavicle.

Phase 1: Perform a transverse scan of the clavicle. Starting at the medial end, apply pressure into the clavicle, moving laterally along the bone in series (figure 17.480). Like in other long bones, the scan tests the ability of the bone to flex. Take note of any specific compacted areas.

Phase 2: Perform a longitudinal test of the clavicle. With one hand, pinch the sternal end, and with the other hand, pinch the acromial end as close as possible to the acromioclavicular joint. Apply a longitudinal tensile force into the bone, twisting it in both directions (figure 17.481). Take note of any compacted patterns or zones.

231

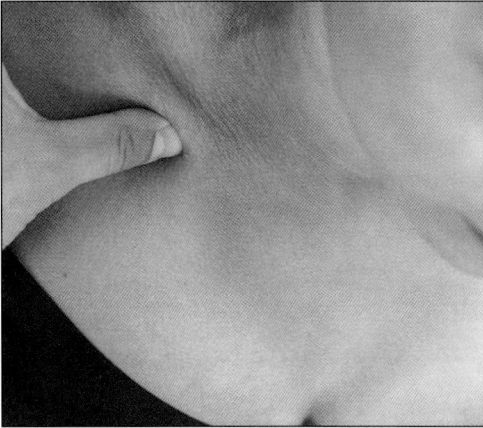

Figure 17.480. Phase 1: Transverse scan of the clavicle. Starting at the medial end, apply pressure into the clavicle moving laterally along the bone.

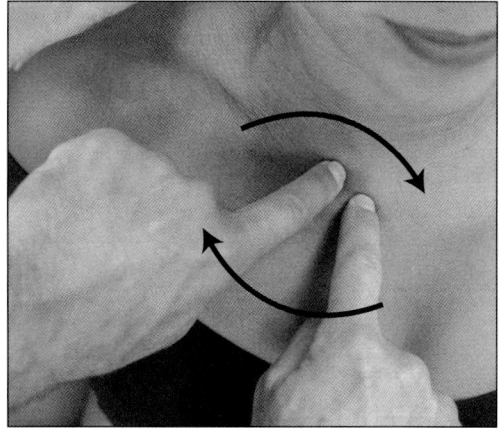

Figure 17.482. Spreading and twisting the connection between the clavicle and the sternum.

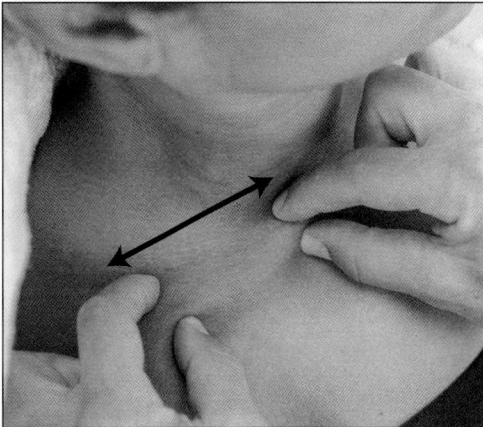

Figure 17.481. Phase 2: Longitudinal test of the clavicle. Apply a longitudinal tensile force into the bone, twisting it in both directions.

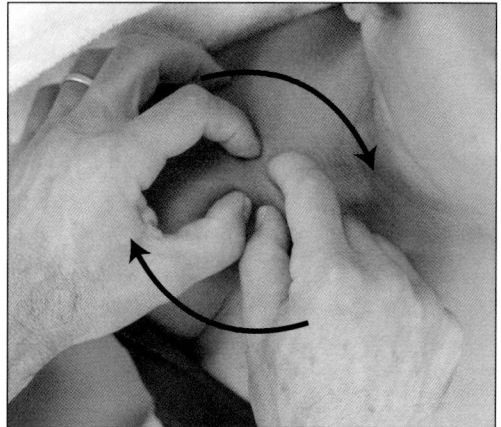

Figure 17.483. Spreading and twisting the connection between the clavicle (right hand) and the acromion process of the scapula (left hand).

Now, test the connections between the clavicle and its neighbors by applying a spreading and twisting force between them (figures 17.482 and 17.483).

If the whole bone and its connections possess elasticity, move to the next bone to be tested. If the entire clavicle, any segments, or any of the connections between the clavicle and its neighbors feel more like concrete than like wood or are fibrotic, proceed to local treatment.

Local treatment

Grasp the clavicle (figure 17.484) and proceed with the six stages of BST treatment (see "Quick Guide to the Six Stages of BST Treatment").

Specific segments: If one or more of the segments of the clavicle is compacted, and if the global approach isn't specific enough, change hand positions to apply the six stages of treatment with corresponding hand

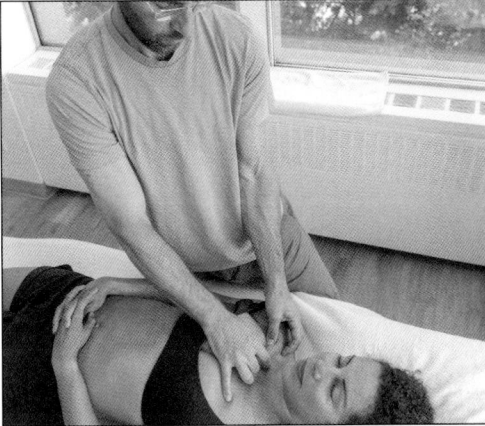

Figure 17.484. Hand and body position for the local treatment of the clavicle.

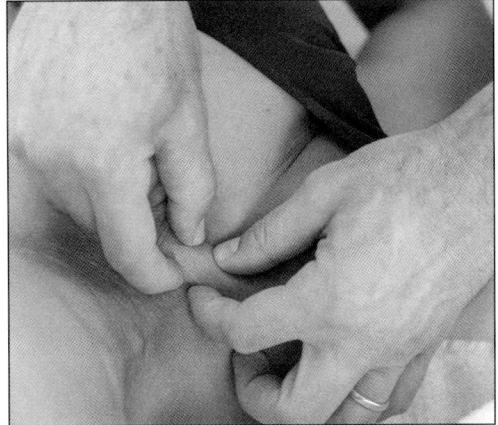

Figure 17.486. Specific treatment of a part of the shaft of the clavicle.

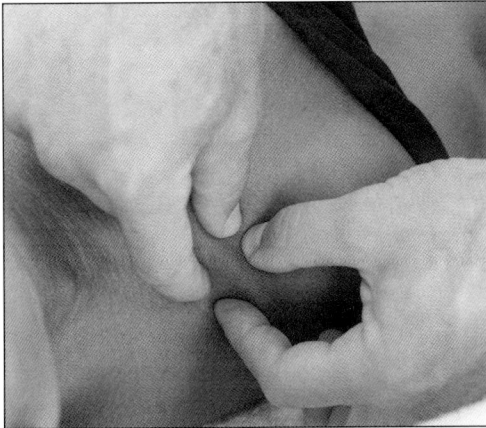

Figure 17.485. Specific treatment of the lateral extremity of the clavicle.

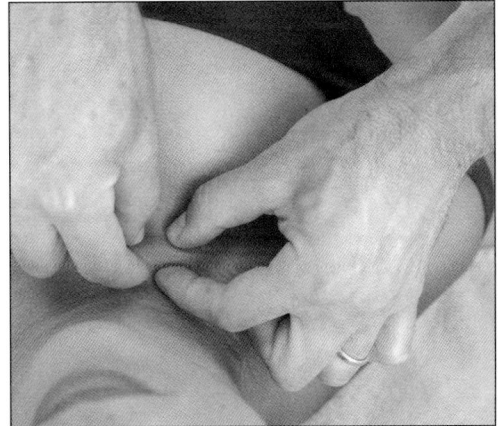

Figure 17.487. Specific treatment of the medial extremity of the clavicle.

positions specifically to the lateral extremity (figure 17.485), specific parts of the shaft (figure 17.486), or the medial extremity (figure 17.487).

Regional treatment

Integrate the local treatment of the clavicle into the region by using the anterior thoracic barrel technique (see "Regional Treatment").

CERVICAL SPINE

There are seven cervical vertebrae (figure 17.488), and like the other vertebrae, each has numerous segments. The body is concave superiorly, convex anteriorly, and is wider than it is deep. The pedicles are projected obliquely outward, and the transverse processes are short, have a double tip, and have a hole through their base, which allows passage of the vertebral arteries, veins, and nerves. The spinous processes are short

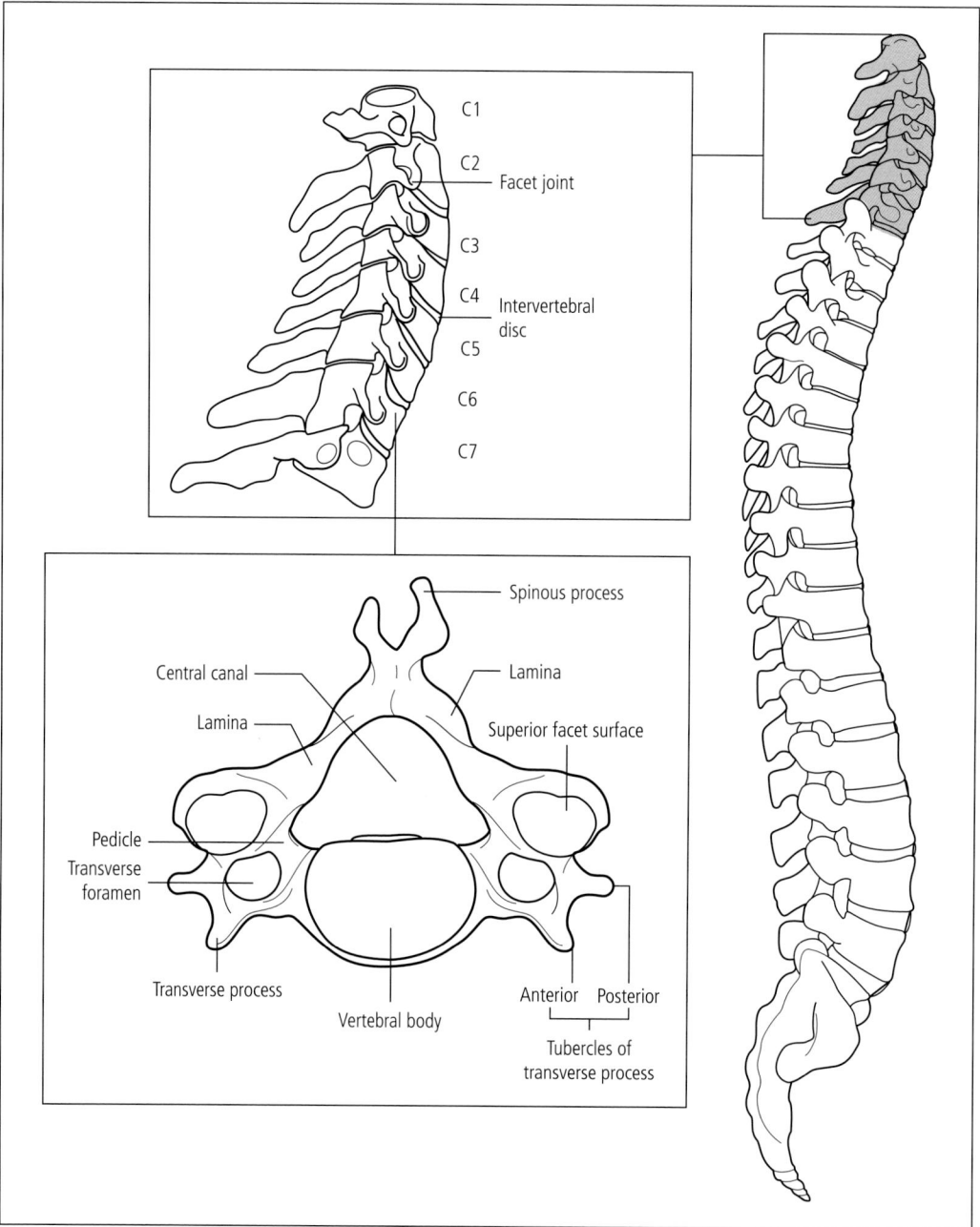

Figure 17.488. Cervical spine.

but increase in length from the fourth cervical vertebra (C4) to the seventh cervical vertebra (C7). Like the lumbars and thoracics, the evaluation of the cervical vertebrae happens in series and is nearly identical from one vertebra to the next. Likewise, the local treatment of the cervical vertebrae is very similar from one to the next. For these reasons, we'll discuss the particulars of C7 and C1, and group the others together.

Seventh cervical vertebra

The fanciest part of C7 (figure 17.489) is its very long spinous process. The transverse processes are also large, but often don't have the split tip as the other cervicals do.

Neighbors

T1
Sixth cervical vertebra (C6)

Palpation

I test and treat the cervicals with the subject in supine. The easiest way to locate C7 is to begin at the second cervical vertebra (C2), and then move distally down the neck. The spinous process of C2 is the first knob distal to the occipital bone. Start at the base of the skull, find C2, then move distally, from spinous process to spinous process, counting—two, three, four, etc.—until you reach C7. Once you arrive at the spinous process of C7, spread your fingers along the posterior ring of the vertebra, including each side of the spinous process, both laminae, and the posterior aspect of each transverse process (figure 17.490).

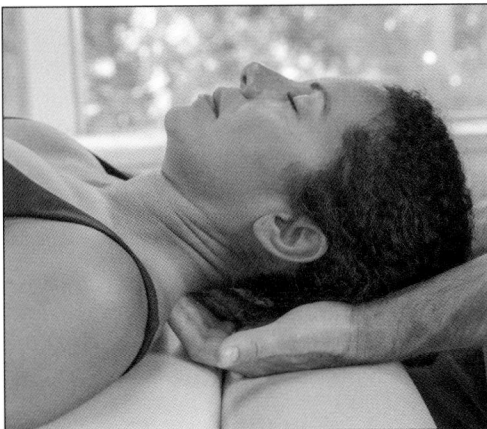

Figure 17.489. C7.

Testing

Phase 1: With the fingers lined up on the bone, spread the fingers (figure 17.491). Does the bone feel like wood or concrete? If the bone feels compacted, fine-tune the spread to identify the torsional pattern of compaction, if any.

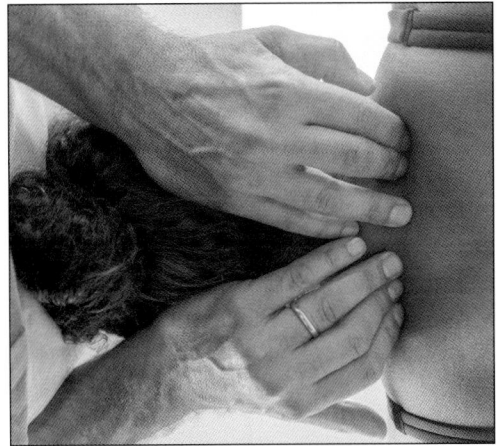

Figure 17.490. Palpating the posterior ring of C7. Normally, this is performed with the patient's head and neck on the table, but here the patient moved back so the neck was past the edge of the table, and the photo was taken from below.

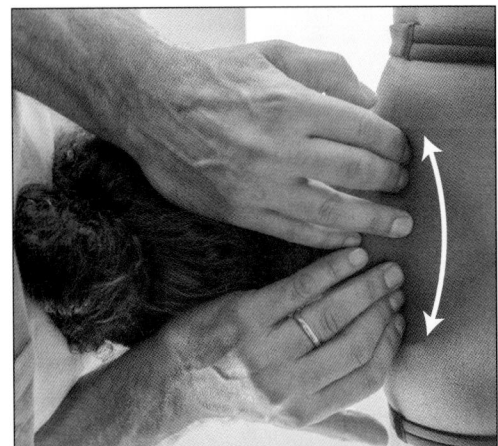

Figure 17.491. Phase 1: Spreading C7. Normally, this is performed with the patient's head and neck on the table, but here the patient moved back so the neck was past the edge of the table, and the photo was taken from below.

Phase 2: Test the micromobility of C7 with T1 by applying a cephalic traction to C7 (figure 17.492). Does the connection have elasticity or is it fibrotic? If the connection is compacted, fine-tune the test to identify the torsional pattern of compaction, if any.

If both the bone and the connection feel normal, move to the next bone to be tested. If either the bone or the connection feels compacted or fibrotic, proceed to local treatment.

Local treatment

We will use C7 as our example, but this general treatment approach can be applied from C7 through to C2. Line the fingers up along each side of the posterior ring of C7 (figure 17.493) and proceed with the six stages of BST treatment (see "Quick Guide to the Six Stages of BST Treatment").

Regional treatment

Integrate the local treatment of C7 into the region by using the cervical gather technique (see "Regional Treatment").

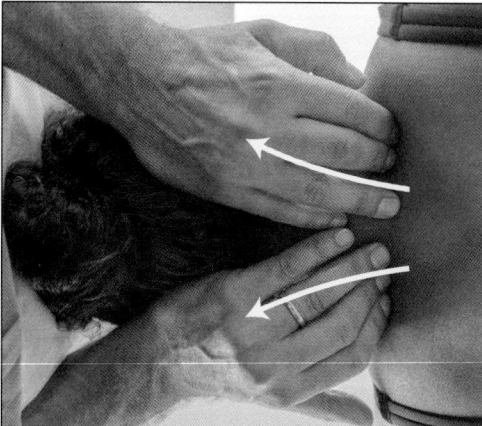

Figure 17.492. Phase 2: Testing the connection between C7 and T1. Normally, this is performed with the patient's head and neck on the table, but here the patient moved back so the neck was past the edge of the table, and the photo was taken from below.

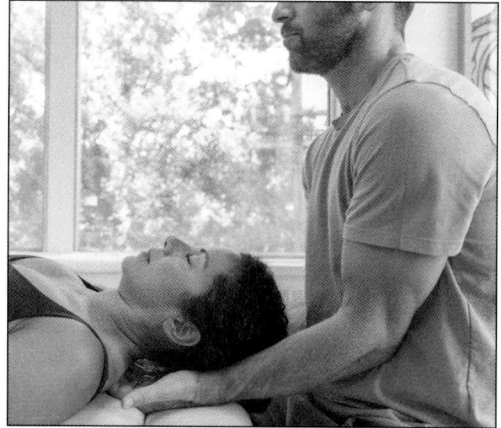

Figure 17.493. Hand and body position for the local treatment of C7.

Sixth to second cervical vertebrae

Neighbors

Vertebra above (C1) and vertebra below (C7).

Palpation, testing, and local treatment

Move up the cervical spine, from C6 to C2, using similar hand positions and repeating the same palpatory, testing, and local treatment protocols as for C7. Test and treat the vertebra itself and its connections with the vertebra below it (for C6, test the connection with C7; for C5, test the connection with C6, etc.)

Regional treatment

Integrate the local treatment of C6 to C2 into the region by using the cervical gather technique (see "Regional Treatment").

First cervical vertebra

The first cervical vertebra (C1; figure 17.494), also known as the atlas, directly supports the weight of the head. Unlike other vertebrae, it lacks a body and has only a rudimentary spinous process. It is ring shaped, with anterior and posterior arches and two

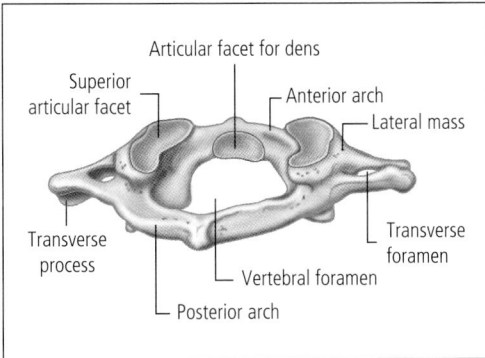

Figure 17.494. C1 (atlas) posterosuperior view.

lateral masses, which articulate with the occipital condyles. The transverse processes are relatively long and the most easily palpable of all the segments.

Neighbors

C2
Occipital

Palpation

To find the transverse processes of C1, place a finger on the bony eminence within the upper neck between the angle of the mandible and the mastoid process (figure 17.495).

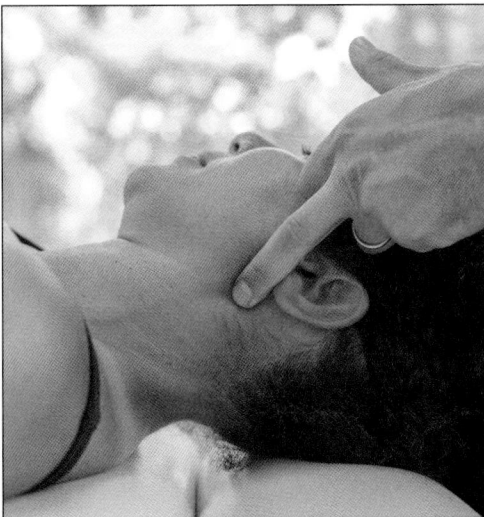

Figure 17.496. Palpating the lateral extremities of the posterior arch of C1.

Once both transverse processes have been located, line up the fingers along the lateral extremities of the posterior arch of C1 (figure 17.496).

Testing

Phase 1: With the fingers lined up on the bone, spread the fingers (figure 17.497). Does the bone feel like wood or concrete? If the bone feels compacted, fine-tune the spread to identify the torsional pattern of compaction.

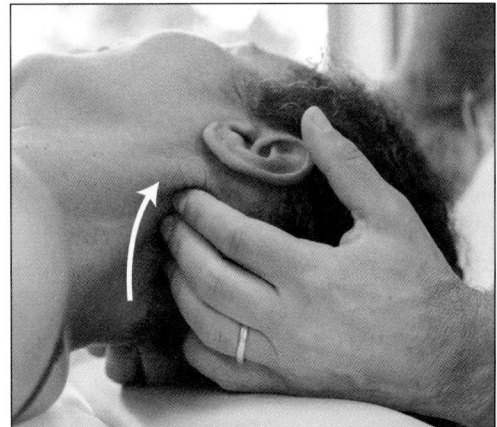

Figure 17.495. Palpating the transverse process of C1.

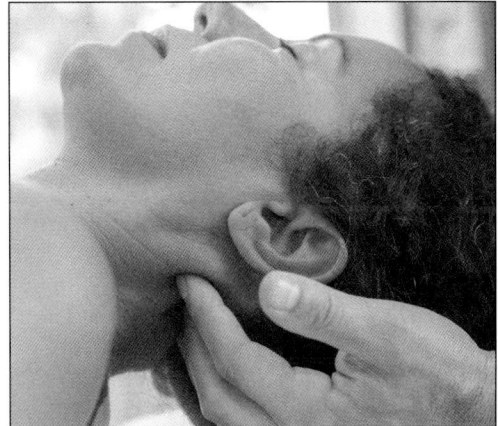

Figure 17.497. Phase 1: Spreading C1. Normally, this is performed with the patient's head flat on the table, but here the patient rotated the head to the right, and the photo was taken from the side.

237

Phase 2a: Grasp C2 with one hand and C1 with the other. Test the micromobility between C1 and C2 by applying cephalic traction to C1 while stabilizing C2 (figure 17.498).

Phase 2b: Grasp C1 with one hand and cup the base of the occipital bone with the other. Test the micromobility of C1 with the occipital bone by applying cephalic traction to the occipital bone while stabilizing C1 (figure 17.499).

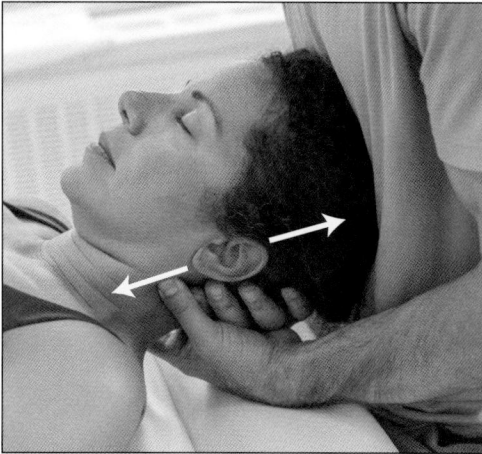

Figure 17.498. Phase 2a: Testing the connection between C1 and C2.

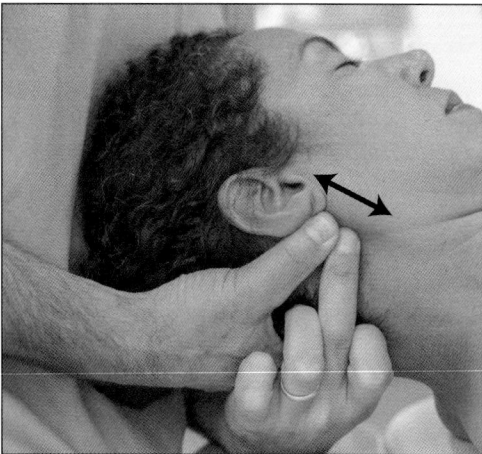

Figure 17.499. Phase 2b: Testing the connection between C1 (left middle finger and thumb) and the occipital bone (right thumb and index finger).

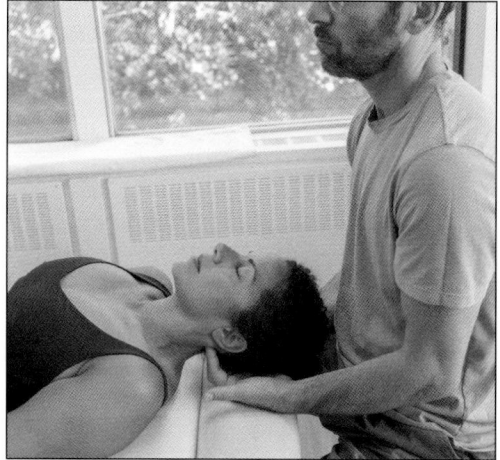

Figure 17.500. Hand and body position for the local treatment of C1.

Do the connections have elasticity or are they fibrotic? If the connections are compacted, fine-tune the test to identify the torsional pattern of compaction. If both the bone and the connections feel normal, move to the next bone to be tested. If either the bone or the connections feel compacted or fibrotic, proceed to local treatment.

Local treatment

Line the fingers along the bone to the lateral extremities of the transverse processes (figure 17.500) and proceed with the six stages of BST treatment (see "Quick Guide to the Six Stages of BST Treatment").

Regional treatment

Integrate the local treatment of C1 into the region by using the cervical gather technique (see "Regional Treatment").

CRANIUM

There are a total of 26 bones in the cranium (figure 17.501), including the small bones in the auditory canal. We'll limit our discussion

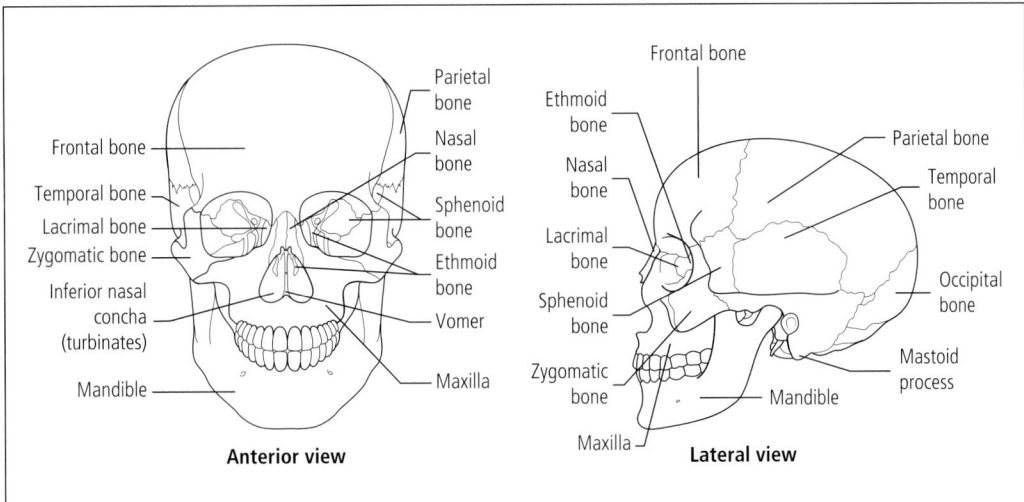

Figure 17.501. Cranium.

to the bones that we can (*a*) easily touch from the outside of the skull and (*b*) easily compress and spread with our hands. These are the occipital, parietals, frontal, temporals, sphenoid, zygomatics, maxillae, and nasal bones, as well as the mandible and hyoid.

Similarly to the carpal bones, we will test and treat the cranial bones *collectively*, as if all of them (except the mandible and hyoid) were parts of one cranial "sphere" divided into five sections: posterior, anterior, inferior, superior, and lateral. Then, we'll discuss separate approaches for the mandible and hyoid. This sectional approach is simple and effective. We'll still discuss the anatomical particulars of the bones so you can find and name them if you have to.

A full description of how to locate and palpate each cranial suture is beyond our scope and not necessary for our sectional BST approach, so details here may be omitted. Also, it will be important to separate the movements happening *within*

the cranium from the movements happening *within the cranial bones*. Remember that inside the skull, the brain pulsates, creating movement within the cranium. Here, you will come into contact with two realities: *brain* motility and *bone* motility. While the two are related, focusing on the latter will help keep our work specific to the motility and texture of osseofascial tissue.

Occipital bone

The occipital bone sits at the posterior and inferior part of the cranium (figure 17.502).

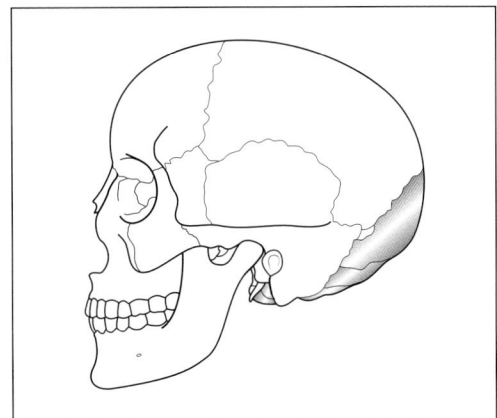

Figure 17.502. Occipital bone, lateral view.

239

The foramen magnum is a large hole in the inferior part of the bone that allows passage of the spinal cord, spinal accessory nerves, and vertebral arteries.

The external occipital protuberance is a prominent lump halfway up the bone. Connecting the foramen magnum to the protuberance is the external occipital crest. There are two sets of curved lines running more or less parallel to each other: the superior lines, which sprout laterally from each side of the protuberance, and the inferior lines, which emerge from the crest.

On each side of the foramen magnum are condyles, which articulate with the lateral masses of C1. The superior border of the occipital bone meets the two parietal bones, forming the lambdoid suture. The inferior border joins the mastoid part of the temporal (forming the occipitomastoid suture) and the petrous part of the temporal (forming the petro-occipital suture).

Neighbors

Both parietals
Both temporals
Sphenoid
C1

Palpation

From the inferior approach, move the fingers up from C2 onto the base of the occipital bone, which is the next bony eminence. By applying slightly more pressure into the musculature toward the front, contact the posterior borders of the condyles and posterior margin of the foramen magnum (figure 17.503).

From the posterior edge of the foramen magnum, follow the central crest up toward the occipital protuberance, and then

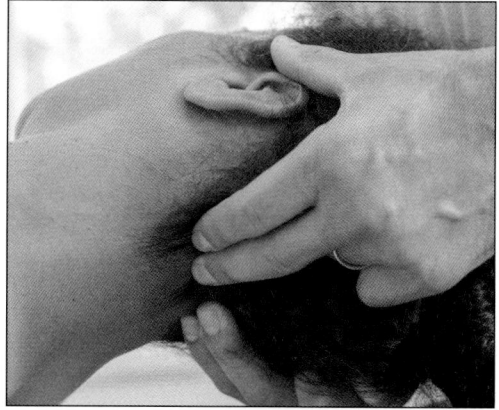

Figure 17.503. Palpating the base of the occipital bone. Normally, this is performed with the patient's head flat on the table, but here the patient rotated the head to the right, and the photo was taken from the side.

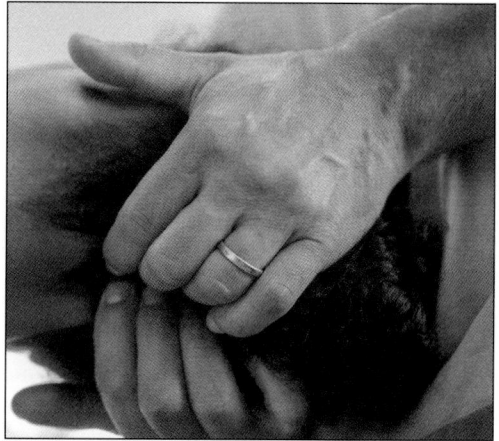

Figure 17.504. Palpating the occipital crest and protuberance of the occipital bone.

laterally along the superior lines on each side (figure 17.504).

Then, continue toward the top of the head to the lambdoid suture, which joins the occipital bone to each parietal (figure 17.505).

Parietals

The two parietal bones form the posterior and superior section of the skull (figure 17.506). Crossing the center of each parietal bone is the temporal ridge, the area above which serves as an attachment for the temporalis fascia and below which serves as an attachment for the temporalis muscle. The superior border of the parietal meets the opposite parietal, forming the sagittal suture. The inferior border of the parietal has three sections: the anterior portion forms the sphenoparietal suture with the great wing of the sphenoid, the middle portion forms the squamosal suture with the squamous portion of the temporal bone, and the posterior section forms the parietomastoid suture with the mastoid part of the temporal. The anterior border of the parietal forms the

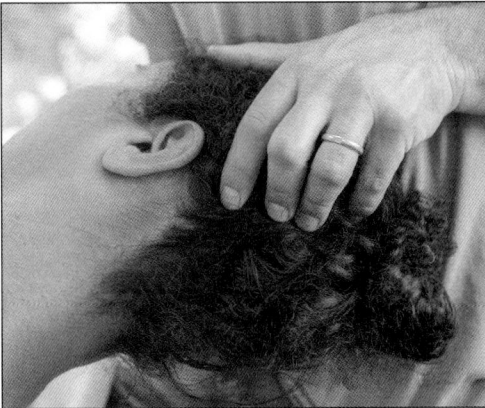

Figure 17.505. Palpating the lambdoid suture with the tips of the fingers.

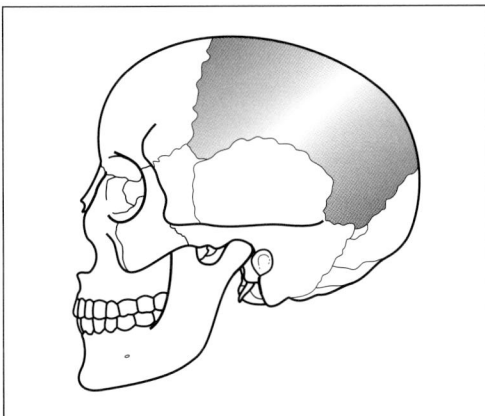

Figure 17.506. Parietal bone, lateral view.

coronal suture with the frontal bone, and the posterior border forms the lambdoid suture with the occipital bone.

Neighbors

Opposite parietal
Occipital
Frontal
Temporal
Sphenoid

Palpation

Have the subject tense and relax the temporal muscle by repetitively biting down. From the side of the cranium, run your finger along the temporal ridge, just below which the temporal muscle will be twitching (figure 17.507). You can also follow the lambdoid suture toward the sagittal suture, which runs from the occipital to the frontal (figure 17.508).

Frontal

The frontal bone is situated at the anterior part of the cranium (figure 17.509). It has a

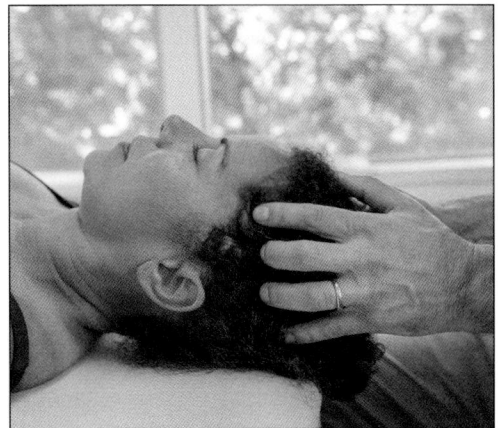

Figure 17.507. Palpating the temporal ridge of the parietal with the tips of the fingers. Have the subject tense and relax the temporal muscle by repetitively biting down to locate the ridge.

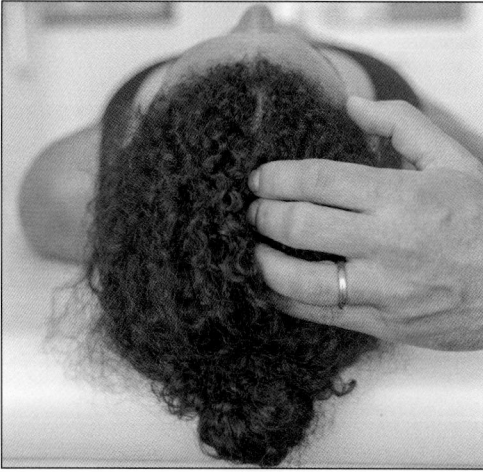

Figure 17.508. Palpating the sagittal suture.

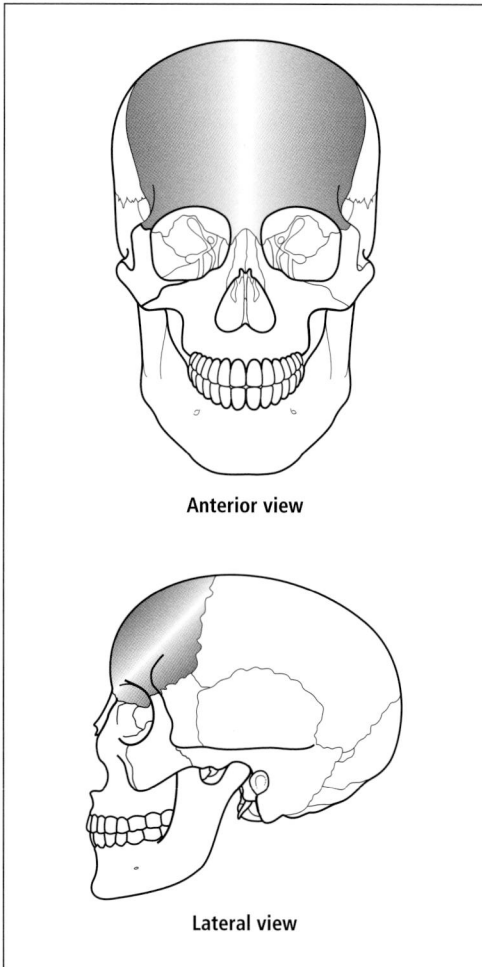

Anterior view

Lateral view

Figure 17.509. Frontal bone.

vertical and a horizontal portion. The vertical portion forms the forehead, and the horizontal portion forms the roof of the orbits and the bridge of the nose. At the top of the vertical portion, the frontal joins both parietals at the coronal suture. The coronal suture is continuous with sphenofrontal suture, the articulation between the frontal and the greater wing of the sphenoid. About halfway between the coronal suture and the horizontal portion exist the two rounded frontal eminences. Just below these, the supraciliary eminences sit just above the eye sockets. The supraorbital arches form the upper angles between the horizontal and vertical portions of the frontal. Within the medial third of each arch is a small, palpable aperture known as the supraorbital notch, which allows passage for the supraorbital artery, vein, and nerve. On each side of the frontal, the anterior portion of the temporal ridge permits attachment of the anterior portion of the temporal fascia. Beneath the ridge, the anterior part of the temporal fossa gives origin to the anterior part of the temporal muscle.

Neighbors

Both parietals
Sphenoid
Ethmoid
Both nasals
Both maxillae
Both lacrimals
Both zygomatics

Palpation

Have the subject tense and relax the temporal muscle by repetitively biting down. From the back and side of the cranium, run your finger along the anterior temporal ridge, from the parietal onto the frontal, where the anterior attachment of the temporal muscle will be twitching (figure 17.510).

From the top of the cranium, locate the sagittal suture running posterior to anterior where it ends at the coronal suture (figure 17.511).

Then, follow the forehead down toward the eyes and over the frontal (figure 17.512) and supraciliary eminences (figure 17.513), and onto the supraorbital arches (figure 17.514).

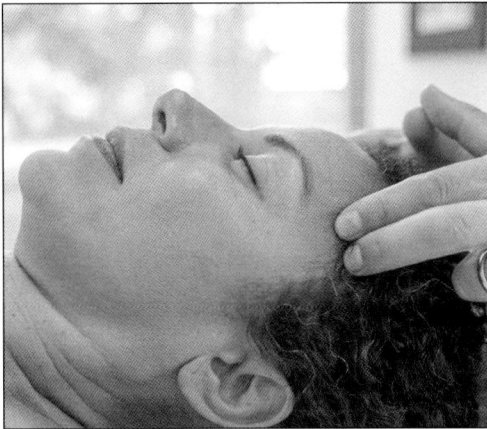

Figure 17.512. Palpating the frontal eminences.

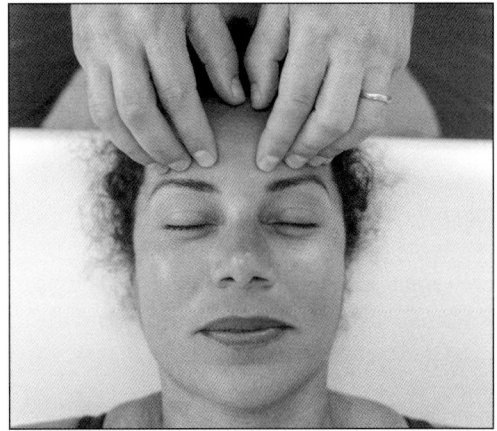

Figure 17.510. Palpating the temporal ridge of the frontal with the tips of the index and middle fingers.

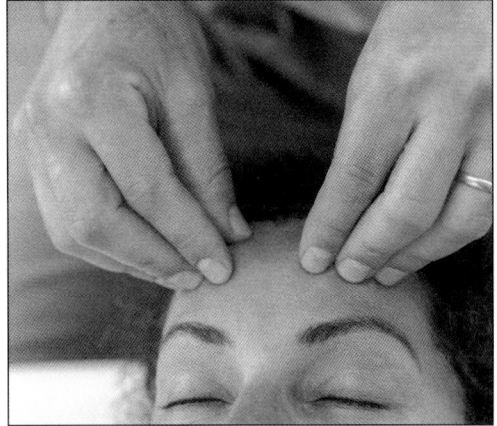

Figure 17.513. Palpating the superciliary eminences with the tips of the fingers.

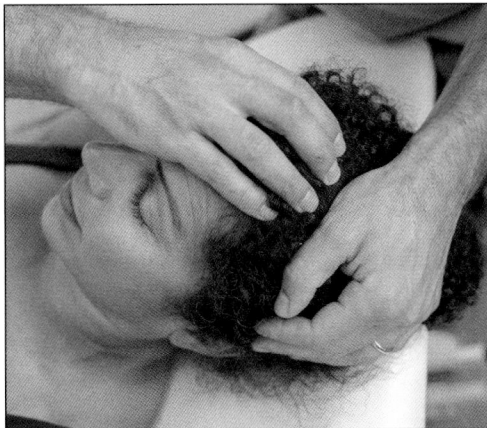

Figure 17.511. Palpating the coronal suture with the tips of the fingers of the right hand.

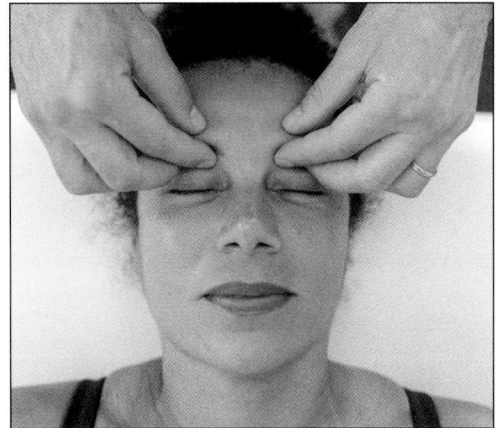

Figure 17.514. Palpating the supraorbital arch with the thumbs and tips of the fingers.

Temporals

The temporals occupy the sides and base of the skull (figure 17.515). Each temporal has three segments: squamous, mastoid, and petrous. The squamous portion is convex and smooth, and is the most anterior and superior part of the bone. The zygomatic process—a long, arched outgrowth—projects from the lower part of the squamous portion and extends toward the face, where it joins the zygomatic bone (zygoma). Just below and behind the base of the zygomatic process are two holes: the glenoid fossa, in which sits the condyle of the mandible, and the auditory canal, which leads to the middle and inner ear.

The superior border of the squamous portion of the temporal articulates with the parietal, and the anterior border joins the greater wing of the sphenoid. The mastoid segment forms the posterior part of the temporal bone, and has a conical projection called the mastoid process. The superior border of the mastoid segment articulates with the parietal bone, and the inferior border joins the occipital bone. The petrous segment of the temporal is a pyramid-shaped process wedged in between the sphenoid and occipital bone at the base of the skull, and contains within it all the hardware involved in hearing.

The styloid process, a long, thin eminence, juts downward, forward, and inward from the inferior portion of the petrous segment.

Neighbors

Occipital
Parietal
Sphenoid
Mandible
Zygoma

Palpation

To palpate the base of the zygomatic arch, follow the vertical ramus of the mandible up to the condyle. Have the subject open and close their mouth. The condyle will move, but the base of the arch will not (figure 17.516).

Follow the arch toward the front of the face (to roughly the level of the internal border of the vertical ramus of the mandible) where it meets the zygoma (figure 17.517).

To palpate the auditory canal, gently place a finger in the subject's ear (figure 17.518). You may want to ask permission first while your subject can still hear you!

Behind and below the ear, the first bony subcutaneous eminence is the mastoid process (figure 17.519).

Now, have the subject bite down repetitively. Follow the twitching temporal muscle along the squamous portion of the bone, to which it attaches (figure 17.520).

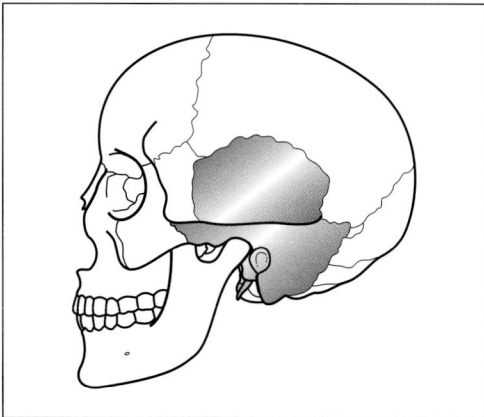

Figure 17.515. Temporal bone, lateral view.

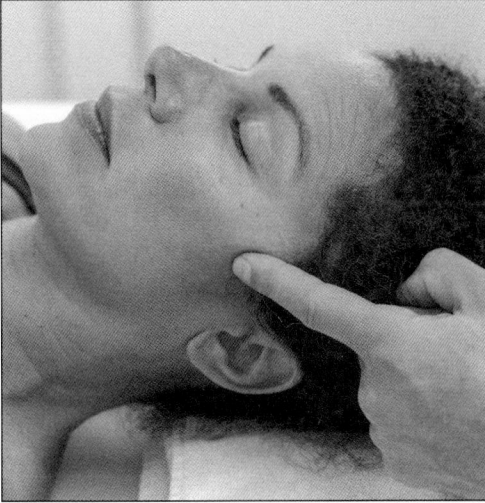

Figure 17.516. Palpating the base of the zygomatic arch of the temporal.

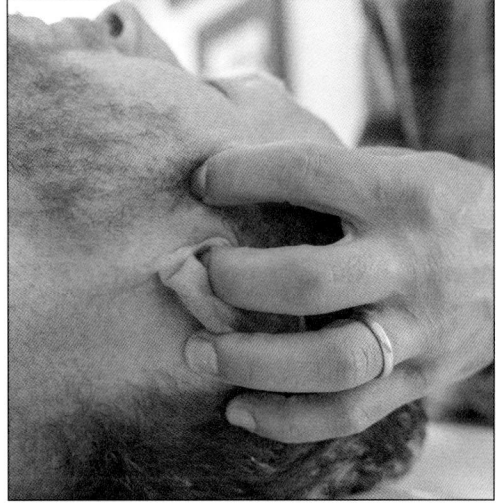

Figure 17.518. Palpating the auditory canal of the temporal with the middle finger.

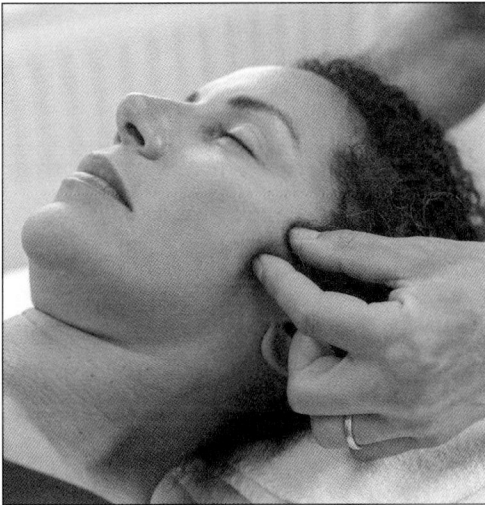

Figure 17.517. Palpating the zygomatic arch of the temporal with the thumb and index finger.

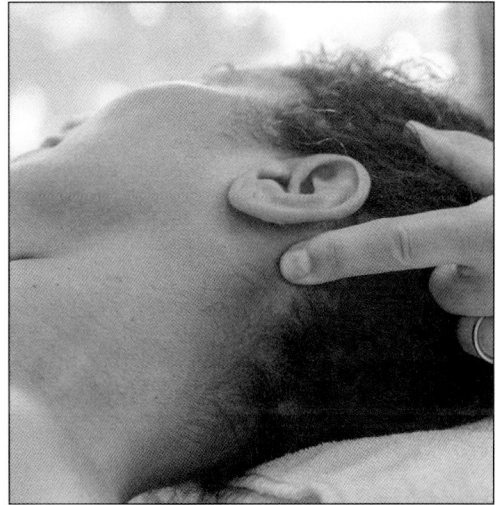

Figure 17.519. Palpating the mastoid process of the temporal with the index finger.

Sphenoid

The sphenoid is sort of shaped like a bat (figure 17.521), with a body and two sets of wings, the greater and lesser. The sphenoid articulates with all the bones of the cranium. The greater wings are the only portions of the sphenoid that are easily and directly accessible, since the other segments are hidden within the base of the skull. The greater wings are exposed on the upper side of the cranium, just behind the lateral edge of the orbit and bordered by the frontal, parietal, and squamous portion of the temporal bone.

245

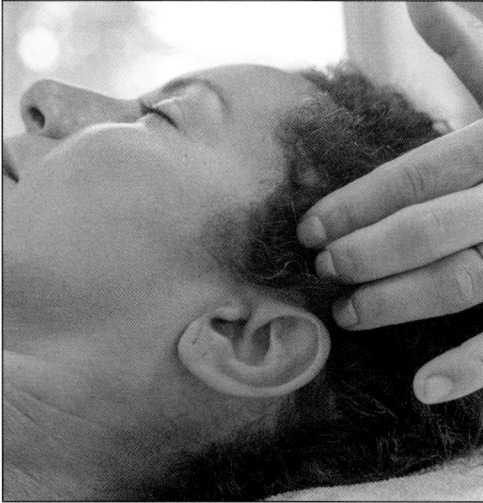

Figure 17.520. Palpating the squamous portion of the temporal with the tips of the fingers.

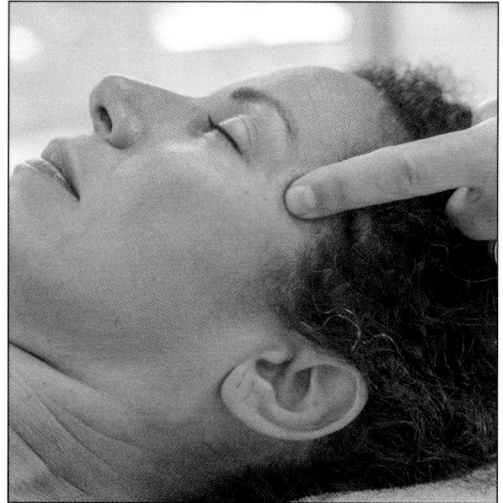

Figure 17.521. Sphenoid bone, lateral view.

Neighbors

All of the cranial bones

Palpation

To palpate the greater wing of the sphenoid, move a finger posteriorly from the lateral edge of the orbit into the small depression (figure 17.522).

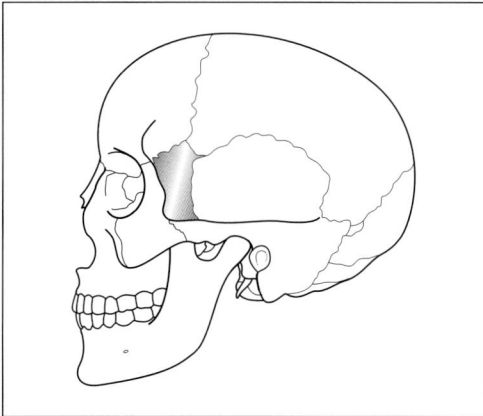

Figure 17.522. Palpating the greater wing of the sphenoid.

Nasals

The two small nasal bones sit side by side, forming the bridge of the nose (figure 17.523).

Neighbors

Frontal
Ethmoid
Opposite nasal
Maxilla

Palpation

To palpate the nasal bones, move a finger inferior from the frontal bone onto the bridge of the nose (figure 17.524).

Maxillae

The maxilla is the largest bone of the face (figure 17.525). Sitting next to each other, the two maxillae form the upper jaw, part of the side of the nose, and the inferior surface of the orbit. Each maxilla has a body and four processes: the zygomatic, nasal, alveolar, and palatine.

Anterior view

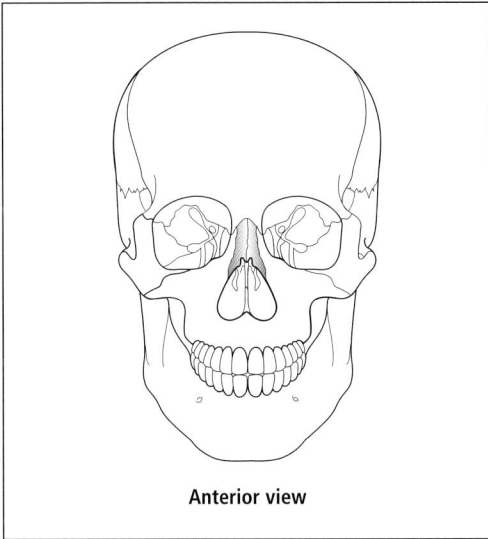

Figure 17.523. Nasals.

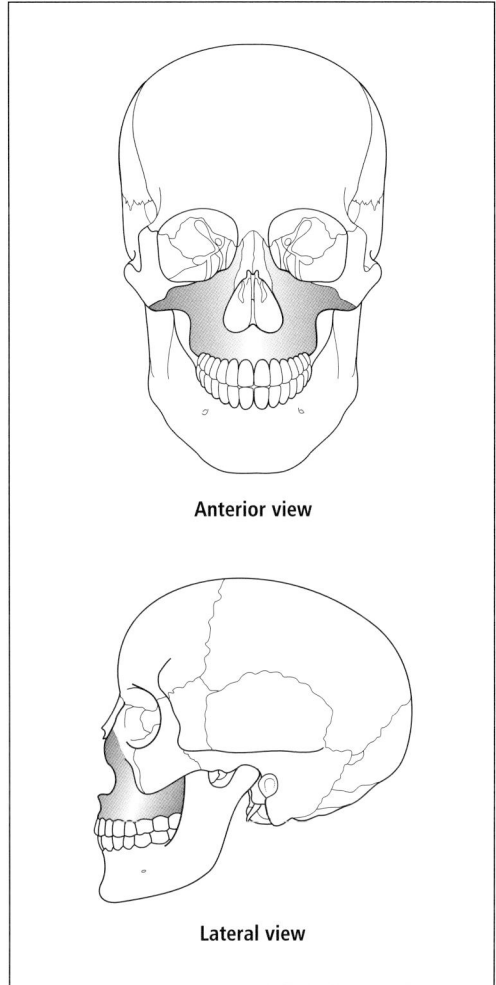

Figure 17.524. Palpating the nasals with the thumb and index finger.

The zygomatic process is triangular in shape and joins the zygomatic process of the temporal. The nasal process forms the part of the side of the nose and part of the circumference of the orbit, and articulates with the nasal bone in front and the lacrimal bone behind.

Anterior view

Lateral view

Figure 17.525. Maxillae.

The alveolar process forms the inferior extremity of the bone and has eight excavations for the upper teeth. The palatine process can only be accessed intrabucally.

The body itself has four surfaces: facial, zygomatic, orbital, and internal. The facial surface of the body is directed forward and upward. The zygomatic surface faces backward and outward, and forms part of the zygomatic fossa. The orbital surface forms part of the floor of the orbit. The internal surface cannot be accessed.

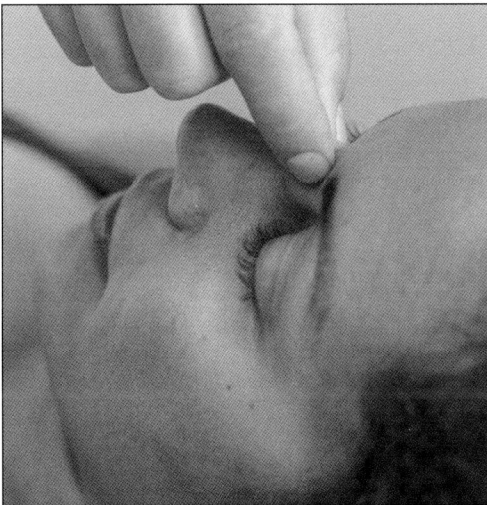

Neighbors

Frontal
Ethmoid
Nasal
Zygomatic
Lacrimal
Palatine
Vomer
Opposite maxilla
Orbital plate of the sphenoid (inconsistent)

Palpation

From the nasal bones, move laterally along the bridge of the nose onto the nasal processes of the maxillae (figure 17.526).

Slide down the sides of the nose to the alveolar processes, where the maxillae meet the teeth (figure 17.527).

Now, move your fingers back up the face to the zygomata and then medially onto the zygomatic processes of the maxillae (figure 17.528).

To palpate the orbital surfaces, move your fingers up toward the eyes and onto the lower bony rims of the orbits (figure 17.529).

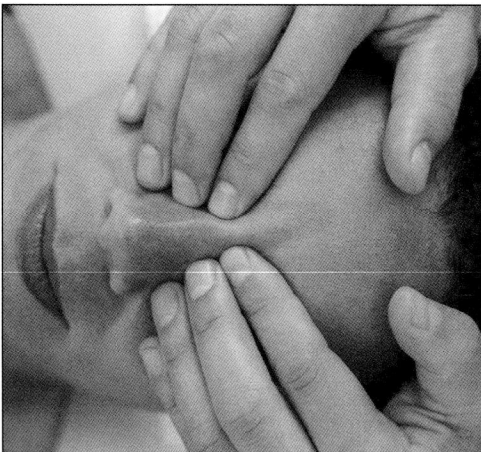

Figure 17.527. Palpating the alveolar processes of the maxillae.

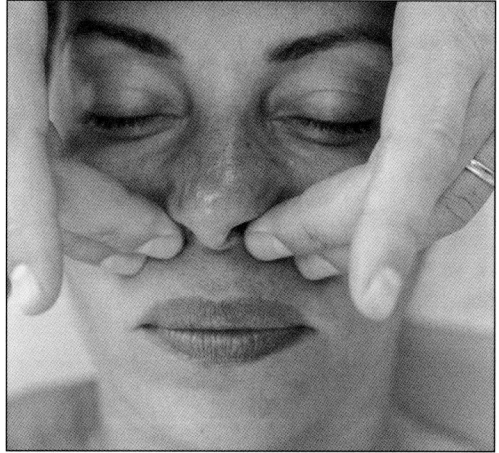

Figure 17.528. Palpating the zygomatic processes of the maxillae.

Zygomata

The zygoma is a four-sided bone that is often called the "cheekbone" (figure 17.530). It forms part of the outer wall of the floor of the orbit and part of the temporal and zygomatic fossa. Each zygomatic bone has four processes: the frontal, orbital, maxillary, and zygomatic.

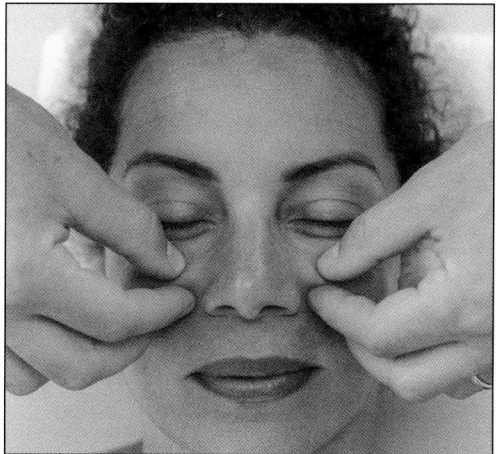

Figure 17.526. Palpating the nasal processes of the maxillae.

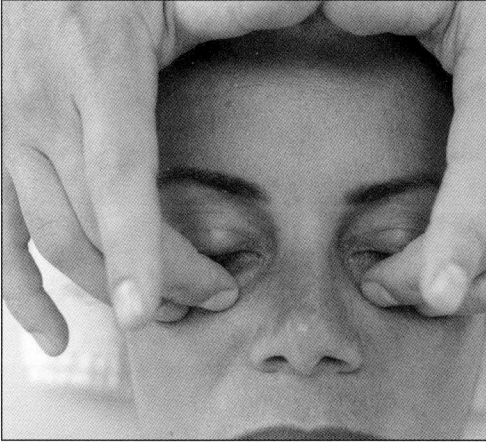

Figure 17.529. Palpating the orbital surfaces of the maxillae.

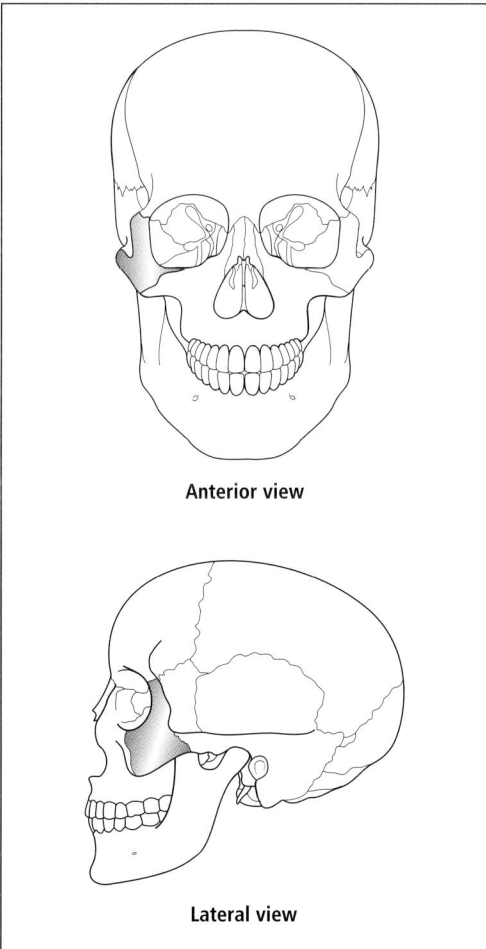

Neighbors

Frontal
Temporal
Sphenoid
Maxilla

Palpation

From the sides, follow the zygomatic processes of the temporal bones onto the zygomatic bones (figure 17.531).

Then, follow the lower rims of the orbits laterally to the orbital processes of the zygomatic bones (figure 17.532).

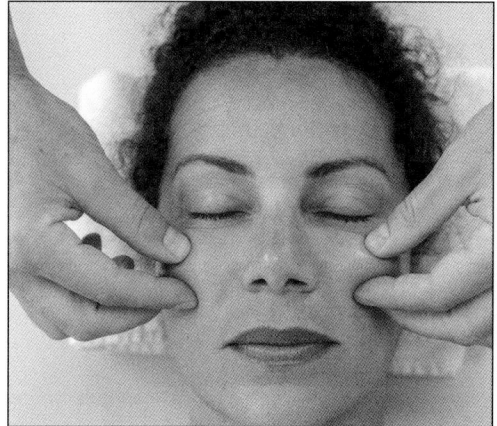

Anterior view

Lateral view

Figure 17.530. Zygomata.

Figure 17.531. Palpating the zygomata from the zygomatic processes of the temporals.

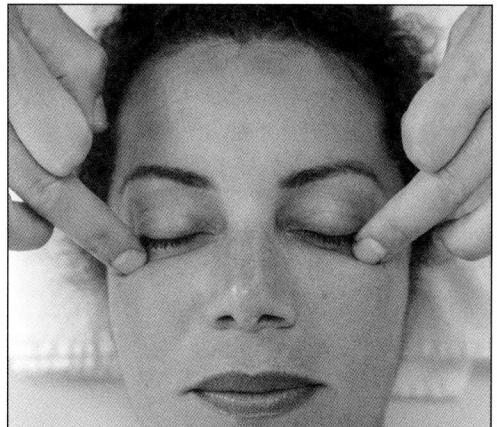

Figure 17.532. Palpating the orbital processes of the zygomata.

249

Cranial Sections

Inferior section

Testing and local treatment

Place your hands on the inferior section of the skull (figures 17.533 and 17.534). Tuck the fingers into the suboccipital musculature. Contact the posterior ridge of the foramen magnum, lining up the fingers along the base of the occipital bone and mastoid portion of the temporals, parallel with the

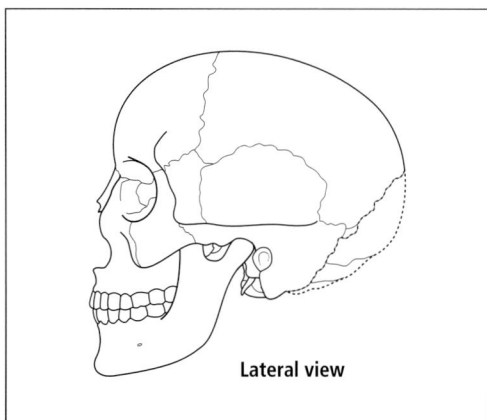

Figure 17.533. Inferior section of the cranium.

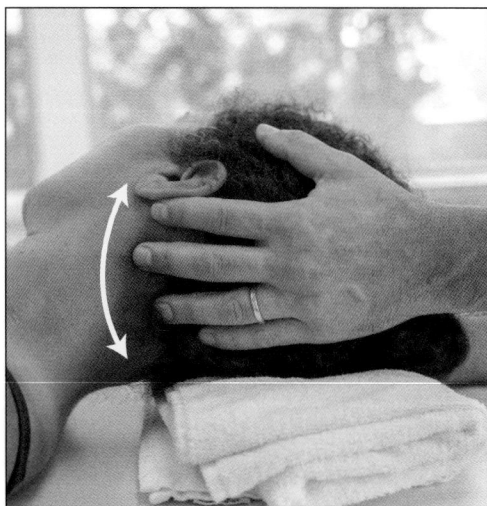

Figure 17.534. Testing and local treatment of the inferior section of the cranium. For this photo, the subject's head is turned to the right.

occipitomastoid sutures. Spread your fingers to test the quality of the bone. Does it feel like wood or concrete? Are there any specific zones that feel more compacted than others? If the bone feels normal, move to the next section to be tested. If the whole section or parts of the section feel compacted, proceed with the six stages of BST treatment (see "Quick Guide to the Six Stages of BST Treatment").

Regional treatment

Integrate the treatment of the inferior cranial section into the region by using the cranial gather technique (see "Regional Treatment").

Posterior section

Testing and local treatment

This section mainly includes the occipital and parietal bones (figure 17.535). Place your hands on the posterior section of the skull (figure 17.536). Spread your fingers to test the quality of the bone. Does it feel like wood or concrete? Are there any specific zones that feel compacted? If the bone feels normal, move to the next section to be tested. If the whole section or parts of the section feel compacted, proceed with the six stages

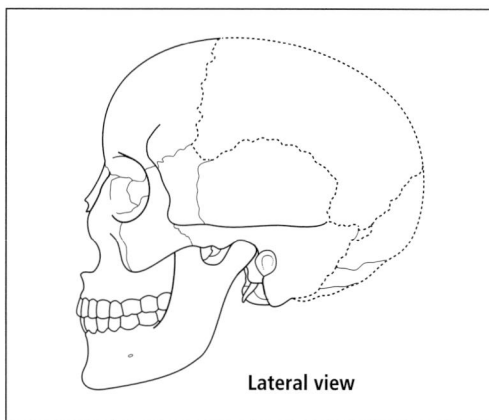

Figure 17.535. Posterior section.

of BST treatment (see "Quick Guide to the Six Stages of BST Treatment").

Regional treatment

Integrate the treatment of the posterior cranial section into the region by using the cranial gather technique (see "Regional Treatment").

Lateral section

Testing and local treatment

This section mainly includes the temporal and parietal bones (figure 17.537). Place

your hands on both lateral sections of the skull (figure 17.538) and spread your fingers to test the quality of the bone. You may choose to test certain zones more specifically (such as the zygomatic arch of the temporal, for example) using both hands (figure 17.539). If using both hands, move to the opposite

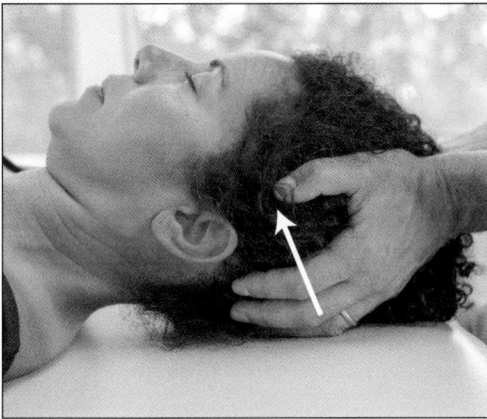

Figure 17.538. Testing and local treatment of the lateral sections of the cranium with one hand on each section.

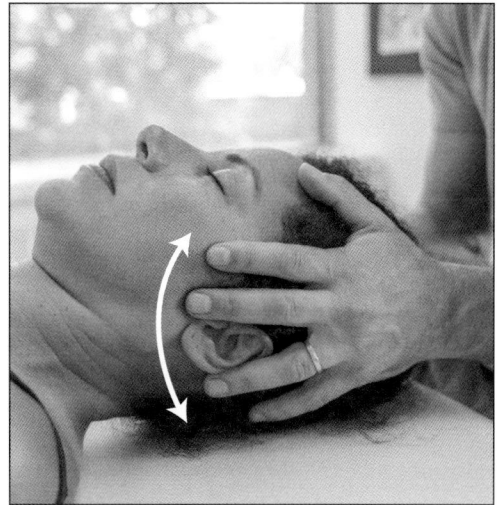

Figure 17.536. Testing and local treatment of the posterior section of the cranium using both hands.

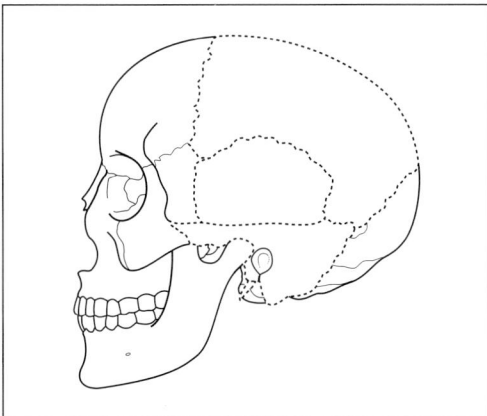

Figure 17.537. Lateral section of the cranium.

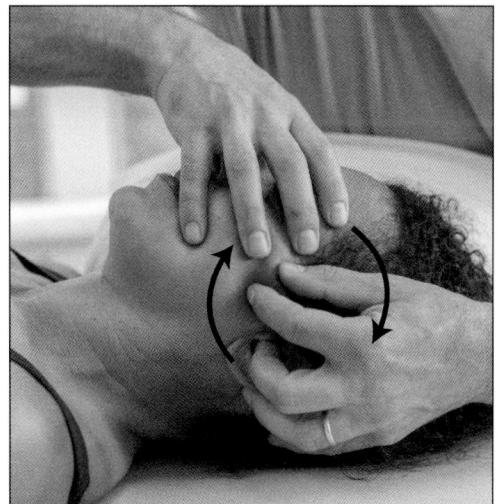

Figure 17.539. Testing and local treatment of specific zones within the lateral section of the cranium using both hands. Use a pillow, if necessary, to stabilize the head of the subject.

side and stabilize the head of the subject with a pillow. Does the section feel like wood or concrete? Are there any specific zones that feel compacted? If the bone feels normal, move to the next section to be tested. If the whole section or parts of the section feel compacted, proceed with the six stages of BST treatment (see "Quick Guide to the Six Stages of BST Treatment").

Regional treatment

Integrate the treatment of the lateral cranial sections into the region by using the cranial gather technique (see "Regional Treatment").

Anterior section

Testing and local treatment

This section mainly includes the bones of the face (figure 17.540). Place your hands on the anterior section of the skull, with thumbs on the bridge of the nose and the fingers pointing down toward the upper teeth (figure 17.541). Once you have descended down through the soft tissue and onto the bony level, spread your fingers to test the quality of each side

of the section. For the testing of specific zones, a two-handed approach may be more efficient (figure 17.542). Does the section feel like wood or concrete? Are there specific zones that feel compacted? If the section feels normal, move to the next section to be tested. If the whole section or parts of the section are compacted, proceed with the six stages of BST treatment (see "Quick Guide to the Six Stages of BST Treatment"). Local treatment can also be done with one or two hands.

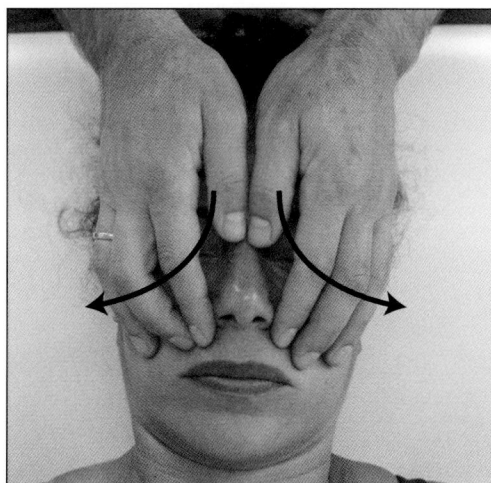

Figure 17.541. Testing and local treatment of both sides of the anterior section of the cranium with one hand on each side.

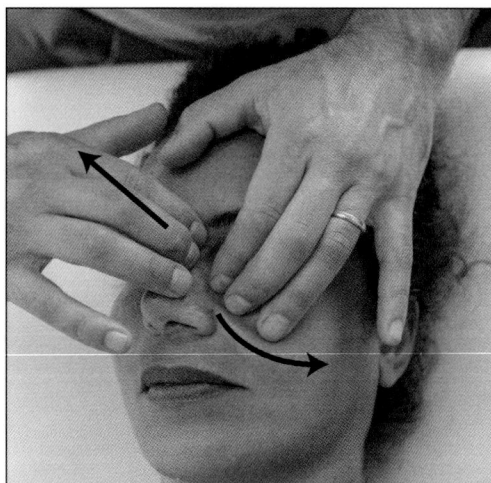

Figure 17.542. Testing and local treatment of specific zones within the anterior section of the cranium using both hands.

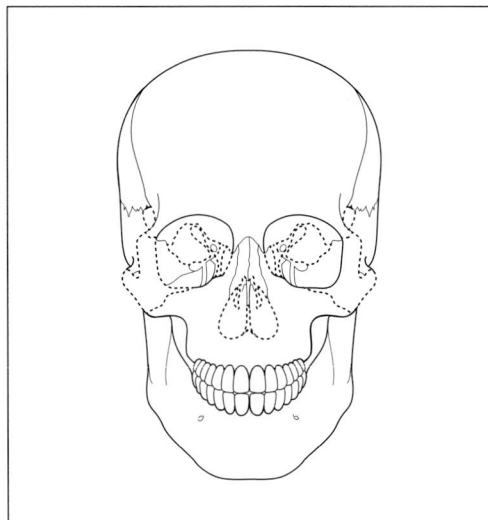

Figure 17.540. Anterior section of the cranium.

Regional treatment

Integrate the treatment of the anterior cranial section into the region by using the cranial gather technique (see "Regional Treatment").

Superior section

Testing and local treatment

This section primarily includes the parietals and the frontal (figure 17.543). Place your hands on the superior section of the skull, with the thumbs lined up along each side of the sagittal suture and the fingers pointing anteriorly (figure 17.544). For those of you

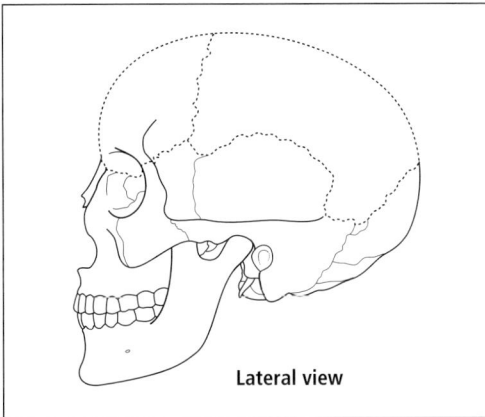

Figure 17.543. Superior section of the cranium.

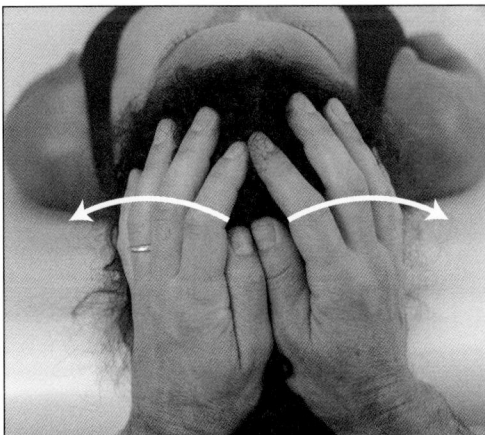

Figure 17.544. Testing and local treatment of the superior section of the cranium. For those of you who have limited extension in the wrists, raising the treatment table may be helpful.

who have limited extension in the wrists (like me), raising the treatment table may be helpful. Spread the bone and the sagittal suture by separating the palms and fingers. Does the section feel like wood or concrete? Are there any specific zones that feel compacted? If the section feels normal, move to the next section or bone to be tested. If the whole section or parts of the section are compacted, proceed with the six stages of BST treatment (see "Quick Guide to the Six Stages of BST Treatment").

Regional treatment

Integrate the treatment of the cranial section into the region by using the cranial gather technique (see "Regional Treatment").

Mandible and Hyoid

Mandible

The mandible is the bone of the lower jaw and is the largest and strongest bone of the face (figure 17.545). It consists of a curved horizontal body and two vertical rami. The rounded prominence at the apex of the body is the mental process, or chin. The alveolar surface of the body contains sixteen holes for the teeth. The upper part of each vertical ramus contains two processes, the coronoid and condyloid, and a deep concavity between them called the sigmoid notch. The condyle articulates with the glenoid fossa of the temporal bone, forming the temporomandibular joint.

Neighbors

Both temporals

Palpation

Have the subject open and close their jaw repetitively. From the auditory canal of the temporal, move the fingers anteriorly onto

253

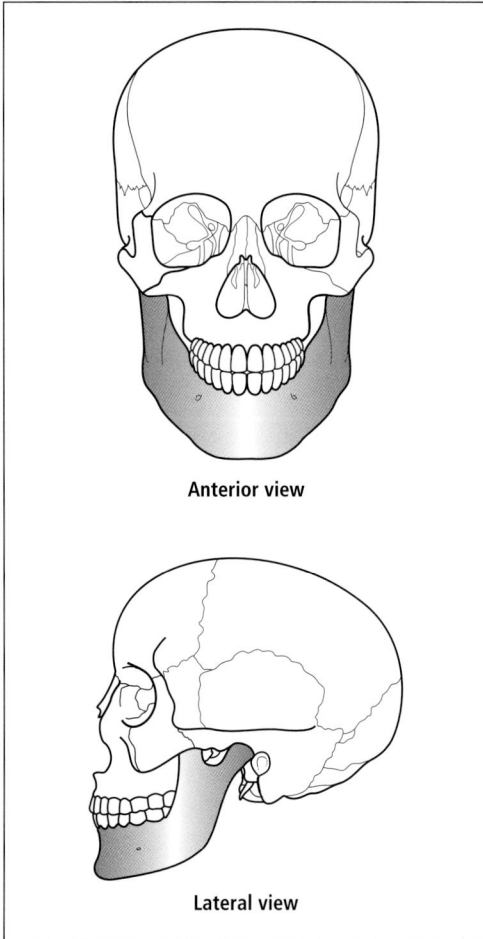

Anterior view

Lateral view

Figure 17.545. Mandible.

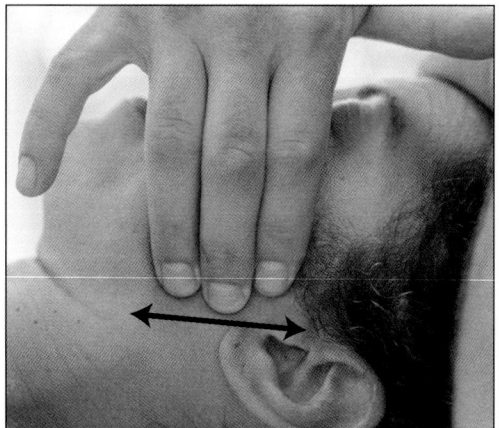

Figure 17.546. Palpating the condyle of the mandible.

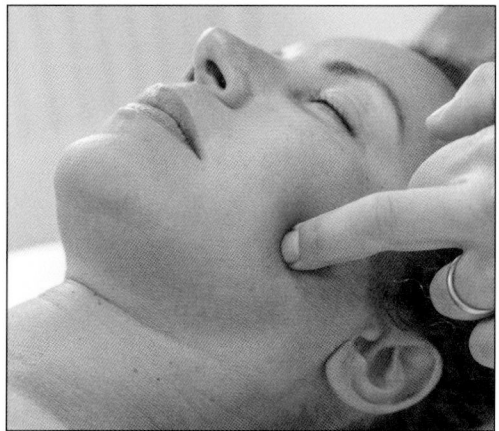

Figure 17.547. Palpating the coronoid process of the mandible.

the condyle of the mandible, which will be moving (figure 17.546).

Follow the zygomatic process of the temporal, and move down onto the coronoid process, which will also be moving (figure 17.547).

Progress down the vertical ramus toward the angle between it and the body (figure 17.548), and then move horizontally along the body to the chin (figure 17.549).

Testing

Phase 1: Curl the fingers of each hand underneath the horizontal body of the

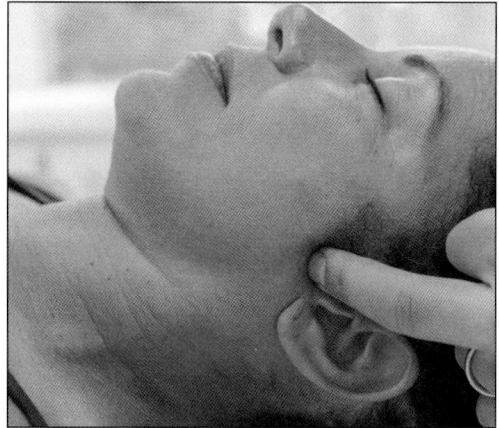

Figure 17.548. Palpating the vertical ramus of the mandible.

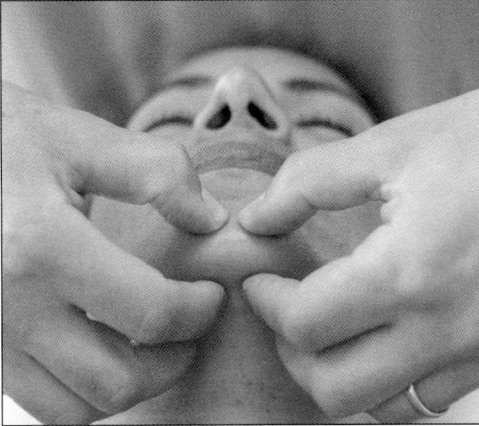

Figure 17.549. Palpating the horizontal body and mental process of the mandible.

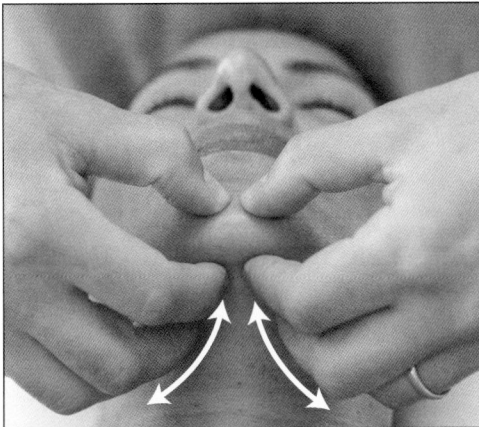

Figure 17.550. Phase 1: Testing the body of the mandible by simultaneously spreading the fingers and opening the elbows.

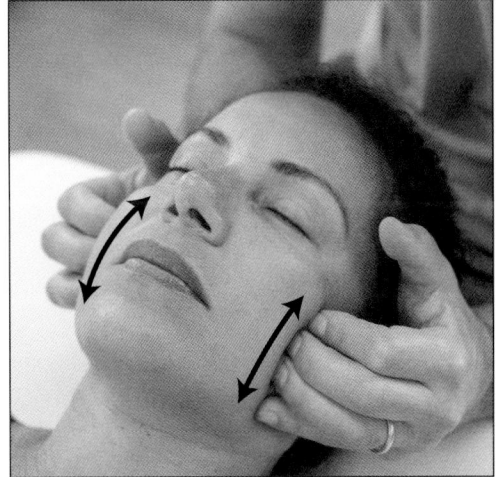

Figure 17.551. Phase 1: Testing the temporomandibular joints, condyloid processes, and vertical rami of the mandible by spreading the fingers.

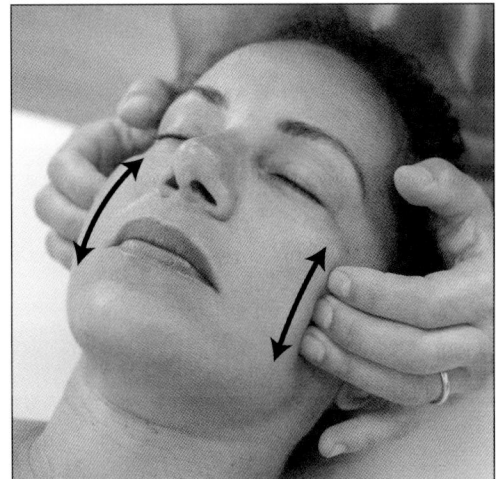

Figure 17.552. Phase 1: Testing the coronoid processes and vertical rami of the mandible by spreading the fingers.

mandible. Test the quality of the body by simultaneously spreading your fingers and opening your elbows (figure 17.550).

Next, line the fingers of each hand along the vertical rami. Test the quality of the condyloid processes, the vertical rami, and the temporomandibular joints by simultaneously spreading your fingers and applying traction to the joint (figure 17.551). Now, adjust your fingers to contact the coronoid processes, and spread the fingers to test the quality of the bone (figure 17.552).

Do the segments feel like wood or concrete? If the bone feels normal, move to the next bone to be tested. If one or more segments are compacted, move to phase 2.

Phase 2: Move to the opposite side to be tested and stabilize the head of the subject with a pillow. Spread and twist the

255

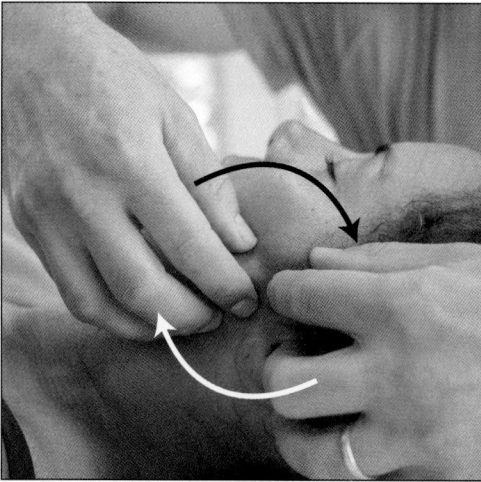

Figure 17.553. Phase 2: Spreading and twisting the temporomandibular joint. Use one hand to stabilize the temporal and the other to grip the vertical ramus of the mandible.

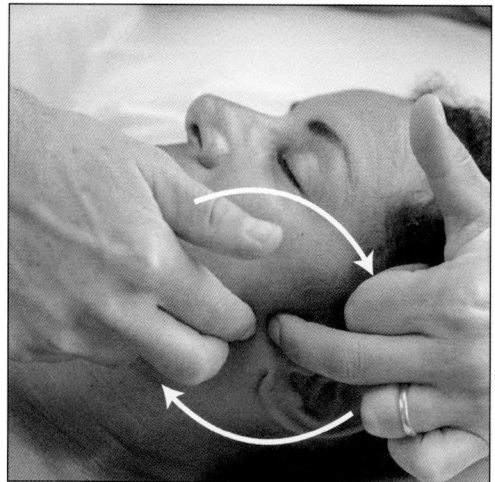

Figure 17.555. Phase 2: Spreading and twisting the condyloid process (and vertical ramus) of the mandible.

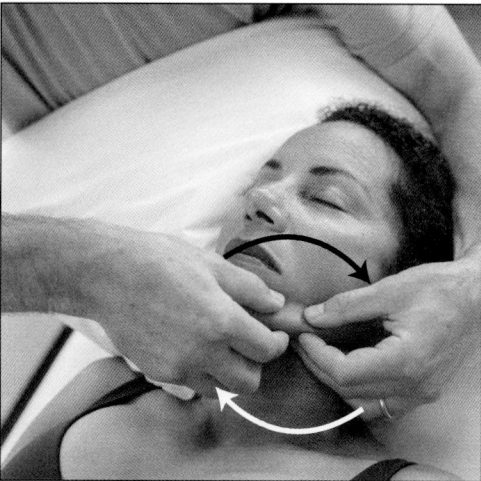

Figure 17.554. Phase 2: Spreading and twisting one side of the body of the mandible.

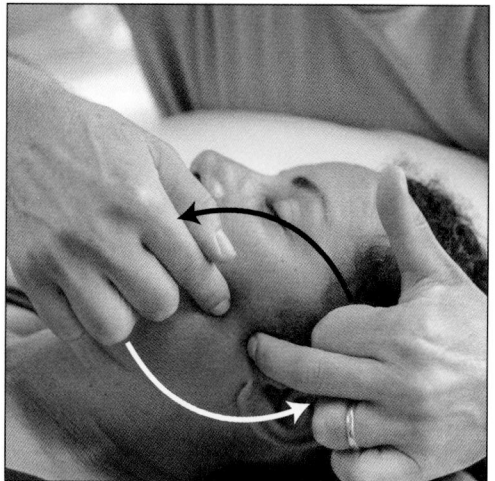

Figure 17.556. Phase 2: Spreading and twisting the coronoid process (and vertical ramus) of the mandible.

temporomandibular joint by contacting the temporal with one hand and grasping the vertical ramus of the mandible with the other (figure 17.553). Remaining on the opposite side of the subject, test the body (figure 17.554), condyloid process (and vertical ramus; figure 17.555),

and coronoid process (and vertical ramus; figure 17.556).

Local treatment

As you did during testing, sit on the opposite side of the subject and stabilize the head with a pillow. Grasp the section of the mandible with both hands (figure 17.557) and proceed with the six stages of BST

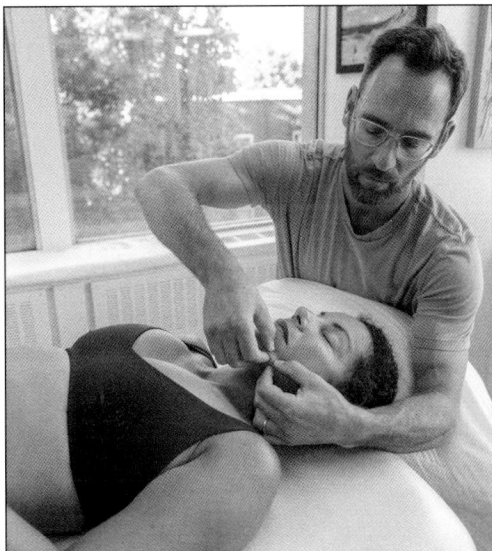

Figure 17.557. Hand and body position for local treatment of the body of the mandible. Adjust the hand position to move to other zones within the bone accordingly.

treatment (see "Quick Guide to the Six Stages of BST Treatment").

Regional treatment

Integrate the treatment of the mandible into the region by using the cranial gather technique (see "Regional Treatment").

Hyoid

The hyoid is a small horseshoe-shaped bone at the anterior midline of the neck between the chin and the thyroid cartilage (figure 17.558). Unlike other bones, the hyoid does not directly articulate with any other bones, but is the site of numerous muscular attachments. It has a body and two sets of bony horns, called the greater and lesser cornua.

Palpation

From the chin, follow the musculature down to the hyoid bone, which is the next bony

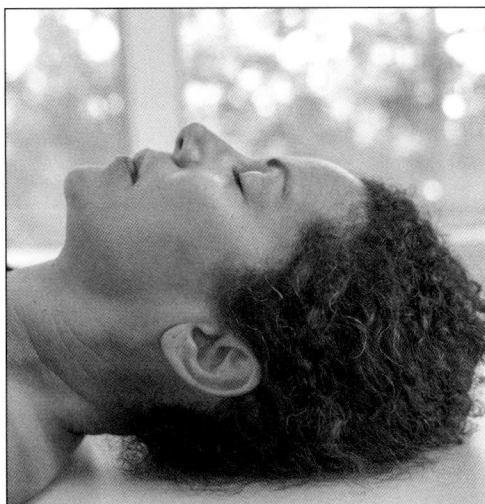

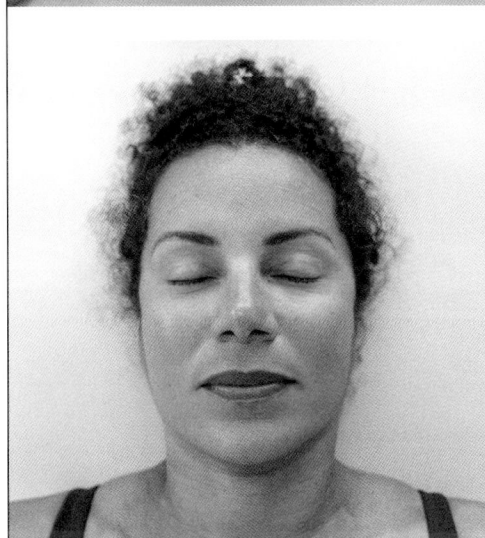

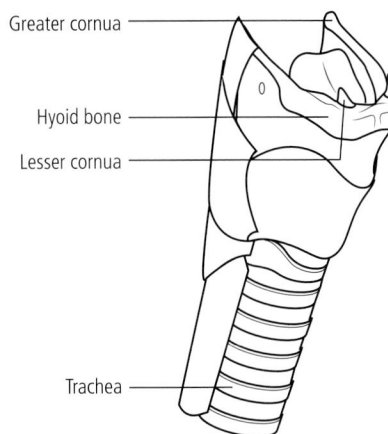

Figure 17.558. Hyoid bone.

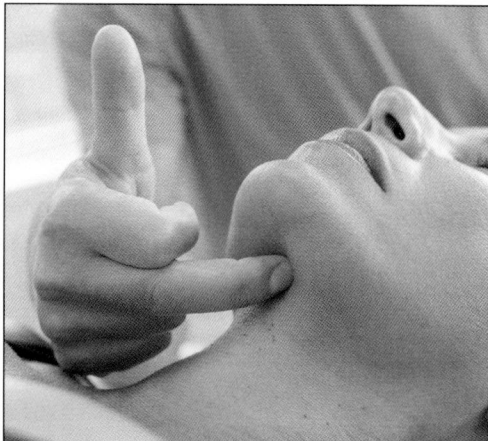

Figure 17.559. Palpating the body of the hyoid.

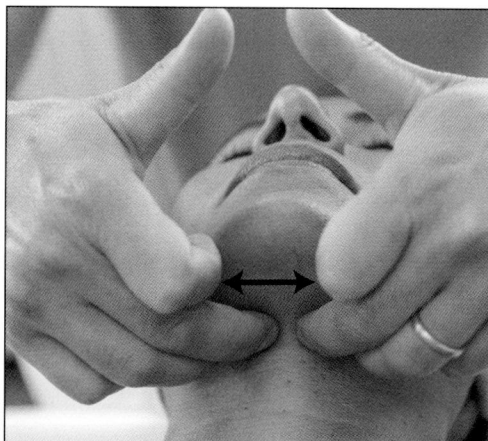

Figure 17.561. Testing the hyoid by spreading the bone.

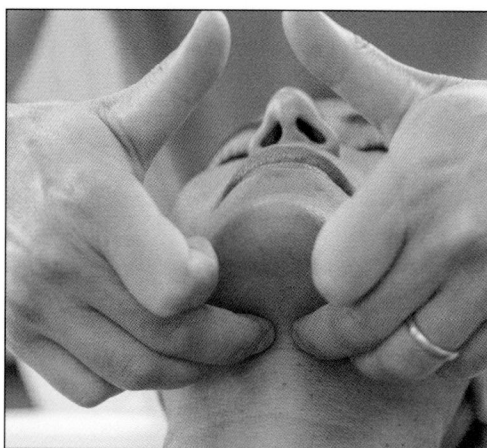

Figure 17.560. Palpating the cornua of the hyoid.

eminence (figure 17.559). Once on the hyoid, follow the bone laterally on each side toward the cornua (figure 17.560).

Testing

Line up two sets of fingers along the hyoid and spread the bone by separating the fingers (figure 17.561). If the bone feels normal, move to the next bone to be tested. If the bone is compacted, proceed to treatment.

Local treatment

With fingers on the bone (figure 17.561), proceed with the six stages of BST treatment (see "Quick Guide to the Six Stages of BST Treatment").

SENSING YOUR PRIMARY RESPIRATION II

Before we look at regional BST treatment, let's take a break and switch gears. This is the second part of the two-part series on sensing your own primary respiration, as it's a neat way to put what you have just learned about testing and local treatment into practice (see also page 77).

Invite a colleague to join you here. During part 1 of this exercise, you simply observed the primary respiration within you. This time, you'll *analyze* the behavior of primary respiration, and see if your findings sync with those of your partner.

Repeat the steps for part 1 (page 78), but instead of simply observing the primary respiration working within you, see if you can identify one or more areas of your body where the expression of the primary respiration is weaker or absent. These inert zones—the "boulders in the stream"—could be anywhere: a small bone in your foot, half of your forehead, an elbow, or the left side of your rib cage, to name a few examples. Regardless of where the compaction exists, take a mental note of it, and be as specific as you can with the location.

For now, don't tell your colleague your findings. Have them evaluate your body, scanning your skeleton for compactions, looking for bones that need help. Once they've completed the evaluation, have them announce their findings and see if they match up with yours. Once complete, switch roles, and repeat the exercise.

REGIONAL TREATMENT

While local BST techniques involve six stages of treatment for one or two bones, regional BST techniques apply the same six stages but to *groups* of bones. Each bone has a corresponding regional technique: a lumbar vertebra has the lumbar gather, a metacarpal bone has the hand and wrist gather, and so on. Local treatment generally precedes regional treatment but does not necessarily have to. Sometimes, I'll start with a regional technique and then hone in on one bone that is compacted, treat that bone locally, and then return to the regional technique to integrate the local work into the region. Regardless of the order, I suggest doing both in the same treatment. Below, I'll describe each regional technique and the six stages of treatment for each one. Some of the techniques are very straightforward, and others are a bit more involved. In either case, take your time here. As each technique unfolds, visualize and sense all the bones in the region coalescing to live and breathe as a single, fluidic entity.

Forefoot Gather

Bones involved

Phalanges
Metatarsals

Regional treatment

With the subject supine, grasp the forefoot (figure 17.562).

1. **Cocooning:** Cocoon the phalanges and metatarsals, imagining them as one viscoelastic structure.
2. **Compression:** Compress the bones together, staying within the fluidic cushion of the region.
3. **Dialogue:** Begin to identify and dialogue with the rhythms of primary respiration (CRI, mid-tide, and long tide) as they emerge from the forefoot. See if you can sense the inertial fulcrum around which some or all of these rhythms are organizing, and then bathe the levers of the region in the stillness of the fulcrum. Wait until the rhythms coalesce, breathing the phalanges and metatarsals with a new resultant oscillation.
4. **Augmentation:** Maintain your compressive dialogue but shift to a slightly more passive contact, allowing

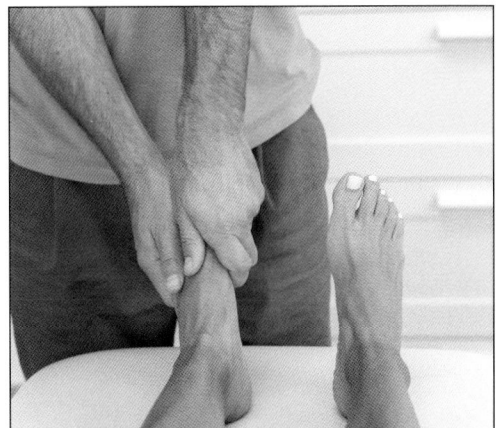

Figure 17.562. Hand position for the forefoot gather.

your fingers to inhale and exhale with the phalanges and metatarsals for a few more complete cycles of primary respiration. If the expression of the long tide is less clear, focus on the CRI and mid-tide.

5. **Spreading:** Without applying too much more force, just *imagine* spreading the phalanges and metatarsals—this will be all the force you need. Stay within the fluidic cushion and wait for the rhythms of primary respiration to reemerge for a few complete cycles. If the expression of the long tide is less clear, focus on the CRI and mid-tide.

6. **Integration:** Sense the primary respiration of the whole body acknowledge and accept the primary respiration within the phalanges and metatarsals. Let your regional work integrate into the whole.

Midfoot Gather

Bones involved

Cuneiforms
Navicular
Cuboid

Regional treatment

With the subject supine, grasp the midfoot (figure 17.563).

1. **Cocooning:** Cocoon the three cuneiforms, cuboid, and navicular, imagining them as one viscoelastic structure.

2. **Compression:** Compress the bones together, staying within the fluidic cushion of the region.

3. **Dialogue:** Begin to identify and dialogue with the rhythms of primary respiration (CRI, mid-tide, and long tide) as they emerge from the midfoot. See if you can sense the inertial fulcrum around which some or all of these rhythms are organizing, and then bathe the levers of

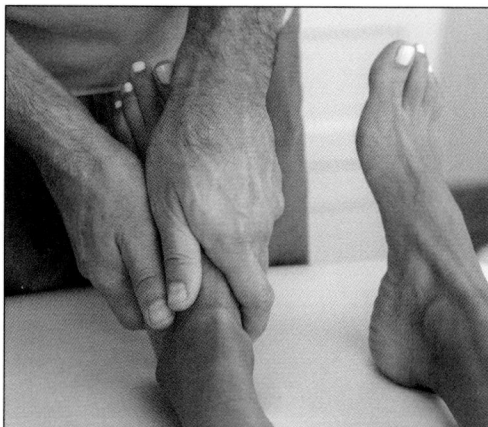

Figure 17.563. Hand position for the midfoot gather.

the region in the stillness of the fulcrum. Wait until the rhythms coalesce, breathing the three cuneiforms, cuboid, and navicular with a new resultant oscillation.

4. **Augmentation:** Maintain your compressive dialogue but shift to a slightly more passive contact, allowing your fingers to inhale and exhale with the three cuneiforms, cuboid, and navicular for a few more complete cycles of primary respiration. If the expression of the long tide is less clear, focus on the CRI and mid-tide.

5. **Spreading:** Without applying too much more force, just *imagine* spreading the three cuneiforms, cuboid, and navicular—this will be all the force you need. Spread the bones by moving your body back and separating your hands. Stay within the fluidic cushion, and wait for the rhythms of primary respiration to reemerge for a few complete cycles. If the expression of the long tide is less clear, focus on the CRI and mid-tide.

6. **Integration:** Sense the primary respiration of the whole body acknowledge and accept the primary respiration within the three cuneiforms, cuboid, and navicular. Let your regional work integrate into the whole.

Hindfoot Gather

Bones involved

Talus
Calcaneus

Regional treatment

With the subject supine, grasp the hindfoot (figure 17.564). The last two fingers of the hand on the talus can rest on the distal end of the tibia.

1. **Cocooning:** Cocoon the talus and calcaneus, imagining them as one viscoelastic structure.
2. **Compression:** Compress the bones together, staying within the fluidic cushion of the region.
3. **Dialogue:** Begin to identify and dialogue with the rhythms of primary respiration (CRI, mid-tide, and long tide) as they emerge from the hindfoot. See if you can sense the inertial fulcrum around which some or all of these rhythms are organizing, and then bathe the levers of the region in the stillness of the fulcrum. Wait until the rhythms coalesce, breathing the talus and calcaneus with a new resultant oscillation.

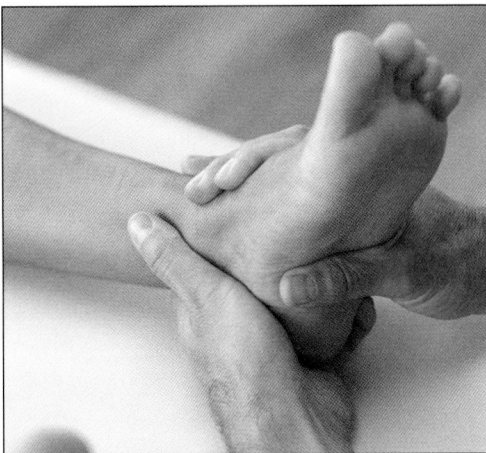

Figure 17.564. Hand position for the hindfoot gather.

4. **Augmentation:** Maintain your compressive dialogue but shift to a slightly more passive contact, allowing your fingers to inhale and exhale with the talus and calcaneus for a few more complete cycles of primary respiration. If the expression of the long tide is less clear, focus on the CRI and mid-tide.
5. **Spreading:** Without applying too much more force, just *imagine* spreading the talus and calcaneus—this will be all the force you need. Spread the region by moving your body backward and separating your hands, suctioning the bones apart. Stay within the fluidic cushion, and wait for the rhythms of primary respiration to reemerge for a few complete cycles. If the expression of the long tide is less clear, focus on the CRI and mid-tide.
6. **Integration:** Sense the primary respiration of the whole body acknowledge and accept the primary respiration within the talus and calcaneus. Let your regional work integrate into the whole.

Lower Extremity Gather

Bones involved

Tibia
Fibula
Femur
Ilium

Regional treatment

Even though this technique involves the three long bones of the lower extremity and the acetabulum, it can be done with contacts on only the tibia and fibula. With the subject supine, place one hand on the tibia and the other hand on the fibula (figure 17.565).

1. **Cocooning:** Cocoon the tibia and fibula and project your contact up through the femur and into the acetabulum, imagining all three long bones as one viscoelastic structure.

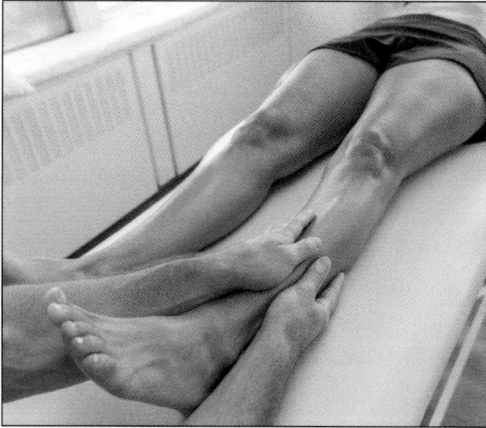

Figure 17.565. Hand positions for the lower extremity gather.

2. **Compression:** Compress the bones together and into the acetabulum, staying within the fluidic cushion of the region.
3. **Dialogue:** Identify and dialogue with the rhythms of primary respiration (CRI, mid-tide, and long tide) as they emerge from the lower extremity. See if you can sense the inertial fulcrum around which some or all of these rhythms are organizing, and then bathe the levers of the region in the stillness of the fulcrum. Wait until the rhythms coalesce, breathing the tibia, fibula, and femur with a new resultant oscillation.
4. **Augmentation:** Maintain your compressive dialogue but shift to a slightly more passive contact, allowing your fingers to inhale and exhale with the tibia, fibula, and femur for a few more complete cycles of primary respiration. If the expression of the long tide is less clear, focus on the CRI and mid-tide.
5. **Spreading:** Without applying too much more force, just *imagine* spreading the tibia, fibula, and femur—this will be all the force you need. Spread the region by moving your body backward and separating your hands, suctioning the tibia and fibula apart. Stay within the fluidic cushion and wait for the rhythms of primary respiration to reemerge for a few complete cycles.

If the expression of the long tide is less clear, focus on the CRI and mid-tide.
6. **Integration:** Sense the primary respiration of the whole body acknowledge and accept the primary respiration within the tibia, fibula, and femur. Let your regional work integrate into the whole.

Knee Gather

Bones involved

Tibia
Patella
Femur

Regional treatment

Place one hand on the patella and the other hand behind the knee within the popliteal fossa and with contact on both the tibia and femur (figure 17.566).

1. **Cocooning:** Cocoon the tibia, femur, and patella, imagining all three bones as one viscoelastic structure.
2. **Compression:** Compress the bones together, staying within the fluidic cushion of the region.
3. **Dialogue:** Identify and dialogue with the rhythms of primary respiration (CRI, mid-tide, and long tide) as they emerge from the knee. See if you can sense the inertial fulcrum around which some or all of these rhythms are organizing, and then bathe the levers of the region in the stillness of the fulcrum. Wait until the rhythms coalesce, breathing the tibia, femur, and patella with a new resultant oscillation.
4. **Augmentation:** Maintain your compressive dialogue but shift to a slightly more passive contact, allowing your fingers to inhale and exhale with the tibia, femur, and patella for a few more complete cycles of primary respiration. If the expression of the long tide is less clear, focus on the CRI and mid-tide.

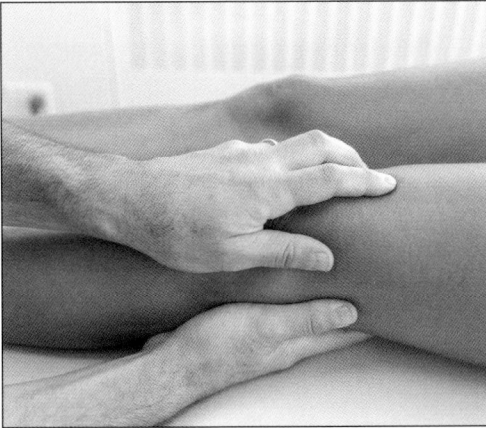

Figure 17.566. Hand positions for the knee gather.

5. **Spreading:** Without applying too much more force, just *imagine* spreading the tibia, femur, and patella—this will be all the force you need. Spread the region by spreading and separating your hands, suctioning the tibia from the femur with one hand and lifting the patella toward the ceiling with the other hand. Stay within the fluidic cushion and wait for the rhythms of primary respiration to reemerge for a few complete cycles. If the expression of the long tide is less clear, focus on the CRI and mid-tide.
6. **Integration:** Sense the primary respiration of the whole body acknowledge and accept the primary respiration within the tibia, femur, and patella. Let your regional work integrate into the whole.

Pelvic Gather

Is there such a thing as a perfect technique?[33] If there is the pelvic gather could be it.

Bones involved

Femurs
Innominates
Sacrum
L5

_____
[33] See chapter 21.

Regional treatment

Place the subject's legs on a pillow so the hips and knees are slightly flexed. Gently squeeze the upper legs of the subject with the forearms and curl the fingers of each hand into each sacroiliac joint (figures 17.567 and 17.568).

1. **Cocooning:** Cocoon the sacrum, innominates, femurs, and L5, imagining all the bones as one viscoelastic structure. Use your arms and wrists to support yourself.
2. **Compression:** Compress the bones together, staying within the fluidic cushion

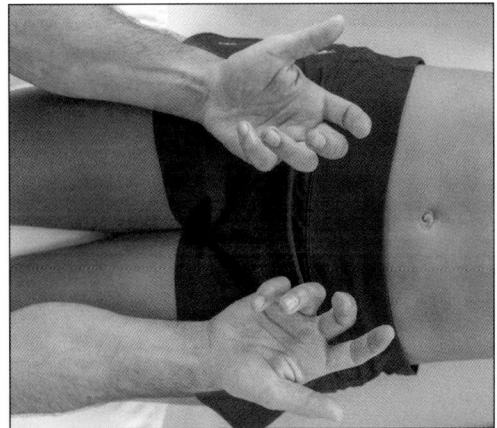

Figure 17.567. Hand positions for the pelvic gather.

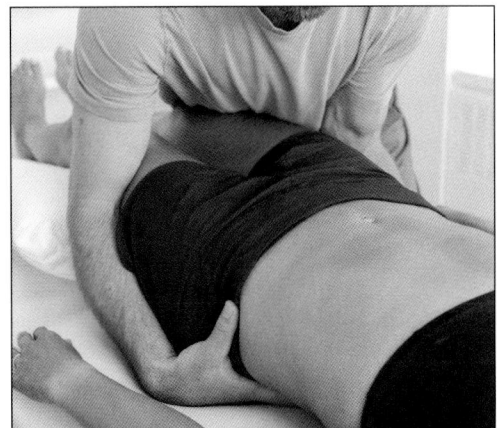

Figure 17.568. Hand and body position for the pelvic gather.

of the region. Simultaneously move the femurs into each acetabulum (honoring the obliquity of the femoral necks) and each ilium up toward the sacrum (honoring the obliquity of the sacroiliac joints), while bringing the sacrum into contact with L5.

3. **Dialogue:** Begin to identify and dialogue with the rhythms of primary respiration (CRI, mid-tide, and long tide) as they emerge from the pelvis and femurs. See if you can sense the inertial fulcrum around which some or all of these rhythms are organizing, and then bathe the levers of the region in the stillness of the fulcrum. Wait until the rhythms coalesce, breathing the sacrum, innominates, femurs, and L5 with a new resultant oscillation.

4. **Augmentation:** Maintain your compressive dialogue but shift to a slightly more passive contact, allowing your fingers to inhale and exhale with the sacrum, innominates, femurs, and L5 for a few more complete cycles of primary respiration. If the expression of the long tide is less clear, focus on the CRI and mid-tide.

5. **Spreading:** Without applying too much more force, just *imagine* spreading the sacrum, innominates, femurs, and L5—this will be all the force you need. Grasping the femurs with the elbows, move your body backward and separate your hands, spreading each innominate bone from the sacrum (honoring the obliquity of the sacroiliac joints) and the sacrum from L5. Stay within the fluidic cushion and wait for the rhythms of primary respiration to reemerge for a few complete cycles. If the expression of the long tide is less clear, focus on the CRI and mid-tide.

6. **Integration:** Sense the primary respiration of the whole body acknowledge and accept the primary respiration within the sacrum, innominates, femurs, and L5. Let your regional work integrate into the whole.

Lumbar Gather

The position for the lumbar gather is almost identical to that for the pelvic gather. With a little practice and some adjustments to hand and body positions, you can even combine both techniques into a hybrid *lumbopelvic* gather.

Bones involved

Sacrum
Lumbars

Regional treatment

Place the subject's legs on a pillow so the hips and knees are slightly flexed. Gently squeeze the innominates above the greater trochanter of the femur with the forearms. With the fingers of each hand, contact the laminae of L1 through L4 and/or L2 through L5, if necessary (having only four fingers has its limitations!) (figures 17.569 and 17.570).

1. **Cocooning:** Cocoon the lumbars, imagining all the bones as one viscoelastic

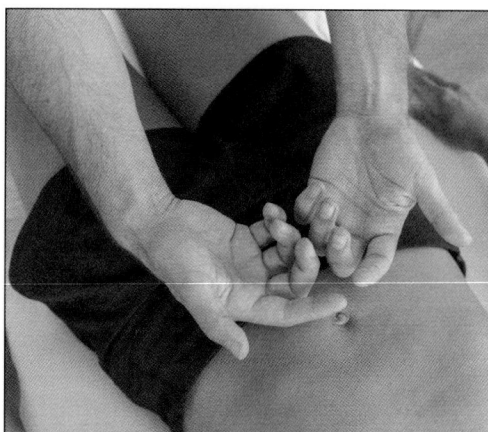

Figure 17.569. Hand positions for the lumbar gather.

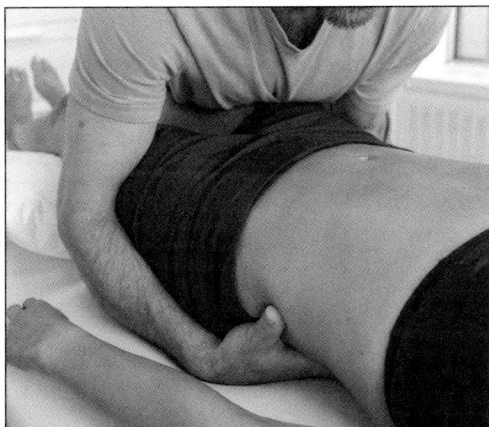

Figure 17.570. Hand and body position for the lumbar gather.

structure. Use your arms and wrists to support yourself.

2. **Compression:** Compress the bones together by moving the pelvis into the lumbar spine and by approximating (with your fingers) the vertebrae, staying within the fluidic cushion of the region.

3. **Dialogue:** Begin to identify and dialogue with the rhythms of primary respiration (CRI, mid-tide, and long tide) as they emerge from the lumbars. See if you can sense the inertial fulcrum around which some or all of these rhythms are organizing, and then bathe the levers of the region in the stillness of the fulcrum. Wait until the rhythms coalesce, breathing the lumbars with a new resultant oscillation.

4. **Augmentation:** Maintain your compressive dialogue but shift to a slightly more passive contact, allowing your fingers to inhale and exhale with the lumbars for a few more complete cycles of primary respiration. If the expression of the long tide is less clear, focus on the CRI and mid-tide.

5. **Spreading:** Without applying too much more force, just *imagine* spreading

the lumbars—this will be all the force you need. Grasping the pelvis with the elbows, move your body backward and separate your fingers, spreading each lumbar vertebra from its neighbors and all of them from T12. Stay within the fluidic cushion and wait for the rhythms of primary respiration to reemerge for a few complete cycles. If the expression of the long tide is less clear, focus on the CRI and mid-tide.

6. **Integration:** Sense the primary respiration of the whole body acknowledge and accept the primary respiration within the lumbars. Let your regional work integrate into the whole.

Thoracic Barrel

This is another wonderful technique. The thoracic barrel involves numerous structures: the ribs, spine, sternum, and clavicles.[34] The thoracic barrel technique can be administered with the subject in either supine or prone, depending on which bones need attention; the bones of the anterior thorax are treated in supine, and the bones of the posterior thorax are treated in prone.

Remember that when treating the thorax, both the rhythms of thoracic respiration *and* those of primary respiration will be present. Try to delineate the two and to remain focused on primary respiration only.

---

[34] The technique was partly inspired by the "cylinder" techniques developed by one of my former teachers, the late French osteopath Robert Rousse, who developed the concept of the *urgences fonctionnels* (functional emergencies) approach. Rousse visualized the thorax as two cohesive rolling cylinders, and my barrel approach is a nod in his direction: the rolling motion also reminds me of rolling barrels, hence the name.

Bones involved

Thoracic vertebrae
Ribs
Costal cartilages
Clavicle
Sternum

Regional treatment

Supine

With the subject supine, place one hand flat on the sternum and the other hand on the inferior (ribs 7 to 10; figure 17.571), middle (ribs 4 to 6; figure 17.572), or superior

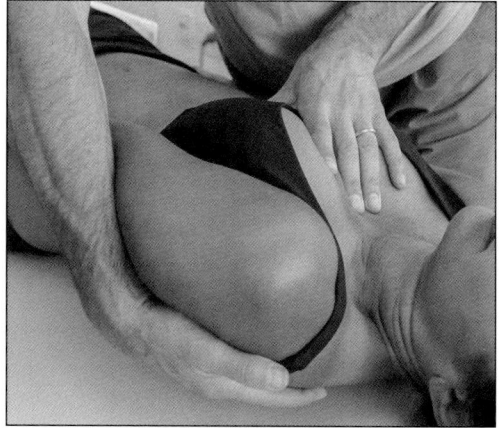

Figure 17.573. Hand positions for the superior supine thoracic barrel.

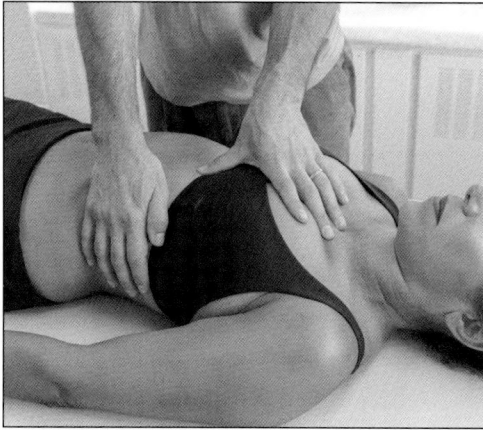

Figure 17.571. Hand positions for the inferior supine thoracic barrel.

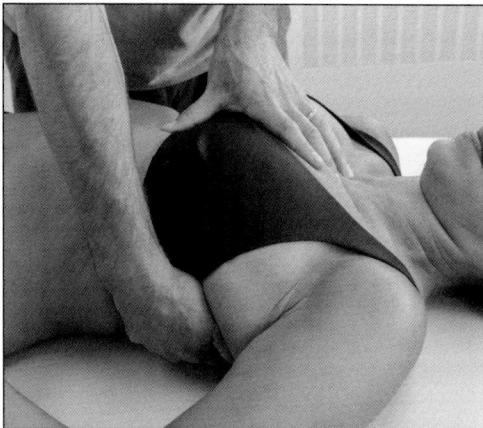

Figure 17.572. Hand positions for the middle supine thoracic barrel.

(ribs 1 to 3; figure 17.573), depending on which section is being treated. While stabilizing the sternum, compress it slightly by approximating the fingers, and roll the ribs toward it, initiating a compressive dialogue between the ribs, cartilages, and sternum itself.

1. **Cocooning:** Roll the thorax (like a barrel) over the sternal hand, cocooning the bones and cartilages of the anterior thorax, imagining all the bones as one viscoelastic structure.
2. **Compression:** Hold the position of the barrel, compressing the bones and cartilages of the anterior thorax together, staying within the fluidic cushion of the region.
3. **Dialogue:** Begin to identify and dialogue with the rhythms of primary respiration (CRI, mid-tide, and long tide) as they emerge from the bones and cartilages of the anterior thorax. You may notice a cephalic–caudal "gliding" or "dissociation" movement between the barrel and the sternum. This is good. See if you can sense the inertial fulcrum around which some or all of these rhythms are organizing, and then bathe the levers of the region in the stillness of the fulcrum. Wait until the

rhythms coalesce, breathing the bones and cartilages of the anterior thorax with a new resultant oscillation.

4. **Augmentation:** Maintain your compressive dialogue but shift to a slightly more passive contact, allowing your fingers to inhale and exhale with the bones and cartilages of the anterior thorax for a few more complete cycles of primary respiration. If the expression of the long tide is less clear, focus on the CRI and mid-tide.

Switch your hand positions so that the heels of both hands are in contact with the sternocostal joint line, with palms on the cartilages, and fingers extended onto the ribs (figure 17.574).

5. **Spreading:** Without applying too much more force, just *imagine* spreading the bones and cartilages of the anterior thorax—this will be all the force you need. Apply a spreading force into the cartilages and ribs along the axis of the ribs. Stay within the fluidic cushion and wait for the rhythms of primary respiration to reemerge for a few complete cycles. If the expression of the long tide is less clear, focus on the CRI and mid-tide.

6. **Integration:** Sense the primary respiration of the whole body acknowledge and accept the primary respiration within the bones and cartilages of the anterior thorax. Let your regional work integrate into the whole.

Prone

With the subject prone, place one hand flat on the opposite side of the inferior (T8 to T12; figure 17.575), middle (T4 to T7; figure 17.576), or superior (T1 to T3; figure 17.577) thoracic spinous processes, and the other hand on the inferior

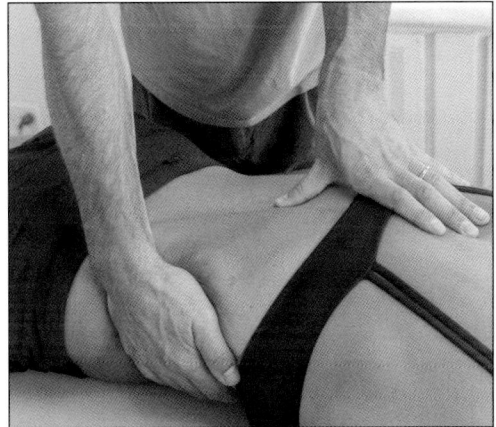

Figure 17.575. Hand positions for the inferior prone thoracic barrel.

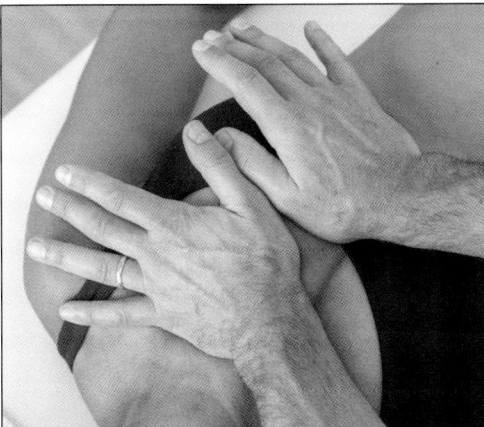

Figure 17.574. Hand positions for the spreading and integration stages of the supine thoracic barrel.

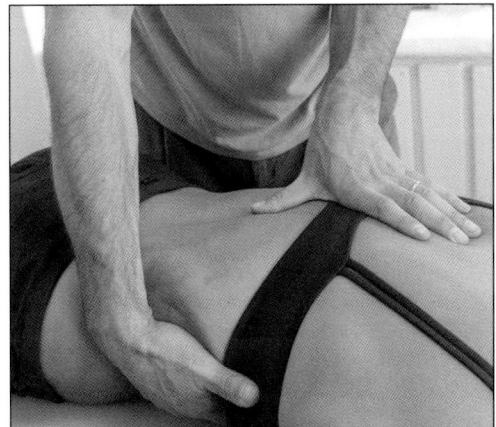

Figure 17.576. Hand positions for the middle prone thoracic barrel.

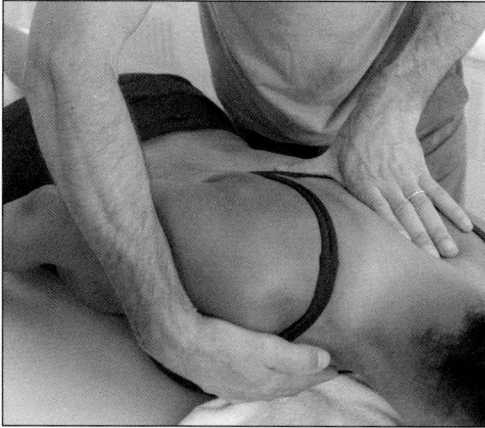

Figure 17.577. Hand positions for the superior prone thoracic barrel.

(ribs 8 to 12; figure 17.575), middle (ribs 4 to 7; figure 17.576), or superior (ribs 1 to 3; figure 17.577) anterior ribs and cartilages, depending on which section is being treated. While stabilizing the spine, compress the vertebrae slightly by approximating the fingers, and roll the thorax toward the other hand, initiating a compressive dialogue between the posterior ribs and the thoracic spine.

1. **Cocooning:** Roll the thorax (like a barrel) toward the vertebral hand, cocooning the posterior ribs and thoracic vertebrae, imagining all the bones as one viscoelastic structure.
2. **Compression:** Maintain the position of the barrel, compressing the posterior ribs and thoracic vertebrae together, staying within the fluidic cushion of the region.
3. **Dialogue:** Begin to identify and dialogue with the rhythms of primary respiration (CRI, mid-tide, and long tide) as they emerge from the posterior ribs and thoracic vertebrae. See if you can sense the inertial fulcrum around which some or all these rhythms are organizing, and then bathe the levers of the region in the stillness of the fulcrum. Wait until the

rhythms coalesce, breathing the posterior ribs and thoracic vertebrae with a new resultant oscillation.

4. **Augmentation:** Maintain your compressive dialogue but shift to a slightly more passive contact, allowing your fingers to inhale and exhale with the posterior ribs and thoracic vertebrae for a few more complete cycles of primary respiration. If the expression of the long tide is less clear, focus on the CRI and mid-tide.

Switch your hand positions so that the heels of both hands are in contact with the costotransverse joint line, with fingers extended onto and in line with the posterior ribs (figure 17.578).

5. **Spreading:** Without applying too much more force, just *imagine* spreading the posterior ribs away from the thoracic vertebrae—this will be all the force you need. Stay within the fluidic cushion and wait for the rhythms of primary respiration to reemerge for a few complete cycles. If the expression of the long tide is less clear, focus on the CRI and mid-tide.
6. **Integration:** Sense the primary respiration of the whole body acknowledge and

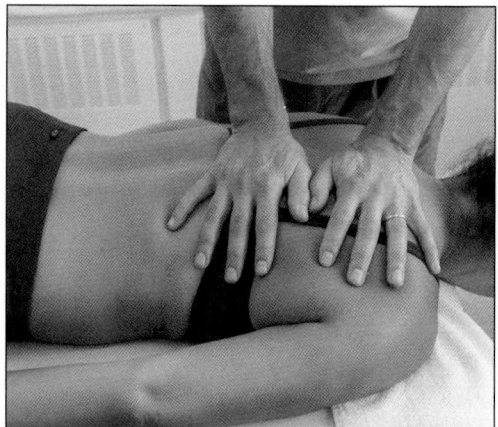

Figure 17.578. Hand positions for the spreading and integration stages of prone thoracic barrel.

accept the primary respiration within the posterior ribs and thoracic vertebrae. Let your regional work integrate into the whole.

Hand and Wrist Gather

Bones involved

Phalanges
Metacarpals
Carpals

Regional treatment

With the subject supine, grasp the hand and wrist (figure 17.579). The index fingers of each hand can rest on the distal ends of the ulna and radius.

1. **Cocooning:** Cocoon the phalanges, metacarpals, and carpals, imagining all the bones as one viscoelastic structure.
2. **Compression:** Compress the phalanges, metacarpals, and carpals together, staying within the fluidic cushion of the region.
3. **Dialogue:** Begin to identify and dialogue with the rhythms of primary respiration (CRI, mid-tide, and long tide) as they emerge from the phalanges, metacarpals, and carpals. See if you can sense the

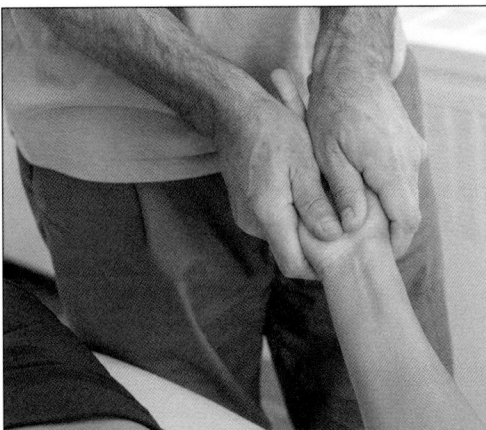

Figure 17.579. Hand position for the hand and wrist gather.

inertial fulcrum around which some or all of these rhythms are organizing, and then bathe the levers of the region in the stillness of the fulcrum. Wait until the rhythms coalesce, breathing the phalanges, metacarpals, and carpals with a new resultant oscillation.

4. **Augmentation:** Maintain your compressive dialogue but shift to a slightly more passive contact, allowing your fingers to inhale and exhale with the phalanges, metacarpals, and carpals for a few more complete cycles of primary respiration. If the expression of the long tide is less clear, focus on the CRI and mid-tide.
5. **Spreading:** Without applying too much more force, just *imagine* spreading the phalanges, metacarpals, and carpals— this will be all the force you need. Stay within the fluidic cushion and wait for the rhythms of primary respiration to reemerge for a few complete cycles. If the expression of the long tide is less clear, focus on the CRI and mid-tide.
6. **Integration:** Sense the primary respiration of the whole body acknowledge and accept the primary respiration within the phalanges, metacarpals, and carpals. Let your regional work integrate into the whole.

Upper Extremity Gather

Bones involved

Radius
Ulna
Humerus

Regional treatment

Even though this technique involves all three long bones of the upper extremity, it can be done with contacts on only the radius and ulna. With the subject supine, place one

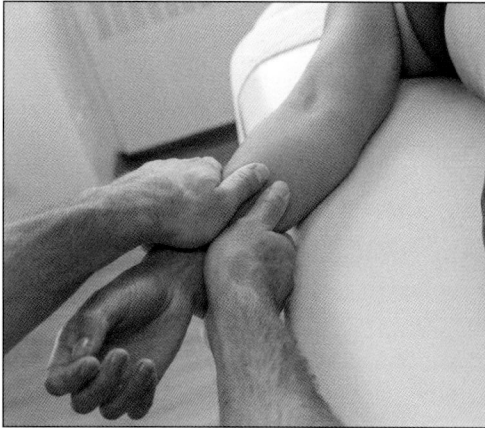

Figure 17.580. Hand positions for the upper extremity gather.

hand on the radius and the other on the ulna (figure 17.580).

1. **Cocooning:** Cocoon the radius and ulna, bringing them into contact with each other and with the humerus and glenoid fossa of the scapula. Imagine all the bones as one viscoelastic structure.
2. **Compression:** Compress the radius and ulna together, compressing them into the humerus, and compressing the humerus into the glenoid fossa. Stay within the fluidic cushion of the region.
3. **Dialogue:** Begin to identify and dialogue with the rhythms of primary respiration (CRI, mid-tide, and long tide) as they emerge from the radius, ulna, and humerus. See if you can sense the inertial fulcrum around which some or all of these rhythms are organizing, and then bathe the levers of the region in the stillness of the fulcrum. Wait until the rhythms coalesce, breathing the radius, ulna, and humerus with a new resultant oscillation.
4. **Augmentation:** Maintain your compressive dialogue but shift to a slightly more passive contact, allowing your fingers to inhale and exhale with the radius, ulna, and humerus for a few more complete cycles of primary respiration.

If the expression of the long tide is less clear, focus on the CRI and mid-tide.

5. **Spreading:** Without applying too much more force, just *imagine* spreading the radius, ulna, and humerus—this will be all the force you need. Stay within the fluidic cushion and wait for the rhythms of primary respiration to reemerge for a few complete cycles. If the expression of the long tide is less clear, focus on the CRI and mid-tide.
6. **Integration:** Sense the primary respiration of the whole body acknowledge and accept the primary respiration within the radius, ulna, and humerus. Let your regional work integrate into the whole.

Shoulder Gather

Bones involved

Humerus
Scapula
Clavicle

Regional treatment

With the subject supine, englobe the scapula, humerus, and clavicle (figure 17.581).

1. **Cocooning:** Cocoon the humerus, scapula, and clavicle, bringing them into

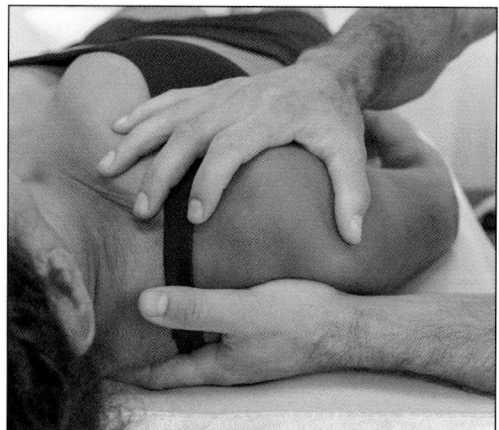

Figure 17.581. Hand positions for the shoulder gather.

contact with each other. Imagine all the bones as one viscoelastic structure.

2. **Compression:** Compress the humerus, scapula, and clavicle. Stay within the fluidic cushion of the region.

3. **Dialogue:** Begin to identify and dialogue with the rhythms of primary respiration (CRI, mid-tide, and long tide) as they emerge from the humerus, scapula, and clavicle. See if you can sense the inertial fulcrum around which some or all of these rhythms are organizing, and then bathe the levers of the region in the stillness of the fulcrum. Wait until the rhythms coalesce, breathing the humerus, scapula, and clavicle with a new resultant oscillation.

4. **Augmentation:** Maintain your compressive dialogue but shift to a slightly more passive contact, allowing your fingers to inhale and exhale with the humerus, scapula, and clavicle for a few more complete cycles of primary respiration. If the expression of the long tide is less clear, focus on the CRI and mid-tide.

5. **Spreading:** Without applying too much more force, just *imagine* spreading the humerus, scapula, and clavicle—this will be all the force you need. "Suction" the bones apart with your hands. Stay within the fluidic cushion and wait for the rhythms of primary respiration to reemerge for a few complete cycles. If the expression of the long tide is less clear, focus on the CRI and mid-tide.

6. **Integration:** Sense the primary respiration of the whole body acknowledge and accept the primary respiration within the humerus, scapula, and clavicle. Let your regional work integrate into the whole.

Cervical Gather

Bones involved

Cervical vertebrae

Regional treatment

With the subject supine, support the base of the cranium with the thenar eminences of both hands, and place the fingers of both hands on either side of the laminae of C7 through C4 (figures 17.582 and 17.583). Since we only have four fingers, repeat the treatment, if necessary, readjusting the fingers to contact C3 through C1.

1. **Cocooning:** Cocoon the cervicals, imagining all the bones as one viscoelastic structure.

2. **Compression:** Move your body forward and approximate the fingers

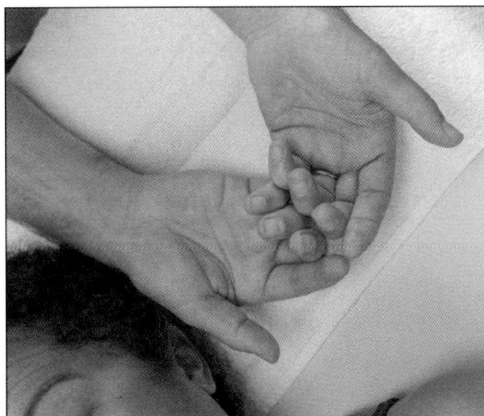

Figure 17.582. Hand and finger positions for the cervical gather.

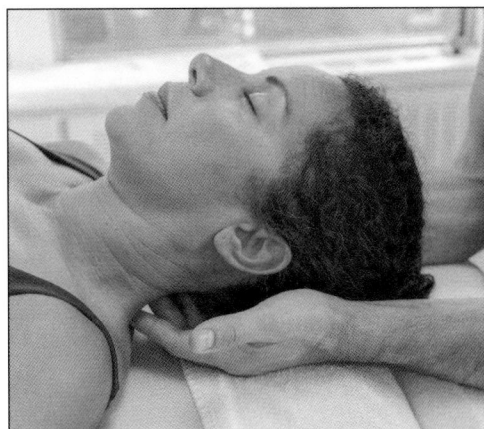

Figure 17.583. Hand positions for the cervical gather.

to approximate the cervicals. As always, stay within the fluidic cushion of the region.

3. **Dialogue:** Begin to identify and dialogue with the rhythms of primary respiration (CRI, mid-tide, and long tide) as they emerge from the cervicals. See if you can sense the inertial fulcrum around which some or all of these rhythms are organizing, and then bathe the levers of the region in the stillness of the fulcrum. Wait until the rhythms coalesce, breathing the cervicals with a new resultant oscillation.

4. **Augmentation:** Maintain your compressive dialogue but shift to a slightly more passive contact, allowing your fingers to inhale and exhale with the cervicals for a few more complete cycles. If the expression of the long tide is less clear, focus on the CRI and mid-tide.

5. **Spreading:** Without applying too much force, just imagine spreading the cervicals. Move your body backward, and using both hands equally, spread the fingers to apply a spreading force to the cervical spine and between each pair of vertebrae. Stay within the fluidic cushion. Wait for the rhythms of primary respiration to reemerge from the region for a few complete cycles before moving to the next stage. If the expression of the long tide is less clear, focus on the CRI and mid-tide.

6. **Integration:** Sense the primary respiration of the whole body acknowledge and accept the primary respiration within the cervicals. Let your regional work integrate into the whole.

Cranial Gather

Bones involved

Cranial bones

Regional treatment

The cranial gather has two hand positions: anteroposterior and lateral. Each time I treat the cranium, I like doing both. When performed together, the two positions allow us to address the region more completely. Furthermore, if any of the facial bones were a priority during local treatment, you could include a third, facial, hand position if necessary. Here, remember to stay tuned to the movements within the bones themselves, not the movements of the brain.

With the subject supine, begin with either the anteroposterior or lateral position, and then switch to the other one. The six stages of treatment are applied to each position.

Anteroposterior hold

For the anteroposterior hold (figure 17.584), cup the base of the occipital bone with one hand and place the other hand on the frontal, with the tips of the fingers lined up along the supraorbital ridges.

1. **Cocooning:** Cocoon the anteroposterior aspects of the cranium, imagining all the bones as one viscoelastic structure.

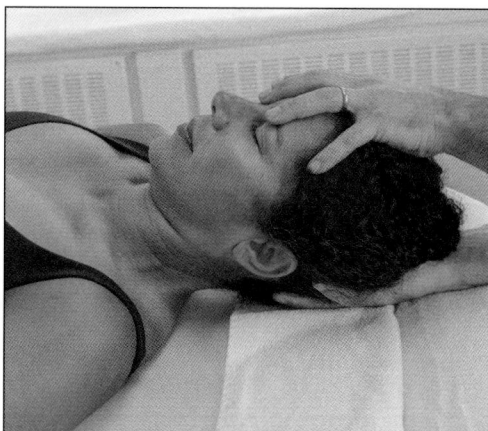

Figure 17.584. Hand positions for the anteroposterior cranial gather.

2. **Compression:** Approximate the fingers and hands with a subtle inferior momentum (toward the subject's feet), compressing the region anteroposteriorly. As always, stay within the fluidic cushion of the region.

3. **Dialogue:** Begin to identify and dialogue with the rhythms of primary respiration (CRI, mid-tide, and long tide) as they emerge from the region. See if you can sense the inertial fulcrum around which some or all of these rhythms are organizing, and then bathe the levers of the region in the stillness of the fulcrum. Wait until the rhythms coalesce, breathing the cranial bones with a new resultant oscillation.

4. **Augmentation:** Maintain your compressive dialogue but shift to a slightly more passive contact, allowing your fingers to inhale and exhale with the cranial bones for a few more complete cycles. If the expression of the long tide is less clear, focus on the CRI and mid-tide.

5. **Spreading:** Without applying too much force, just *imagine* spreading the region. Cup the occipital bone and frontal by gripping the bones with the tips of the fingers. Simultaneously separate both hands and move backward, securing the occipital bone to the table and lifting the frontal. As always, stay within the fluidic cushion of the region. Wait for the rhythms of primary respiration to reemerge from the region for a few complete cycles before moving to the next stage. If the expression of the long tide is less clear, focus on the CRI and mid-tide.

6. **Integration:** Now, sense the primary respiration of the whole body acknowledge and accept the primary respiration within the cranial bones. Let your regional work integrate into the whole.

Lateral hold

For the lateral hold (figure 17.585), place a hand on each side of the cranium, with index fingers on the lateral borders of the vertical rami of the mandible, middle fingers on the medial borders of the mastoid processes, and the last two fingers resting on the lateral base of the occipital bone.

1. **Cocooning:** Cocoon the lateral aspects of the cranium, including the mandible, imagining all the bones as one viscoelastic structure.

2. **Compression:** Approximate the fingers and hands, compressing the region laterally. As always, stay within the fluidic cushion of the region.

3. **Dialogue:** Begin to identify and dialogue with the rhythms of primary respiration (CRI, mid-tide, and long tide) as they emerge from the region. See if you can sense the inertial fulcrum around which some or all of these rhythms are organizing, and then bathe the levers of the region in the stillness of the fulcrum. Wait until the rhythms coalesce, breathing the cranial bones with a new resultant oscillation.

4. **Augmentation:** Maintain your compressive dialogue but shift to a

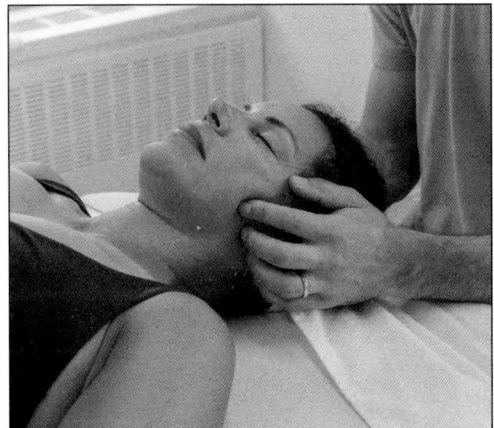

Figure 17.585. Hand positions for the lateral cranial gather.

slightly more passive contact, allowing your fingers to inhale and exhale with the cranial bones for a few more complete cycles. If the expression of the long tide is less clear, focus on the CRI and mid-tide.

5. **Spreading:** Without applying too much force, just *imagine* spreading the region. Separate the fingers, spreading the mandible from the glenoid fossa and mastoid process of the temporal, the frontal from the greater wing of the sphenoid, and with the palm, the parietals from the posterior squamous portion of the temporal. As always, stay within the fluidic cushion of the region. Wait for the rhythms of primary respiration to reemerge from the region for a few complete cycles before moving to the next stage. If the expression of the long tide is less clear, focus on the CRI and mid-tide.

6. **Integration:** Now, sense the primary respiration of the whole body acknowledge and accept the primary respiration within the cranial bones. Let your regional work integrate into the whole.

BALANCING THE THREE SPHERES

We've now learned how to find and treat osseofascial compactions throughout the body. We've discussed local BST treatment (compactions within a bone or between two bones) and regional BST treatment (broader lesional fields involving larger groups of bones). Now, we'll integrate the local and regional work into the whole through an approach I call "balancing the three spheres." This idea considers the pelvis, thorax, and cranium as three separate primary anatomical "spheres," hence the name.[35]

---

[35]I use the word *primary* for good reason. In the body (and based on my experience), we often (but not always) find important "primary" osteopathic lesions in these three areas.

Usually, I use this technique at the end of a session to integrate the work. Occasionally, I implement it at the beginning to get a general impression of how the body on my table is living. I also sometimes use it at the beginning *and* at the end of a treatment. The approach still incorporates potency, fulcrums, and levers, but veers somewhat from the habitual six stages of BST treatment. The three spheres is more about listening than about compressing or spreading, but it's not totally passive, either. Before we review the specs of the technique, understanding the concept of the functional midline will help situate it within our protocol.

The functional midline arises from a formative stillness within the human embryo, and remains present within us from conception until death. Druelle speaks of a series of visceral structures he calls the central chain. According to Druelle, the nature of and relationship between the structures of the central chain—organs arranged up and down the midline—hold special importance. The midline is a natural fulcrum, of sorts, and like other fulcrums, the functional midline is a column-shaped reservoir of health.

During the three spheres technique, we balance the levers around the midline, bathing them in its stillness. By doing this, we encourage the health from the midline to permeate the periphery, enhancing the biodynamic interchange. When Becker sensed an optimal interchange between stillness and body physiology, his treatment was complete.

This technique uses two hand positions that we've already seen—those used for the pelvic gather and for the lateral cranial gather—and one we haven't, a posterolateral thoracic hug-type hold.

When balancing the spheres, try to include more than just the bones and connective tissues in your awareness; hold the total physiology of each region—bone, fascia, viscera, blood, and nerve. Hug and help all of it at once.

Pelvis

You can treat any of the three spheres in any order you choose, but it's nice to address all three in the same session, if possible. Here, we'll start with the pelvis.

Use the hand positions for the pelvic gather (figure 17.586). Gently compress each innominate bone toward the sacrum, respecting the obliquity of the sacroiliac joints. Establish a dialogue between each side of the pelvis and the midline. Bathe the levers in the fulcrum, optimizing the interchange between the stillness and the total physiology of the pelvis. Evaluate the relationship between the midline and each side of the pelvis. If one side feels less harmonious, compress that side a little more toward the midline, staying within the fluidic cushion of the region. Wait until the interchange

between the stillness and each side of the sphere becomes softer and smoother.

By placing each side in dialogue with the midline, see if you can encourage a deeper symmetry. Spend as much time as you need balancing the pelvic sphere before moving to the thorax.

Thorax

Sit at the head of the subject and slide each hand underneath the rib cage onto the inferolateral ribs (figure 17.587). Engage each side of the thorax in light compression while simultaneously bringing the ribs in toward the spine and approximating the inferior ribs to the superior ribs.

As you did with the pelvis, evaluate the interchange between the stillness of the midline and each side of the thorax. Feel each thoracic barrel rolling internally and externally, being breathed by primary respiration. Are the movements symmetrical? If the relationship between the stillness of the midline and one or other side of the thorax seems strained, put that side into

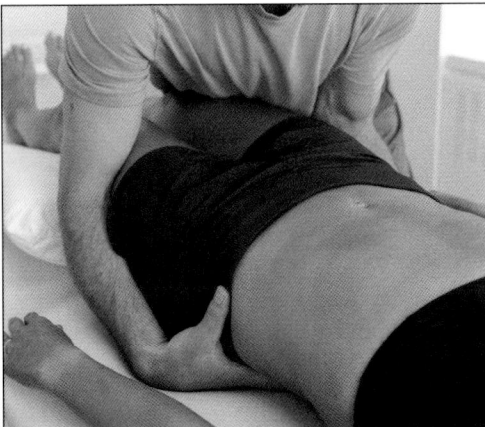

Figure 17.586. Hand and body position for the treating the pelvic sphere.

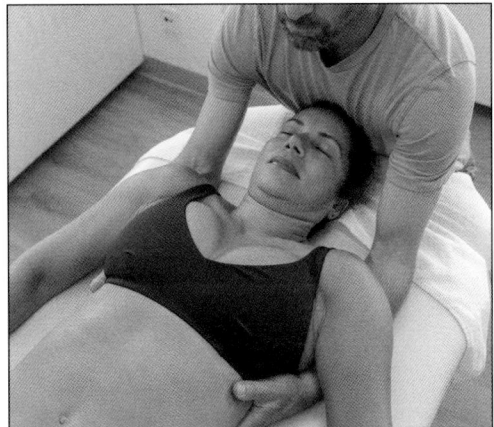

Figure 17.587. Hand and body position for the treating the thoracic sphere.

closer contact with the midline, bathing it in health. Spend as much time as you need until each side of the thorax finds its symmetry around the center.

Cranium

Still at the head of the subject, place your hands on each side of the cranium as you did for the lateral cranial gather technique (figure 17.588). Establish a dialogue between each side of the cranium and the midline. Bathe the levers in the fulcrum in the midline, optimizing the interchange between the stillness and the total physiology of the cranium.

Unlike during the local and regional BST work, become aware of all the movements in your hands; the primary respiration of the brain and of the cranial bones themselves. Evaluate the relationship between the midline and each side of the cranium. If one side feels less harmonious, compress that side a little more toward the midline, staying within the fluidic cushion of the region. Wait until the

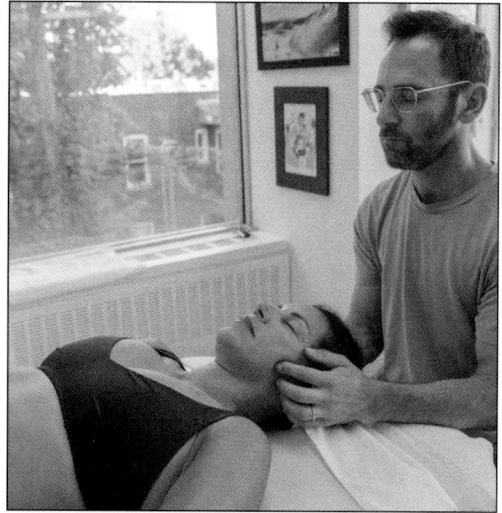

Figure 17.588. Hand and body position for the treating the cranial sphere.

interchange between the stillness and each side of the sphere becomes smoother.

By placing each side in dialogue with the midline, see if you can encourage a deeper symmetry, balancing the cranial sphere before removing the hands.

CHAPTER 18

Martha's Cranium

One day, while I was treating Martha's cranium, I drifted into a kind of dream, but it really wasn't a dream at all. A scene emerged of Martha and her father arguing. I opened my eyes and asked her about her family.

Martha described, in detail, a lifetime of hardship related to her dad. Until that day, I had never had such an experience with any other patient. Thousands of treatments later, I have not had another one since.

Sensing II

We are brilliant enough machines that we can sense when something is genuine.

—Michael Stipe

Gut, Brain, and Bone

The information in this book is based on testimony from my predecessors and on my own clinical experience. As I sit writing these words, there are a total of zero studies examining the impact of BST on the human body, so hopefully this text is an opening in this regard. Aside from compiling more evidence on how BST impacts the musculoskeletal system, another compelling avenue for further scientific exploration may be how BST affects the three-way body conversation known as the *gut-brain-bone axis*.

THE GUT-BRAIN-BONE AXIS AND BIODYNAMIC SKELETAL THERAPY

Together with the central nervous system and the gastrointestinal tract, bone tissue is an integral part of a crucial multidirectional exchange. With its gazillions of neurons, the central nervous system is the undisputed commander in chief of the body. The gastrointestinal tract, which contains the second-largest number of (intestinal) neurons, is the "brain" of the gut, and is commonly referred to as our second brain.

Our two brains get along swimmingly; the gut transmits information to the brain about X, and the brain responds by doing Z, or the brain tells the gut something important, and

the gut reacts in appropriate (and sometimes inconvenient) ways. The pathways of these conversations are traditionally referred to as the gut-brain axis. But this axis connects to a third pole: bone.

Besides providing structure to the body, bone possesses important organ-like endocrine functions, splicing the gut-brain conversation into a three-way visceral chat. In this triad, bone is more often the customer than it is the delivery person—it receives information more often than it transmits it—but it participates nonetheless. For example, the neurotransmitter serotonin is produced in the brain, but resides mainly in the gut. Serotonin impacts both the brain and the gut in diverse ways, affecting things like mood and memory and vomiting. Curiously, serotonin also exists in bone tissue, where it plays a role in bone development. But serotonin in bone is not produced by bone cells—it flows downstream from the brain to the gut and *then* to bone.

Bone has been shown to impact organs upstream from it, too. It was recently discovered that LCN2, a bone-derived mediator, can pass from bone into the blood and then into the hypothalamus, influencing the gut by suppressing appetite. Bone fracture can impact the central nervous system, exacerbating inflammation associated with traumatic brain injury, and so on. The conversations along the gut-brain-bone axis swing both ways—from brain to gut to bone and back again.

Therefore, bone supports and protects our two brains *and* is a "third" brain, of sorts. Could BST impact this exchange? To find out, let's look at the role of bone tissue within the gut-brain-bone axis from two specific angles: as offering physical support to the axis through key bony landmarks, and as an organ—a third brain—participating in a multipronged drive toward homeostasis.

BONE SUPPORTING THE GUT-BRAIN AXIS THROUGH BONY LANDMARKS

The gut-brain axis involves organs and nerves that are attached to, lean on, bump up against, or pass through bone tissue. The vagus and splanchnic nerves, for instance, are essential components of the gut-brain axis.

The vagus nerve exits the base of the skull through the jugular foramen, an aperture formed between the mastoid process of the temporal bone and the occipital bone. It then travels down through the thorax and abdomen, piercing the diaphragm on its way to numerous visceral targets. If either the mastoid process or occipital bone is compacted, the mobility of the bones and even the jugular foramen itself could be compromised. By treating these local compactions with BST, the vitality of the region can be restored, and the vagus nerve enabled to exit the skull undisturbed, free to wander about and spread its vagal charm.

The splanchnic nerves are paired autonomic nerves that supply the abdominal and pelvic viscera. They are composed of motor nerve fibers passing to and sensory nerve fibers originating from these organs, making the splanchnics an essential conduit within the gut-brain axis.

On each side of the body, there are thoracic, lumbar, and sacral splanchnic nerves. The thoracic branch splits to form the greater, lesser, and least branches, which, via the celiac and mesenteric ganglia, collectively innervate the organs of the gastrointestinal tract. But before synapsing with the ganglia, the branches emerge from the T5 to T12 spinal nerve roots, which themselves had to wiggle out from between vertebrae. As with the occipitomastoid suture, dysfunction within the T5 to T12 vertebrae could impact bone quality and function and, in turn, the trajectory and function of the nerve. This dysfunctional cascade could theoretically scramble the coherence of the gut-brain axis.

Key bony landmarks are associated not only with nerves, but with the gastrointestinal viscera themselves. Obvious examples are the skull, which houses the brain; the vertebrae, which guide and protect the spinal cord and the spinal nerves; the pelvic bowl, which helps support the sigmoid colon and cecum; and the sacrum and coccyx, which guide and protect the lower digestive tract. Two other specific examples are L2 and the right sacroiliac joint, both of which are in close contact with the attachments of the root of the mesentery. Compactions within any of these landmarks could theoretically impact the viscera with which they mingle, potentially compromising important brain-gut cross-talk.

BONE IMPACTING THE BRAIN THROUGH AN AFFERENT LOOP

The second way bone can impact the gut-brain-bone axis is via bones' afferent communication with the central nervous system. The efferent stream of communication between the brain and bone tissue is well known; anxiety, depression, and Alzheimer's disease can all lead to skeletal change. The flow of information in the opposite direction remains less investigated, but evidence is beginning to emerge in this regard. While the former is fascinating, it is the latter that interests us most.

Through its impact on compacted bone tissue, could BST indirectly affect the brain? And if so, could our work with bones affect the incidence or severity of common neurological or psychological conditions like anxiety, depression, and Alzheimer's disease?

There is emerging evidence that skeletal injury or disease can exacerbate certain neuropathologies. Some patients with cleidocranial dysplasia (a birth defect that mostly affects bones and teeth) additionally suffer from delayed brain development. Coffin-Lowry syndrome, a genetic skeletal disorder, is often associated with brain malfunction. In rare instances, bone trauma due to injury or routine surgery leads to complex regional pain syndrome (CRPS), which affects the nervous system and bone simultaneously. It has also been demonstrated that, compared to women with limited hip bone loss, women with high levels of bone loss have an increased probability of developing dementia.

Bone talks to the brain in two ways: indirectly, through the peripheral nervous system, and directly, by releasing molecules able to cross the blood-brain barrier, that handy semipermeable border of endothelial cells that regulates the passage of chemicals between blood and cerebrospinal fluid. Once stimulated, bone cells secrete chemical mediators called osteokines, which can cross the blood-brain barrier and elicit a response in the brain. Osteocalcin is one such mediator, and once in the brain, it has been shown to influence the production of several neurotransmitters, which in turn promote spatial learning and memory and prevent anxiety and depression. Physical exercise has been shown to stimulate the release of osteocalcin, and it has been hypothesized that some of the beneficial effects of exercise on neurological conditions are associated with this bone-to-brain process. Could the release and transfer of osteocalcin from bone be why aerobic and resistance exercise has been shown to prevent certain neurological disorders?

Besides osteocalcin, other molecules reside and function in both the brain and bone, including irisin, receptor activator of NF-κB ligand, bone morphogenic protein, and brain-derived neurotrophic factor, to name a few. Irisin, for instance, has neuroprotective effects *and* enhances bone development. Clearly, bone and brain are linked in more ways than one.

Research has shown that osteopathic manipulative therapy, including spinal mobilizations and cranial work, reduces symptoms of depression, anxiety, sleep disturbances, headaches, and migraines. Could BST, applied either alone or in tandem with other modalities, do the same? Could BST even amplify the impact of these modalities? If so, how? Future research could shed light on these questions.

The Perfect Technique

The only perfect technique
is one which transmits the

CELEBRATION

of our mutual imperfection.

The Breath of Life

Go outside and listen as far away
as you can, then listen even further.
A beautiful surprise awaits.

—James Jealous

CHAPTER 23

Listen

Epilogue: Let Us Compare Meteorologies

Brian Arthur, a Belfast-born economist, reminds us that economics, as it's usually practiced, operates in a deductive mode: a problem is translated into mathematics and then solved through analytical reasoning. In the late 1980s, Arthur met John Holland, a pioneer in the field of genetic engineering, who introduced Arthur to a new way of seeing economics, called induction. Induction is a way of reasoning where pieces of information are used to form a model. It's when one starts with observations, and then develops a rule based on those observations. For instance, induction allows one to infer that a cat belongs to the tail vanishing in a flash around a corner. The cat itself was never seen, but the sight of its tail was enough to induce that a cat was attached to it.

Compellingly, the image that often crystallizes from induction—from the fusing together of fragments of knowledge—is often more vivid and more realistic than the one that simply appears when we have all the information at hand. Some of the most moving works of art consist only of sparse lines of poetry or minimal streams of sounds or suggestive bits of line or color on canvas. These fragments of information force us to complete the artist's message with our minds, leading to an image often more profound and extraordinary. Reading the book before seeing the movie *based* on the book is important, since reading provides a special opportunity to fill in the missing details of the unfolding story. "Filling in the blanks" and "reading between the lines" in these ways are both examples of using induction to better understand and even transcend the bits and pieces of data we actually see or hear. Thanks to our remarkable cognitive abilities, the image generated of the cat from the mere sight of its tail may turn out to be even more "catlike" than the image of the cat itself, and if read prior to viewing, the book often ends up making the story (and movie) better.

According to Arthur, problems in economics are often missing crucial bits of information or clearly repeating patterns, so as opposed to deductive reasoning, one often has to use inductive reasoning to infer solutions. With his new insight, Arthur realized that economics worked less like math and more like the weather: ever evolving and changing and often hard to predict. Weather is a component of the biosphere, and we use induction—through the science of meteorology—to predict its patterns. In the body, potency is a component of our internal biosphere, and like the weather, its patterns are difficult to predict. Is there a "meteorology" we can use to help us better understand, predict, and explain potency, biodynamic manual therapy, and BST?

In his 2007 essay "The Numbers of Our Nature: Is There a Math of Style?," Daniel Rockmore reports that in the late nineteenth century Wincenty Lutoslawski developed stylometry, a method for finding mathematical patterns in works of literature. By analyzing the usage of letters, words, and sentences, Lutoslawski developed the science of stylometry to better understand an otherwise nonscientific phenomenon.

Fast-forward to the early 2000s, when computer scientist Bill Manaris at the College of Charleston did the same for music. Manaris tabulated note usage over a range of musical compositions, and used his analysis to extract statistical features from musical scores. His work allowed for the scientific classification of music—another nonscientific phenomenon—from classical to jazz to rock.

By analyzing fragmented pieces of information—letters, words, and musical notes—Lutoslawski and Manaris used induction to infer mathematical patterns where they didn't exist before, and then used these patterns to better understand art. Perhaps we can do the same for BST.

To do so, we must first compile similar fragments of information, and then use induction to identify emerging patterns from the data. Perhaps the best way to accomplish this is not by performing isolated experiments with a few subjects at a time, but rather by sharing a large number of anecdotal reports.

Lessons learned from one case study can be profound; lessons learned from one thousand case studies even more so. I'm sure Bill Manaris would agree that, compared to being played alone, musical notes sound differently when arranged into a melody. Likewise, when compiled, our $n = 1$ case studies become much more than the sum of their parts.

With this goal in mind, please find, follow, and join our BST social media pages and groups, and begin sharing *your* BST stories today. The form of the report is unimportant. Describe what you feel, what you do, and your results. Talk about whether or not your client or patient returned feeling better, worse, or the same. Include details about texture and rhythm. Tell us how you incorporated BST into your own practice and how it complemented other forms of manual therapy, and so on. Ask questions, share answers, and be as specific and detailed as you can.

Together, we can help the science—the meteorology—of BST emerge to help us better understand the awesome potential of our work.

Adrian Burhop, my closest friend since I was 13 years old, always encouraged me to write. As he was a talented scribe himself, I always took this as high praise. While I was putting this book together, on Wednesday, December 6, 2023, Adrian died after falling through the ice while cross-country skiing on a frozen lake in Morin Heights, Quebec. He was 48 years old.

Sometime later, a group of us hiked Adrian's ashes up a mountain in Vermont. Following months of disbelief, letting the bone fragments of my best friend sift through my fingers like sand made Adrian's death feel real. After each saying a few words, we took turns scattering a cup of Adrian's ashes into the air. Once aloft, the smaller particles of bone dust twisted upward before vaporizing into silk-blue prism. With gravity, the larger pieces of bone fell to the ground. Enlivened by the seasons to come, these larger bone shards will dissolve into dirt, their calcium and phosphorus nourishing the lichen and mosses of those high alpine meadows for generations. In this way, the bones of this creative, passionate, caring, hilarious, talented, and beloved man—formed by the forces acting upon them during Adrian's life and now unwound, reorganized, and redistributed by the forces acting upon them after his death—will remain very much alive. And since our bones reflect who we are, custom-tailored throughout our lives via their remodeling and renewal, a part of Adrian will also live on up there. That thought brings me comfort.

Acknowledgments

I am grateful to so many people. Thanks to Jon Hutchings from Lotus Books for seeing the potential in a little blue book with a bone on the cover and helping me turn it into this. Jon, your trust and guidance over the last two years have been invaluable. Thank you, Jason Muzinic and the team at Human Kinetics for believing in BST (and in me), and for bringing biodynamics to the big stage! Thank you to my editor, Maia Vaswani, for your precision and professionalism.

To Amanda Williams, thanks for your expertise and artistry in illustrating the book. Thank you to my photographer, Emily Gan, for those grueling (and fun) photo shoots with our (very patient) models Byron and Alissa. Emily, your skill as a photographer shines through in every photograph, and will hopefully make learning BST even more enjoyable. To my dear friend and running buddy (and the most talented writer this side of the Mississippi), Eleni Schirmer, who read a few sections of the book and provided me with advice on how to make them (much) better.

Anthony "Tones" Wexler (who I have known for over 30 years), thank you for your friendship, your sense of humor, your support, and your lifelong appreciation for the written word.

To the legendary Tom Myers, for reading an early draft of this manuscript and providing your honest review. Tom, it goes without saying but I'll say it anyway—your contributions to the field of manual therapy and anatomy are without compare, and I am honored that you took the time for us.

Thank you to another legend, Sharon Wheeler. Sharon, I enjoyed our chat about BoneWork and BST. Hopefully, we'll eventually cross paths and compare notes.

Thank you to my miraculous wife, Tasha, and my two incredible kids, Frida and Sarah, for all of your love and support over the last few years while I toiled away at this project. I love you guys and will forever.

To my late friend, Adrian Burhop, who passed away while I was writing this book. Adrian, thanks for always inspiring me to create.

Finally, to all of my teachers, colleagues, and patients—thank you for helping me learn.

Glossary

Biodynamics describes the nature of the forces at work that organize our mind-body system from embryological development throughout life.

Biodynamic skeletal therapy (BST) is a manual therapy approach developed by the author, which combines craniosacral biodynamics and structural manual therapy into the same maneuvers. It involves a local dialogue with the fluid tissue matrix to help the body reorganize the bone tissue from within, and then makes those same bones move better within their environment.

Biomechanical fulcrum-lever systems involve mobility of levers such as bones upon a fulcrum such as a joint.

Biotensegrity is tensegrity in biological systems.

Birdcaging is the separation of individual substrands of pure collagen under compression.

Compression is what happens when forces push an object inward on itself.

Cranial rhythmic impulse is the local movement within the craniosacral mechanism that is reflected through the body via the interconnectedness of the dural-fascial and musculoskeletal systems as rotations and other movements within individual bones, and can be perceived anywhere in the body as a wavelike impulse of approximately 12 cycles per minute.

Cushion test is a way to orient to the right amount of compressive and tensile force to use within any given bone.

Elasticity describes how materials can return undamaged to their original shape after being stretched or compressed.

External fulcrum-lever system is a point of dynamic stability offered by the therapist from outside the body, and upon which an inertial fulcrum-lever system can balance.

Fibrosis is a palpable thickening of fascial tissue.

Floating bone principle describes Levin's observations regarding the counterintuitive separation of bones under compression.

Fulcrum describes the point on which a lever rests or is supported and about which it pivots.

Fulcrum-lever system is a system that consists of a fulcrum and levers.

Gut-brain-bone axis is a three-way body conversation between the gastrointestinal tract, the central nervous system, and bone tissue.

Heterarchy is where each component, regardless of size or scale, carries equal importance within a network.

Holistic shift is a term coined by Rollin Becker and describes what happens when the practitioner's awareness shifts from the variable waveforms of the cranial rhythmic impulse to the deeper rhythms of the primary respiratory mechanism. From a biodynamic craniosacral perspective, it is once the holistic shift occurs that true healing can begin.

Homeostasis refers to an innate drive toward a narrow range of balance, despite changing circumstances in the external environment.

Induction is a way of reasoning where pieces of information are used to form a model.

Inertial fulcrum-lever system is a point of unresolved conditional forces that cannot shift as easily with the respiratory cycles of primary respiration and contains within it the unresolved conditional forces as well as the organizational and protective forces of potency.

Interstitium is a body-wide network of fluid-filled interstitial spaces.

Intraosseous dysfunction or *intraosseous compaction* or *osseofascial compaction* is zones within bones that have lost their elasticity and vitality.

Long tide describes the intrinsic health of the human system and manifests as a stable cycle of 50-second inhalation and 50-second exhalation phases.

Mechanotransduction is a process where cells sense mechanical stimuli and then translate the information into signals, which can elicit a response.

Mid-tide is a term coined by Sills that reflects an interplay and interchange among potency, fluids, and tissues. It can be felt as a welling-up-and-receding rhythm of one to three cycles per minute within all tissues of the body.

Mobility is the ability to move freely or be easily moved.

Modularity accounts for how each part or group of parts integrates into a tensegrity structure.

Motility means to possess spontaneous movement.

Natural fulcrum-lever system describes a point of balance within the body that moves freely with the inhalation and exhalation phases of primary respiration and can automatically shift to compensate for unresolved conditions in the body.

Neutral is a term coined by Jealous to describe when the central nervous system, cerebrospinal fluid, all other fluids and tissues merge into the fluid body.

Nonlinear dynamics is a way to understand how a large number of different parts organize themselves into a coherent system with properties that cannot be understood by studying each part in isolation.

Ordering field or matrix is a general term that describes a quantum-level energy field established at conception, within which the embryo forms and develops.

Osseofascial compaction see *Intraosseous dysfunction.*

Osseofascial continuum is the living ecosystem of collagen-rich connective tissue, including bone and fascia.

Piezoelectricity is the inherent ability of materials to generate electric fields in response to external strain.

Plasticity is the nonreversible deformation of a material.

Potency is the word Sutherland used to describe the intelligence found in our fluids. It is through the fluids that the action of potency is transmitted to the tissues, creating tissue motility.

Primary respiration is the palpable expression of fluid and tissue motility, the embodied manifestation of a potent drive toward homeostasis and health.

Primary respiratory mechanism has five elements: fluctuation of the cerebrospinal fluid, mobility of the intracranial and intraspinal membranes and the function of the reciprocal tension membrane, inherent mobility of the central nervous system, articular mobility of the cranial bones, and the involuntary mobility of the sacrum between the iliac bones. The five elements of the primary respiratory mechanism work together synchronistically, flexing and extending as a cohesive mechanism in a respiratory-type rhythm.

Sharpey's fibers are expansions of the periosteum that penetrate the bone matrix, connecting the periosteum to the endosteum.

Somatic dysfunction is the altered function of the somatic system.

Strain is a term used to describe deformation, or how materials change their shape when they are under stress.

Stress is a physical quantity that describes forces present during deformation.

Stylometry is a method for finding mathematical patterns in works of literature.

Tensegrity describes how compression struts and tension cables collectively maintain the coherence of a structure.

Tension is a pulling force that is transmitted in the opposite direction of compression.

Three bodies is a concept that describes the physical, fluid, and tidal bodies. The physical body is suspended in the fluid body, and is the densest of all three. The fluid body is suspended in the tidal body, and includes all fluids. The tidal body refers to the wider tidal presence of the primary respiratory mechanism, and it can be sensed as a steady suspensory force that supports both the physical and fluid bodies.

Touch-testing is the evaluation method used within the biodynamic skeletal therapy approach, which involves briefly contacting a structure to determine its mobility and micromotility.

Twisted rope theory helps explain how twisted substrands of collagen unwind during compression.

Viscoelasticity is a property of materials that possess both viscosity and elasticity.

Viscosity is the thickness of a liquid.

Wolff's law says that a bone will adapt to the loads placed upon it; an increase in load leads to the strengthening of bone, while a decrease in load will cause bone to weaken.

References

Aaron, Jean E. 2012. "Periosteal Sharpey's Fibers: A Novel Bone Matrix Regulatory System?" *Frontiers in Endocrinology* 3 (98): https://doi.org/10.3389/fendo.2012.00098.

Armstrong, C. 2021. "Unity, Continuity, Structure, and Function: The Ongoing Search for a Deeper Understanding of the Many Roles Attributed to Fascia in the Living Human Body—An Osteopathic Perspective." *OBM Integrative and Complementary Medicine* 6 (3): 26. https://doi.org/10.21926/obm.icm.2103026.

Becker, Rollin E. 2023. *Stillness of Life*. Edited by Rachel E. Brooks. Stillness Press.

Bellow, Saul. 1976. *Humboldt's Gift*. Penguin Books.

Benias, Petros C., Rebecca G. Wells, Bridget Sackey-Aboagye, Heather Klavan, Jason Reidy, Darren Buonocore, Markus Miranda, Susan Kornacki, Michael Wayne, David L. Carr-Locke, and Neil D. Theise. 2018. "Structure and Distribution of an Unrecognized Interstitium in Human Tissues." *Scientific Reports* 8 (1): 4947. https://doi.org/10.1038/s41598-018-23062-6.

Bicalho, E. 2020. "The Intraosseous Dysfunction in the Osteopathic Perspective: Mechanisms Implicating the Bone Tissue." *Cureus* 12 (1): e6760. https://doi.org/10.7759/cureus.6760.

Blechschmidt, Erich, and Erich Gasser. 2012. *Biokinetics and Biodynamics of Human Differentiation*. North Atlantic Books.

Bordoni, Bruno, Andrea R. Escher, Federico Tobbi, Luca Pianese, Alessio Ciardo, Jorge Yamahata, Stefano Hernandez, and Oscar Sanchez. 2022. "Fascial Nomenclature: Update 2022." *Cureus* 14 (6): e25904. https://doi.org/10.7759/cureus.25904.

Bordoni, Bruno, Andrea R. Escher, Federico Tobbi, Andrea Pranzitelli, and Luca Pianese. 2021. "Fascial Nomenclature: Update 2021, Part 1." *Cureus* 13 (2): e13339. https://doi.org/10.7759/cureus.13339.

Bordoni, Bruno, Stevan Walkowski, Bruno Ducoux, and Filippo Tobbi. 2020a. "The Cranial Bowl in the New Millennium and Sutherland's Legacy for Osteopathic Medicine: Part 1." *Cureus* 12 (9): e10410. https://doi.org/10.7759/cureus.10410.

———. 2020b. "The Cranial Bowl in the New Millennium and Sutherland's Legacy for Osteopathic Medicine: Part 2." *Cureus* 12 (9): e10435. https://doi.org/10.7759/cureus.10435.

Bose, Sayan, Shuang Li, Elisa Mele, and Vadim V. Silberschmidt. 2022. "Exploring the Mechanical Properties and Performance of Type-I Collagen at Various Length Scales: A Progress Report." *Materials* 15 (8): 2753. https://doi.org/10.3390/ma15082753.

Bozec, Laurent, Greta van der Heijden, and Michael Horton. 2007. "Collagen Fibrils: Nanoscale Ropes." *Biophysical Journal* 92 (1): 70–75. https://doi.org/10.1529/biophysj.106.085704.

Brooks, Rodney. 2022. "The Chain Reaction That Propels Civilization: What Do Living Cells, Britain's Canals, and Deep Learning Have in Common?" *IEEE Spectrum*, April 19, 2022. https://spectrum.ieee.org/why-autocatalysis-matters.

Canarelli, Anne. 2016. *Osteopaths: The Philosophy, the Spirit, and the Art of Osteopathy*. Anima Mundi Editions.

Chaitow, Leon. 2014. "Somatic Dysfunction and Fascia's Gliding-Potential." *Journal of Bodywork and Movement Therapies* 18 (1): 1–3. https://doi.org/10.1016/j.jbmt.2013.11.019.

Currey, John D. 2008. *Bones: Structure and Mechanics*. Princeton University Press.

Cyron, Christopher J., and Jay D. Humphrey. 2017. "Growth and Remodeling of Load-Bearing Biological Soft Tissues." *Meccanica* 52 (3): 645–64. https://doi.org/10.1007/s11012-016-0472-5.

Dietrich, Michael R. 2015. "Explaining the Pulse of Protoplasm: The Search for Molecular Mechanism of Protoplasmic Streaming." *Journal of Integrative Plant Biology* 57 (1): 14–22. https://doi.org/10.1111/jipb.12317.

Granke, Mathilde, Mark D. Does, and Jeffry S. Nyman. 2015. "The Role of Water Compartments in the Material Properties of Cortical Bone." *Calcified Tissue International* 97 (3): 292–307. https://doi.org/10.1007/s00223-015-9977-5.

Gray, Henry. 2010. *Gray's Anatomy*. 2nd ed. Arcturus Publishing.

Harry Potter and the Sorcerer's Stone. 2001. Directed by Chris Columbus.

Hart, Nicolas H., Sophia Nimphius, Timo Rantalainen, Alex Ireland, Aris Siafarikas, and Robert U. Newton. 2017. "Mechanical Basis of Bone Strength: Influence of Bone Material, Bone Structure and Muscle Action." *Journal of Musculoskeletal & Neuronal Interactions* 17 (3): 114–39. https://doi.org/10.5281/zenodo.835582.

Jealous, James. 2015. *An Osteopathic Odyssey*. Edited by Jennifer Weiss. Tame Prepress.

Lesondak, David. 2022. *Fascia: What It Is, and Why It Matters*. 2nd ed. Handspring Publishing.

Liem, Torsten. 2016. "A.T. Still's Osteopathic Lesion Theory and Evidence-Based Models Supporting the Emerged Concept of Somatic Dysfunction." *Journal of the American Osteopathic Association* 116 (10): 654–61. https://doi.org/10.7556/jaoa.2016.129.

McPartland, John M., and Erik Skinner. 2005. "The Biodynamic Model of Osteopathy in the Cranial Field." *Explore* 1 (1): 21–32. https://doi.org/10.1016/j.explore.2004.10.005.

Morgan, Elise F., Gopinath U. Unnikrisnan, and Amr I. Hussein. 2018. "Bone Mechanical Properties in Healthy and Diseased States." *Annual Review of Biomedical Engineering*

20: 119–43. https://doi.org/10.1146/annurev-bioeng-062117-121139.

Peacock, Christopher, Edward Lee, Thomas Beral, Radoslaw Cisek, Daniel Tokarz, and Laurent Kreplak. 2020. "Buckling and Torsional Instabilities of a Nanoscale Biological Rope Bound to an Elastic Substrate." *ACS Nano* 14 (10): 12877–84. https://doi.org/10.1021/acsnano.0c03695.

Pearson, O. M., and D. E. Lieberman. 2004. "The Aging of Wolff's 'Law': Ontogeny and Responses to Mechanical Loading in Cortical Bone." *American Journal of Physical Anthropology* Suppl. 39: 63–99. https://doi.org/10.1002/ajpa.20155.

Rieu, Sophie. 2022. "Potency: The Winged Messenger." *Fulcrum*, no. 85. https://www.craniosacral.co.uk/blog/potency-the-winged-messenger.

Rockmore, Daniel. 2007. "The Numbers of Our Nature: Is There a Math of Style?" In *Worlds Hidden in Plain Sight: The Evolving Idea of Complexity at the Santa Fe Institute, 1984–2019*, edited by David C. Krakauer, Murray Gell-Mann, Kenneth Arrow, W. Brian Arthur, John H. Holland, Richard Lewontin, Harold Morrowitz, Jessica C. Flack, Jennifer Dunne, and Geoffrey West, 147–59. Santa Fe, NM: SFI Press.

Sanet, Steven. 2020. *Talking with Healers: Insights and Answers*. Kindle. Independently published.

Scarr, Graham. 2018. *Biotensegrity: The Structural Basis of Life*. Handspring Publishing.

Shea, Michael. 2006. "What Does 'Biodynamic' Mean? Implications for Manual Therapists." https://bti.edu/pdfs/Shea_The-Meaning-of-Biodynamic.pdf.

Schleip, R., G. Hedley, and C. A. Yucesoy. 2019. "Fascial Nomenclature: Update on Related Consensus Process." *Clinical Anatomy* 32 (7): 929–33. https://doi.org/10.1002/ca.23423.

Sills, Franklyn. 2011. *Foundations in Craniosacral Biodynamics*. Vol. 1, *The Breath of Life and Fundamental Skills*. Kindle. North Atlantic Books.

Stecco, Carla, Carmelo Pirri, Caterina Fede, Can Yucesoy, Raffaele Caro, and Antonio Stecco. 2020. "Fascial or Muscle Stretching? A Narrative Review." *Applied Sciences* 11: 307. https://doi.org/10.3390/app11010307.

Still, Andrew T. 2004. *Philosophy of Osteopathy*. American Academy of Osteopathy.

Surowiec, Rachel K., Matthew R. Allen, and Joseph M. Wallace. 2021. "Bone Hydration: How We Can Evaluate It, What Can It Tell Us, and Is It an Effective Therapeutic Target?" *Bone Reports* 16: 101161. https://doi.org/10.1016/j.bonr.2021.101161.

Sutherland, William Garner. 1990. *Teachings in the Science of Osteopathy*. Sutherland Cranial Teaching Foundation.

Tozzi, Paolo. 2015a. "A Unifying Neuro-fasciagenic Model of Somatic Dysfunction: Underlying Mechanisms and Treatment—Part I." *Journal of Bodywork and Movement Therapies* 19 (2): 310–26. https://doi.org/10.1016/j.jbmt.2015.01.001.

———. 2015b. "A Unifying Neuro-fasciagenic Model of Somatic Dysfunction: Underlying Mechanisms and Treatment—Part II." *Journal of Bodywork and Movement Therapies* 19 (3): 526–43. https://doi.org/10.1016/j.jbmt.2015.03.002.

Verzella, Massimo, Eleonora Affede, Luca Di Pietrantonio, Valentina Cozzolino, and Laura Cicchitti. 2022. "Tissutal and Fluidic Aspects in Osteopathic Manual Therapy: A Narrative Review." *Healthcare* 10 (6): 1014. https://doi.org/10.3390/healthcare10061014.

Waldrop, Mitchell M. 1993. *Complexity: The Emerging Science at the Edge of Order and Chaos.* Simon and Schuster.

Walker, Sara Imari. 2024. *Science as No One Knows It: The Physics of Life's Emergence.* Riverhead Books.

Walker, Thomas. 2014. "Bones to Fluids: A Path to Understanding Wholeness." In *2014 IASI Yearbook of Structural Integration.* https://listeninghandsseminars.com/wp-content/uploads/Bones-to-Fluids-A-Path-to-Understanding-Wholeness-Walker.pdf.

Bibliography

Abrahams, Peter, ed. 2009. *A Complete Guide to How the Body Works*. Amber Books.

Ameta, Shubham, Yusuke J. Matsubara, Nilay Chakraborty, Sandeep Krishna, and Shashi Thutupalli. 2021. "Self-Reproduction and Darwinian Evolution in Autocatalytic Chemical Reaction Systems." *Life (Basel)* 11 (4): 308. https://doi.org/10.3390/life11040308.

Andriotis, Orestis G., Marc Nalbach, and Philipp J. Thurner. 2023. "Mechanics of Isolated Individual Collagen Fibrils." *Acta Biomaterialia* 163: 35–49. https://doi.org/10.1016/j.actbio.2022.12.008.

Behnke, Robert S. 2012. *Kinetic Anatomy*. 3rd ed. Human Kinetics.

Biswas, L., J. Chen, J. De Angelis, A. Singh, C. Owen-Woods, Z. Ding, J. M. Pujol, N. Kumar, F. Zeng, S. K. Ramasamy, and A. P. Kusumbe. 2023. "Lymphatic Vessels in Bone Support Regeneration after Injury." *Cell* 186 (2): 382–97.e24. https://doi.org/10.1016/j.cell.2022.12.031.

Bliziotes, M. 2010. "Update in Serotonin and Bone." *Journal of Clinical Endocrinology and Metabolism* 95 (9): 4124–32. https://doi.org/10.1210/jc.2010-0861.

Blokhuis, Alex, Damien Lacoste, and Pierre Nghe. 2020. "Universal Motifs and the Diversity of Autocatalytic Systems." *Proceedings of the National Academy of Sciences of the United States of America* 117 (41): 25230–36. https://doi.org/10.1073/pnas.2013527117.

Bordoni, Bruno, Annalisa R. Escher, Filippo Castellini, Jorge Vale, Fabio Tobbi, Luca Pianese, Marco Musorrofiti, and Emiliano Mattia. 2024. "Fascial Nomenclature: Update 2024." *Cureus* 16 (2): e53995. https://doi.org/10.7759/cureus.53995.

Bordoni, Bruno, and Maria Giulia Lagana. 2019. "Bone Tissue Is an Integral Part of the Fascial System." *Cureus* 11 (1): e3824. https://doi.org/10.7759/cureus.3824.

Boussard, A., A. Fessel, C. Oettmeier, L. Briard, H. G. Döbereiner, and A. Dussutour. 2021. "Adaptive Behaviour and Learning in Slime Moulds: The Role of Oscillations." *Philosophical Transactions of the Royal Society of London, Series B: Biological Sciences* 376 (1820): 20190757. https://doi.org/10.1098/rstb.2019.0757.

Breeland, Grant, Madison A. Sinkler, and Ritesh G. Menezes. 2023. "Embryology, Bone Ossification." *StatPearls*. https://www.ncbi.nlm.nih.gov/books/NBK539718/.

Buehler, Markus J. 2007. "Molecular Nanomechanics of Nascent Bone: Fibrillar Toughening by Mineralization." *Nanotechnology* 18: 295102. https://doi.org/10.1088/0957-4484/18/29/295102.

Ching, Lisa M., Brett A. Benjamin, Eric G. Stiles, and Henry H. Shaw. 2023. "Enabling Health Potential: Exploring Nonlinear and Complex Results of Osteopathic Manual Medicine through Complex Systems Theory." *Journal of Osteopathic Medicine* 123 (4): 207–13. https://doi.org/10.1515/jom-2022-0118.

Ciani, Cesare, Stephen B. Doty, and Susannah P. Fritton. 2005. "Mapping Bone Interstitial Fluid Movement: Displacement of Ferritin Tracer during Histological Processing." *Bone* 37 (3): 379–87. https://doi.org/10.1016/j.bone.2005.04.004.

Clarke, Bart. 2008. "Normal Bone Anatomy and Physiology." *Clinical Journal of the American Society of Nephrology* 3 (Suppl. 3): S131–39. https://doi.org/10.2215/CJN.04151206.

Cowan, Peter T., Maria V. Launico, and Praveen Kahai. 2024. "Anatomy, Bones." *StatPearls*. https://www.ncbi.nlm.nih.gov/books/NBK539788/.

Cowin, Scott C., and Luis Cardoso. 2015. "Blood and Interstitial Flow in the Hierarchical Pore Space Architecture of Bone Tissue." *Journal of Biomechanics* 48 (5): 842–54. https://doi.org/10.1016/j.jbiomech.2014.12.013.

DiGiovanna, Eileen L., Stanley Schiowitz, and Dennis J. Dowling, eds. 2005. *An Osteopathic Approach to Diagnosis and Treatment.* 3rd ed. Lippincott Williams and Wilkins.

Dixon, Lauren, Katerina Fotinos, Edona Sherifi, Sam Lokuge, Alan Fine, Matthew Furtado, Lorraine Anand, Kira Liberatore, and Mark A. Katzman. 2020. "Effect of Osteopathic Manipulative Therapy on Generalized Anxiety Disorder." *Journal of the American Osteopathic Association* 120 (3): 133–43. https://doi.org/10.7556/jaoa.2020.026.

Frost, Harold M. 1994. "Wolff's Law and Bone's Structural Adaptations to Mechanical Usage: An Overview for Clinicians." *Angle Orthodontist* 64 (3): 175–88. https://doi.org/10.1043/0003-3219.

Gachon, Edouard, and Pierre Mesquida. 2022. "Mechanical Properties of Collagen Fibrils Determined by Buckling Analysis." *Acta Biomaterialia* 149: 60–68. https://doi.org/10.1016/j.actbio.2022.06.044.

Gao, Huajian. 1970. "Application of Fracture Mechanics Concepts to Hierarchical Biomechanics of Bone and Bone-like Materials." *International Journal of Fracture* 138: 101–37. https://doi.org/10.1007/978-1-4020-5423-5_8.

García-Castellano, José Manuel, Pedro Díaz-Herrera, and José A. Morcuende. 2000. "Is Bone a Target Tissue for the Nervous System? New Advances on the Understanding of Their Interactions." *Iowa Orthopaedic Journal* 20: 49–58. PMID: 10934625; PMCID: PMC1888751.

Gerosa, Luca, and Giovanni Lombardi. 2021. "Bone-to-Brain: A Round Trip in the Adaptation to Mechanical Stimuli." *Frontiers in Physiology* 12: 623893. https://doi.org/10.3389/fphys.2021.623893.

Gilbert, Scott F. 2000. *Developmental Biology.* 6th ed. Sinauer Associates.

Guyton, Arthur C., and John E. Hall. 1996. *Textbook of Medical Physiology*. 9th ed. W. B. Saunders.

Hordijk, Wim. 2013. "Autocatalytic Sets: From the Origin of Life to the Economy." *BioScience* 63 (11): 877–81. https://doi.org/10.1525/bio.2013.63.11.6.

Huang, Sui, Cornel Sultan, Donald Ingber, and Evangelia Micheli-Tzanakou. 2006. "Tensegrity, Dynamic Networks, and Complex Systems Biology: Emergence in Structural and Information Networks within Living Cells." In *Complex Systems Science in Biomedicine*, edited by T. S. Deisboeck and J. Y. Kresh, 283–310. Springer. https://doi.org/10.1007/978-0-387-33532-2_11.

Ibrahim, Idris, S. Syamala, John A. Ayariga, Jia Xu, B. K. Robertson, S. Meenakshisundaram, and O. S. Ajayi. 2022. "Modulatory Effect of Gut Microbiota on the Gut-Brain, Gut-Bone Axes, and the Impact of Cannabinoids." *Metabolites* 12 (12): 1247. https://doi.org/10.3390/metabo12121247.

Klineberg, Ian, and George Murray. 1999. "Osseoperception: Sensory Function and Proprioception." *Advances in Dental Research* 13: 120–29. https://doi.org/10.1177/08959374990130010101.

Krakauer, David C., Murray Gell-Mann, Kenneth Arrow, W. Brian Arthur, John H. Holland, Richard Lewontin, Harold Morrowitz, Jessica C. Flack, Jennifer Dunne, and Geoffrey West. 2019. *Worlds Hidden in Plain Sight: The Evolving Idea of Complexity at the Santa Fe Institute, 1984–2019*. SFI Press.

Kumar, Vijay, Zobia Umair, Shiv Kumar, Ravi Shankar Goutam, Soochul Park, and Jaebong Kim. 2021. "The Regulatory Roles of Motile Cilia in Cerebrospinal Fluid Circulation and Hydrocephalus." *Fluids and Barriers of the Central Nervous System* 18 (31): https://doi.org/10.1186/s12987-021-00265-0.

Lane, Nick. 2016. *The Vital Question*. W. W. Norton.

Langevin, Helene M., Patricia Keely, Jun Mao, Lisa M. Hodge, Robert Schleip, Gary Deng, Boris Hinz, Melody A. Swartz, Beverley A. de Valois, Suzanna Zick, and Thomas Findley. 2016. "Connecting (T) issues: How Research in Fascia Biology Can Impact Integrative Oncology." *Cancer Research* 76 (21): 6159–62. https://doi.org/10.1158/0008-5472.CAN-16-0753.

Levin, Michael, and Christopher J. Martyniuk. 2018. "The Bioelectric Code: An Ancient Computational Medium for Dynamic Control of Growth and Form." *Biosystems* 164: 76–93. https://doi.org/10.1016/j.biosystems.2017.08.009.

Levin, Simon, Sonia de Solórzano, and Graham Scarr. 2017. "The Significance of Closed Kinematic Chains to Biological Movement and Dynamic Stability." *Journal of Bodywork and Movement Therapies* 21 (3): 664–72. https://doi.org/10.1016/j.jbmt.2017.03.012.

Libretti, Sabrina, and Yvonne Puckett. 2023. "Physiology, Homeostasis." *StatPearls*. https://www.ncbi.nlm.nih.gov/books/NBK539778/.

Liu, Hongyu, Kai Fu, Xiaojie Cui, Hui Zhu, and Bo Yang. 2023. "Shear Thickening Fluid and Its Application in Impact Protection: A Review." *Polymers* 15 (10): 2238. https://doi.org/10.3390/polym15102238.

Maas, Mary C. 2009. "Histology of Bones and Teeth." In *Encyclopedia of Marine Mammals*,

2nd ed., edited by William F. Perrin, Bernd Würsig, and J.G.M. Thewissen, 124–29. Academic Press. https://doi.org/10.1016/B978-0-12-373553-9.00034-1.

Maes, Christa, Tetsuya Kobayashi, Martin K. Selig, Sofie Torrekens, Shunichi Roth, Susan Mackem, Geert Carmeliet, and Henry M. Kronenberg. 2010. "Osteoblast Precursors, but Not Mature Osteoblasts, Move into Developing and Fractured Bones along with Invading Blood Vessels." *Developmental Cell* 19 (2): 329–44. https://doi.org/10.1016/j.devcel.2010.07.010.

Magoun, Harold I., ed. 2011. *Osteopathy in the Cranial Field.* 3rd ed. Cranial Academy.

Marenzana, Marco, and Timothy R. Arnett. 2013. "The Key Role of the Blood Supply to Bone." *Bone Research* 1 (3): 203–15. https://doi.org/10.4248/BR201303001.

McCredie, John. 2007. "Nerves in Bone: The Silent Partners." *Skeletal Radiology* 36 (6): 473–75. https://doi.org/10.1007/s00256-006-0253-7.

Meltzer, Kate R., and Paul R. Standley. 2007. "Modeled Repetitive Motion Strain and Indirect Osteopathic Manipulative Techniques in Regulation of Human Fibroblast Proliferation and Interleukin Secretion." *Journal of the American Osteopathic Association* 107 (12): 527–36. PMID: 18178762.

Mercier, Andrée-Anne. 2020. "Effets du traitement ostéopathique à visée intra-osseuse sur un ex-joueur de soccer ayant des douleurs aux genoux." Postgraduate case study, Collège d'Etudes Ostéopathique de Montréal.

Mooallem, Jon. 2023. "Michael Stipe Is Writing His Next Act. Slowly." *New York Times*, December 3. https://www.nytimes.com/2023/12/03/magazine/michael-stipe-solo-album.html.

Nahian, Arif, and Poonam R. Chauhan. 2023. "Histology, Periosteum and Endosteum." *StatPearls.* https://www.ncbi.nlm.nih.gov/books/NBK557584/.

Nakagaki, Toshiyuki, Hiroyasu Yamada, and Agota Toth. 2000. "Maze-Solving by an Amoeboid Organism." *Nature* 407: 470. https://doi.org/10.1038/35035159.

O'Connell, Judith A. 2003. "Bioelectric Responsiveness of Fascia: A Model for Understanding the Effects of Manipulation." *Techniques in Orthopaedics* 18 (1): 67–73. https://doi.org/10.1097/00013611-200303000-00012.

Oftadeh, Ramin, Miguel Perez-Viloria, Juan C. Villa-Camacho, Ashkan Vaziri, and Ara Nazarian. 2015. "Biomechanics and Mechanobiology of Trabecular Bone: A Review." *Journal of Biomechanical Engineering* 137 (1): 010802. https://doi.org/10.1115/1.4029176.

Otto, Elmar, Philipp R. Knapstein, Daniel Jahn, Jutta Appelt, Karl-Heinz Frosch, Serafeim Tsitsilonis, and Jürgen Keller. 2020. "Crosstalk of Brain and Bone-Clinical Observations and Their Molecular Bases." *International Journal of Molecular Sciences* 21 (14): 4946. https://doi.org/10.3390/ijms21144946.

Peng, Zhiyuan, Zachary R. Adam, Albert C. Fahrenbach, and Betül Kaçar. 2023. "Assessment of Stoichiometric Autocatalysis across Element Groups." *Journal of the American Chemical Society* 145 (41): 22483–93. https://doi.org/10.1021/jacs.3c07041.

Phillips, Carl. 2022. *My Trade Is Mystery.* Yale University Press.

Powers, Richard. 2007. *The Echo Maker.* Picador.

Reznikov, Natalia, Ron Shahar, and Steve Weiner. 2014. "Bone Hierarchical Structure in Three Dimensions." *Acta Biomaterialia* 10 (9): 3815–26. https://doi.org/10.1016/j.actbio.2014.05.024.

Ricard-Blum, Sylvie. 2011. "The Collagen Family." *Cold Spring Harbor Perspectives in Biology* 3 (1): a004978. https://doi.org/10.1101/cshperspect.a004978.

Roberts, Lindsey. 2011. "Effects of Patterns of Pressure Application on Resting Electromyography during Massage." *International Journal of Therapeutic Massage & Bodywork* 4 (1): 4–11. https://doi.org/10.3822/ijtmb.v4i1.25.

Rowe, Peter, Alexander Koller, and Suman Sharma. 2023. "Physiology, Bone Remodeling." *StatPearls.* https://www.ncbi.nlm.nih.gov/books/NBK499863/.

Scarr, Graham. 2018. *Biotensegrity: The Structural Basis of Life.* Handspring Publishing.

Schleip, Robert, Gil Hedley, and Can A. Yucesoy. 2019. "Fascial Nomenclature: Update on Related Consensus Process." *Clinical Anatomy* 32 (7): 929–33. https://doi.org/10.1002/ca.23423.

Seifriz, William. 1954. *Seifriz on Protoplasm.* Lowen Foundation. YouTube, June 24, 2015. https://www.youtube.com/watch?v=_ihSxAn4WR8.

Sharkey, John. 2021. "Should Bone Be Considered Fascia: Proposal for a Change in Taxonomy of Bone—a Clinical Anatomist's View." *International Journal of Biological and Pharmaceutical Sciences*, archive 1: 01-010. https://doi.org/10.30574/ijbpsa.2021.1.1.0001.

Sharma, A., Colby Adams, Benjamin D. Cashdollar, Zheng Li, Nam V. Nguyen, Himsari Sai, Jiachun Shi, Gautham Velchuru, Kevin Z. Zhu, and Gerald H. Pollack. 2018. "Effect of Health-Promoting Agents on Exclusion-Zone Size." *Dose-Response* 16: 1559325818796937. https://doi.org/10.1177/1559325818796937.

Sharma, A., and Gerald H. Pollack. 2020. "Healthy Fats and Exclusion-Zone Size." *Food Chemistry* 316: 126305. https://doi.org/10.1016/j.foodchem.2020.126305.

Shen, Zhi-Li, Harris Kahn, Robert Ballarini, and Steven J. Eppell. 2011. "Viscoelastic Properties of Isolated Collagen Fibrils." *Biophysical Journal* 100 (12): 3008–15. https://doi.org/10.1016/j.bpj.2011.04.052.

Shoulders, Matthew D., and Ronald T. Raines. 2009. "Collagen Structure and Stability." *Annual Review of Biochemistry* 78: 929–58. https://doi.org/10.1146/annurev.biochem.77.032207.120833.

Stock, S. R. 2015. "The Mineral-Collagen Interface in Bone." *Calcified Tissue International* 97 (3): 262–80. https://doi.org/10.1007/s00223-015-9984-6.

Tomlinson, Ryan E., Blaine A. Christiansen, Andrew A. Giannone, and Damian C. Genetos. 2020. "The Role of Nerves in Skeletal Development, Adaptation, and Aging." *Frontiers in Endocrinology (Lausanne)* 11: 646. https://doi.org/10.3389/fendo.2020.00646.

Tomlinson, Ryan E., and Matthew J. Silva. 2013. "Skeletal Blood Flow in Bone Repair and Maintenance." *Bone Research* 1 (4): 311–22. https://doi.org/10.4248/BR201304002.

Tonk, Christian, Markus Witzler, Margit Schulze, and Edda Tobiasch. 2020. "Mesenchymal Stem Cells." In *Advances in Experimental Medicine and Biology*, edited by Sabine Wislet-Gendebien, 21–39. Springer. https://doi.org/10.1007/978-3-030-33923-4_2.

Tramontano, Marco, Francesco Tamburella, Fabio Dal Farra, Andrea Bergna, Chiara Lunghi, Marco Innocenti, Francesco Cavera, Fabio Savini, Vittoria Manzo, and Giuseppe D'Alessandro. 2021. "International Overview of Somatic Dysfunction Assessment and Treatment in Osteopathic Research: A Scoping Review." *Healthcare (Basel)* 10 (1): 28. https://doi.org/10.3390/healthcare10010028.

Uniyal, Prashant, Sukhdeep Kaur, Vikas Dhiman, Sanjay Kumar Bhadada, and Neeraj Kumar. 2023. "Effect of Inelastic Deformation on Strain Rate-Dependent Mechanical Behaviour of Human Cortical Bone." *Journal of Biomechanics* 161: 111853. https://doi.org/10.1016/j.jbiomech.2023.111853.

Valeryevich, Novoseltsev Svyatoslav, Reshetnikov Alexey Germanovich, Vyunov Vladislav Dmitrievich, Suleymanov Timur Rasimovich, Nefedova Anastasia Maksimovna, and Solomatov Petr Grigorievich. 2023. "Mechanotransduction and Biomechanical Properties of Bone Tissue as a Basis for the Use of Intraosseous Osteopathic Techniques." *International Journal of Membrane Science and Technology* 10 (3): 692–700. https://doi.org/10.15379/ijmst.v10i3.1589.

Vercher-Martínez, Antonio, Eugenio Giner, Carlos Arango, and Francisco J. Fuenmayor. 2015. "Influence of the Mineral Staggering on the Elastic Properties of the Mineralized Collagen Fibril in Lamellar Bone." *Journal of the Mechanical Behavior of Biomedical Materials* 42: 243–56. https://doi.org/10.1016/j.jmbbm.2014.11.022.

Verzella, Marco, Erika Affede, Luca Di Pietrantonio, Vincenzo Cozzolino, and Luca Cicchitti. 2022. "Tissutal and Fluidic Aspects in Osteopathic Manual Therapy: A Narrative Review." *Healthcare* 10 (6): 1014. https://doi.org/10.3390/healthcare10061014.

Wang, Liyun, Cesare Ciani, Stephen B. Doty, and Susannah P. Fritton. 2004. "Delineating Bone's Interstitial Fluid Pathway In Vivo." *Bone* 34 (3): 499–509. https://doi.org/10.1016/j.bone.2003.11.022.

White, Tim D., Michael T. Black, and Pieter A. Folkens. 2011. *Human Osteology*. Academic Press.

Williams, John. L., and John. L. Lewis. 1982. "Properties and an Anisotropic Model of Cancellous Bone from the Proximal Tibial Epiphysis." *Journal of Biomechanical Engineering* 104 (1): 50–56. https://doi.org/10.1115/1.3138303.

Yeung, Alice Y., Thomas C. Arbor, and Rahul Garg. 2023. "Anatomy, Sesamoid Bones." *StatPearls*. https://www.ncbi.nlm.nih.gov/books/NBK567773/.

Zhang, Shaoqi, Danielle S. Bassett, and Beth A. Winkelstein. 2016. "Stretch-Induced Network Reconfiguration of Collagen Fibers in the Human Facet Capsular Ligament." *Journal of the Royal Society Interface* 13 (114): 20150883. https://doi.org/10.1098/rsif.2015.0883.

Zimmerman, Elizabeth A., Bjorn Busse, and Robert O. Ritchie. 2015. "The Fracture Mechanics of Human Bone: Influence of Disease and Treatment." *Bonekey Reports* 4 (743): https://doi.org/10.1038/bonekey.2015.112.

Index

About the Author

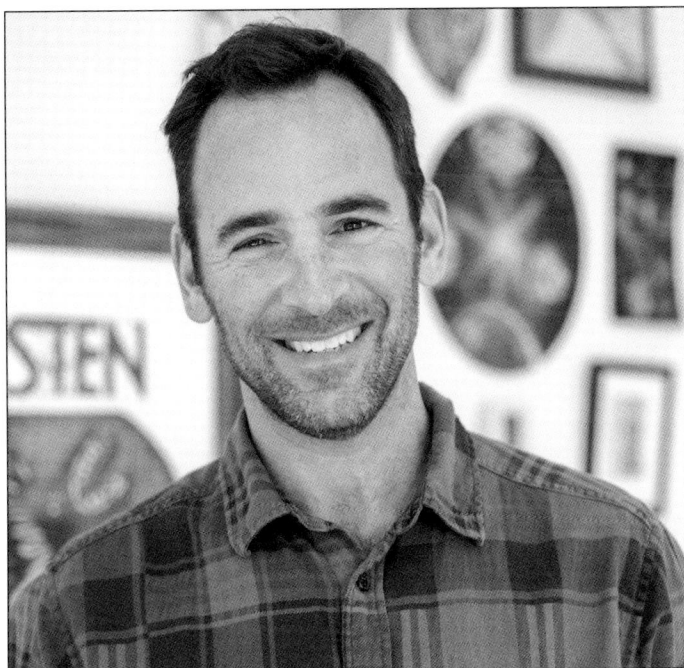

Scott Sternthal, D.O. (Diploma of Osteopathy) is a Canadian osteopath, writer, and teacher. He is the founder of Le Collectif d'Ostéopathie, a multidisciplinary clinic in Westmount, Quebec, and the developer of biodynamic skeletal therapy (BST). Sternthal teaches BST to myofascial and manual therapists worldwide at conferences, clinics, and workshops. His BST Level 1 course is approved by the National Certification Board for Therapeutic Massage & Bodywork (NCBTMB) in the United States and the Canadian Massage & Manual Osteopathic Therapists Association (CMMOTA) in Canada. He introduced the BST Level 2 course in September 2025. He is also the self-published author of *Melting Bone, Healing Tide*.

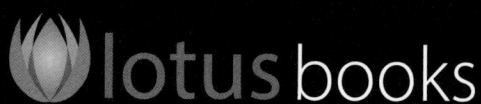